Cardiothoracic Surgery: Recent Advances and Techniques

Cardiothoracic Surgery: Recent Advances and Techniques

Editor: Daniel Willson

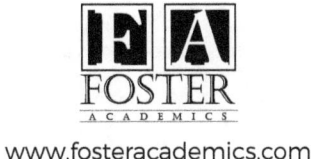

www.fosteracademics.com

www.fosteracademics.com

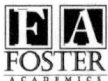

Cataloging-in-Publication Data

Cardiothoracic surgery : recent advances and techniques / edited by Daniel Willson.
    p. cm.
Includes bibliographical references and index.
ISBN 978-1-63242-596-6
1. Heart--Surgery. 2. Chest--Surgery. 3. Surgical technology. I. Willson, Daniel.
RD598 .C37 2019
617.412--dc23

Foster Academics,
118-35 Queens Blvd., Suite 400,
Forest Hills, NY 11375, USA

ISBN 978-1-63242-596-6 (Hardback)

Contents

Preface

Over the recent decade, advancements and applications have progressed exponentially. This has led to the increased interest in this field and projects are being conducted to enhance knowledge. The main objective of this book is to present some of the critical challenges and provide insights into possible solutions. This book will answer the varied questions that arise in the field and also provide an increased scope for furthering studies.

The field of medicine targeted at the surgical treatment of the organs within the thorax and the treatment of heart and lung diseases is known as cardiothoracic surgery. Some of the surgical procedures involving cardiac and thoracic surgery are open heart surgery, modern beating-heart surgery, pleurectomy, lung volume reduction surgery, lobectomy, pneumonectomy, video-assisted thoracoscopic surgery (VATS) lobectomy, etc. Cardiovascular surgery when performed on children is known as pediatric cardiovascular surgery. Infection constitutes the principal non-cardiac complication from cardiothoracic surgery. Some common infections are mediastinitis, endocarditis cardiac device infection, empyema, infectious myo- or pericarditis, etc. This book contains some path-breaking studies in the area of cardiothoracic surgery. It unravels the recent advances and modern techniques of cardiothoracic surgery. For all readers who are interested in this domain, the case studies included in this book will serve as an excellent guide to develop a comprehensive understanding.

I hope that this book, with its visionary approach, will be a valuable addition and will promote interest among readers. Each of the authors has provided their extraordinary competence in their specific fields by providing different perspectives as they come from diverse nations and regions. I thank them for their contributions.

Editor

Surgical strategies protecting against right ventricular dilatation following tetralogy of Fallot repair

Amr A. Arafat[1*†], Elatafy E. Elatafy[1†], Sahar Elshedoudy[2], Mahmoud Zalat[3], Neamet Abdallah[4] and Ahmed Elmahrouk[1]

Abstract

Background: Right ventricular (RV) volume overload increases morbidity and mortality after tetralogy of Fallot (TOF) repair. Surgical strategies like pulmonary leaflets sparing and tricuspid valve repair at time of primary repair may decrease RV overload. Our objective is to evaluate early and midterm results of pulmonary leaflets sparing with infundibular preservation and tricuspid valve repair in selected TOF patients with moderate pulmonary annular hypoplasia.

Methods: From 2011 to 2016; 46 patients with TOF and moderate pulmonary annular hypoplasia had surgical repair with sparing of the pulmonary valve leaflets. Concomitant tricuspid valve repair was performed in 33 patients (71.8%). Mean age was 13.1 ± 4.8 months, 68% were males ($n = 31$) and mean weight was 9.5 ± 2.3 kg. Preoperative McGoon ratio was 1.9 ± 0.4 and pulmonary valve z-score ranges from -2 to -3. Preoperative pressure gradient of RVOT was 80.9 ± 7.7 mmHg and 10.9% had minor coronary anomalies ($n = 5$).

Results: All repairs were performed through trans-atrial trans-pulmonary approach. 87% had pulmonary valve commissurotomy ($n = 40$). Mean cardiopulmonary bypass time was 71 ± 6.3 min and ischemic time 42.4 ± 4.9 min. Hospital mortality occurred in 4.3% ($n = 2$). Mean RVOT pressure gradient decreased significantly postoperatively (28.8 ± 7.2 mmHg, p-value< .001) and at the last follow up (23.6 ± 1.8 mmHg, p-value< .001). Pulmonary regurgitation progressed by one grade in 2 patients compared to the postoperative grade. 1 patient (2.5%) had late mortality and reintervention was required in 5 patients (12.5%).

Conclusion: Pulmonary leaflets sparing, and tricuspid valve repair are safe for TOF repair with no added morbidity or mortality. These procedures could contribute to reducing right ventricular volume overload over time after TOF repair.

Keywords: Tetralogy of Fallot repair, Pulmonary leaflets sparing, Infundibular preservation, Tricuspid valve repair

Background

Severe pulmonary valve regurgitation following tetralogy of Fallot (TOF) repair leads to right ventricular (RV) volume overload. Volume overload of the right ventricle is aggravated with any associated tricuspid regurgitation and it is considered the major cause of function impairment and increased morbidity and mortality in those patients [1–3]. Several techniques have been proposed to alleviate the acute and chronic right ventricular volume overload after TOF repair and recently pulmonary valve sparing procedure has gained popularity [4–7]. Pulmonary valve sparing could decrease right ventricular volume overload with the benefit of preserving the growth potential of the pulmonary valve. However, it bears the risk of residual pulmonary valve stenosis with increased right ventricular pressure afterload especially when performed in patients with moderate and severe annular hypoplasia. Recently repair of more than moderate degree of tricuspid valve regurgitation at time of pulmonary valve replacement was found to be associated with improved patients' functional status [8]. The objective of this study is to evaluate early

* Correspondence: amr.arafat@med.tanta.edu.eg
†Equal contributors
[1]Cardiothoracic Surgery Department, Tanta University, Al-Geish Street, Tanta 31527, Gharbya, Egypt
Full list of author information is available at the end of the article

and midterm effects of pulmonary leaflets sparing and tricuspid valve repair in TOF repair in selected patients with moderate pulmonary annular hypoplasia on right ventricular outflow tract (RVOT) pressure gradient, degree of pulmonary regurgitation, tricuspid valve regurgitation and reoperation.

Methods

Patients population

This retrospective cohort study included 46 patients with tetralogy of Fallot who were operated by the same surgical team from January 2011 to March 2016. Selection of patients was based on the preoperative pulmonary annulus z-score, the study included all consecutive TOF patients who had moderate pulmonary annular hypoplasia with z score ranges from – 2 to – 3 and amenable for pulmonary leaflets preservation. Patients with severe pulmonary annular hypoplasia, pulmonary atresia, absent pulmonary valve or discontinuation of the pulmonary arteries were excluded from the study. Moreover, patients with moderate annular hypoplasia (z-score from – 2 to – 3) with dysplastic pulmonary valve had mono-cusp pulmonary valve reconstruction and were excluded from the study. The study was approved by the ethical committee and patients' consent was waived due to the retrospective nature of the study.

Preoperative data collection

Patients' charts and preoperative echocardiography were retrospectively reviewed to collect the preoperative patients' characteristics, pulmonary annulus z-score, RVOT pressure gradient, associated lesions, prior shunts and the preoperative rhythm. McGoon ratio were measured by echocardiography as the sum of the diameters of immediately pre-branching left and right pulmonary arteries to descending aorta just above level of diaphragm.

Surgical technique

Surgical repair of TOF was performed through full median sternotomy whether primary or redo sternotomy. After aorto-bicaval cannulation, cardiopulmonary bypass was commenced with cardioplegic arrest and cold blood cardioplegia was repeated every 25 min. All operations were performed through a trans-atrial trans-pulmonary approach. Right atriotomy was performed and venting was done through the inter-atrial septum. Splitting of the obstructing bundles in the infundibulum with very minimal resection was performed to preserve the right ventricular outflow tract geometry. Closure of the ventricular septal defect was done with Gore-Tex patch using polyprolene 6/0 continuous sutures. Pulmonary arteriotomy was performed to complete the resection of the obstructing bundles. Pulmonary valvotomy was done in most patients and in case of borderline annulus not passing 2 sizes less than the expected Hegar dilator for the body surface area, the incision

was extended few mms though the annulus keeping the valve in situ. Pulmonary valvotomy was performed at the site of the fused leaflets. Commissural suspension was performed in 2 patients. Closure of the incision was performed using glutaraldehyde treated pericardial patch. In patients with more than mild degree of tricuspid regurgitation identified by the preoperative echocardiography and confirmed by intraoperative saline test, tricuspid repair was performed. Tricuspid repair was done by closing the commissure between anterior and septal leaflets in case of sufficient septal leaflet tissues or by bicuspidization technique in case of rudimentary septal leaflet. RV and PA pressures were directly measured after weaning from cardiopulmonary bypass and pressure gradient of 30–35 mmHg was accepted.

Postoperative clinical data

Postoperative clinical data including duration of intensive care unit (ICU) and hospital stay were collected. Patients were followed clinically and echocardiography after discharge and mean duration of follow up was collected.

Echocardiographic follow up

Transesophageal echocardiography (TEE) was performed after TOF repair in all patients to evaluate the adequacy of the repair. All patients had transthoracic echocardiography pre-discharge. Further follow up was performed by the cardiologists and the last echocardiographic data were collected including the degree of pulmonary and tricuspid valve regurgitation and RVOT pressure gradient. Time to reintervention, causes and types "whether surgical or catheter based intervention" were reported.

Study outcomes

Pulmonary regurgitation (PR) was recorded and graded from 0 to 4 (0, none; 1, trivial; 2, mild; 3, moderate and 4, severe). RVOT pressure was reported from last echocardiographic evaluation and compared to the preoperative and pre-discharge values. Recurrence of tricuspid regurgitation was reported at follow up.

Statistical analysis

Continuous variables were presented as mean ± standard deviation, median and range and categorical variables as numbers and percent. Continuous variables were compared using paired t-test for normally distributed variables and categorical variables with Fisher's exact test. Changes in RVOT pressure were plotted against time and random effect model was used to test the significance of the change. Logistic regression was used to identify predictors of the use of trans-annular patch and odds ratio were reported. All analyses were performed using STATA 14 statistical software (Statacorp, Texas, USA). P-value less than 0.05 was considered significant.

Results

Patients' characteristics and operative data

Forty- Six patients had TOF repair with pulmonary leaflets sparing and infundibular preservation. All patients had moderate pulmonary annular hypoplasia with z-score ranged from − 2 to − 3. Mean age at time of repair was 13.1 ± 4.8 months (median age = 11 months). Trans-annular patch (TAP) was required in 23.9% ($n = 11$) and pulmonary valve commissurotomy in 86.96% ($n = 40$) patients. Five patients had minor coronary anomaly defined as small conal branch crossing the RVOT and 1 patients had the left anterior descending artery originating from the right coronary artery. Most common pulmonary valve morphology was bicuspid valve in 56.5% ($n = 26$) and tricuspid valve in 37% ($n = 17$). Tricuspid valve repair was performed concomitantly in 72% patients ($n = 33$) to reduce postoperative right ventricular volume overload (Table 1).

Clinical outcomes

Mean ICU stay was 3.1 ± 1.2 days. Hospital mortality occurred in 4.4% ($n = 2$) patients, 4 patients lost for follow up and late mortality occurred in 1 patient. Reintervention either surgical or catheter based was performed in 5 patients and indications of reintervention were: RVOT obstruction, restrictive ventricular septal defect (VSD), complete heart block, left pulmonary artery stenosis and diaphragmatic paralysis. The interventions performed were resection of the right ventricular obstructing bundle, open VSD closure, trans-venous pacing, trans-catheter stenting of the left pulmonary artery and diaphragmatic plication respectively. Mean time from primary repair to reintervention was 0.94 ± 0.6 years (median = 1.2 years) (Table 2).

Pulmonary valve and RVOT

Mean time to the latest echocardiographic follow up was $3.85 \pm .85$ years. RVOT pressure gradient dropped significantly postoperatively compared to the preoperative gradient (p-value < 0.0001). The decline continued during follow up (Table 3). The decrease in RVOT pressure between patients with and without TAP was comparable ($p = .59$) (Fig. 1).

Pulmonary regurgitation regressed by one grade in 10 patients compared to the pre-discharge echocardiography and progressed by one grade in 2 patients, both had TAP. (p-value < 0.001) (Table 4).

Low body weight at time of repair predicted of the use of the TAP ($p = 0.03$) (Table 5) and the use of TAP was significantly associated with postoperative PR ($p = .003$).

Tricuspid valve

Tricuspid valve repair was performed in 71.8% of the patients for moderate and severe degree of tricuspid regurgitation at time of primary TOF repair ($n = 33$). All patients had no degree of tricuspid regurgitation postoperatively. During follow up, 8 patients (20%) developed mild degree of tricuspid regurgitation and 1 patient (2.5%) had moderate tricuspid regurgitation. Tricuspid regurgitation significantly occurred in patients with no prior tricuspid valve repair (p-value = 0.002).

Discussion

Since the first repair of tetralogy of Fallot which was performed through a large right ventricular incision with the use of trans-annular patch, [9] several surgical strategies have been developed to reduce the drawbacks of TOF repair especially right ventricular volume overload. The deleterious effect of chronic pulmonary regurgitation following TOF repair has shifted the paradigm of TOF management from strategy aiming mainly to relieve pulmonary stenosis to one aiming at preserving the pulmonary valve. The monocusp valve reconstruction with autologous pericardium or polytetrafluoroethylene was attempted to decrease the degree of pulmonary regurgitation postoperatively [10]. Despite the reported success of the technique by some authors, [11, 12] it doesn't gain a wide acceptance because of lack of growth potential of the prosthetic material and the high reoperation rate. Biological material was used to reconstruct the monocusp pulmonary valve to preserve the growth potential however, progressive pulmonary regurgitation was noted during follow up [5]. Our conservative technique is based on preserving the native pulmonary valve leaflets in patients presenting with moderate annular hypoplasia (z-score − 2 to − 3) by performing pulmonary valvotomy, limited arteriotomy and keeping the valve in place to preserve its natural geometry. This strategy was not associated with residual pulmonary valve stenosis and RVOT pressure gradient was effectively reduced both postoperatively and at follow up. Pulmonary regurgitation has been reduced by one grade over the follow up compared to the pre-discharge grade and no reoperation on pulmonary valve was required in a mean follow up of $3.85 \pm .85$ years although long term follow up is recommended. The changes of pulmonary regurgitation in our series could be explained by the growth potential of preserved pulmonary valve leaflets. Pulmonary valve z-score 4 or less was found to be a predictor of recurrent RVOT obstruction in other series [13] and our current strategy is to preserve the pulmonary valve in patients without severe annular hypoplasia. Hoashi et al., [14] found that pulmonary valve z-score was not a predictor of recurrent

Table 1 Preoperative and operative data

Patients' characteristic	Value
Age (months)	
Mean ± SD	13.1 ± 4.8
Median	11
Range	8–26
Male	31 (67.4%)
Weight (Kg)	
Mean ± SD	9.5 ± 2.3
Median	9
Range	6–16
Associated lesions:	
ASD	4 (8.7%)
PDA	7 (15.2%)
PLSVC	1 (2.2%)
McGoon Ratio	
Mean ± SD	1.9 ± 0.14
Median	1.9
Range	1.7–2.2
RVOT pressure Gradient (mmHg)	
Mean ± SD	80.9 ± 7.7
Median	80
Range	65–97
Prior MBT shunt	8 (17.4%)
Coronary anomalies	
No	40 (86.96%)
Minor	5 (10.87%)
Major	1 (2.17%)
Preoperative Rhythm	
Sinus	44 (95.66%)
Partial HB	1 (2.17%)
Complete HB	1 (2.17%)
TAP	11 (23.9%)
Cardiopulmonary bypass time (min)	
Mean ± SD	71.2 ± 6.3
Median	70
Range	55–94
Ischemic time (min)	
Mean ± SD	42.4 ± 4.9
Median	42
Range	35–62
Pulmonary valve morphology	
Unicuspid	1 (2.17%)
Bicuspid	26 (56.52%)
Tricuspid	17 (36.96%)
Indeterminate	2 (4.35%)

Table 1 Preoperative and operative data *(Continued)*

Patients' characteristic	Value
Pulmonary valve commissurotomy	40 (86.96%)
TV repair	33 (71.74%)

(Continuous variables are expressed as mean ± SD, median and range) Categorical variables are presented as number and (percent)) *ASD* Atrial septal defect, *PDA* Patent ductus arteriosus, *PLSVC* Persistent left superior vena cava, *RVOT* Right ventricular outflow tract, *MBT* Modified Blalock Taussig shunt, *HB* Heart block, *TAP* Trans-annular patch

ROVT obstruction but z-score less than − 2 was a predictor of progressive pulmonary regurgitation which was not found in our study, the degree of pulmonary regurgitation regressed by one grade in 10 patients during the follow up. The most common pulmonary valve morphology encountered was a bicuspid valve followed by tricuspid morphology. This finding is in concordance with Vida et al., [7] who found that bicuspid and tricuspid pulmonary valve morphology were amenable for preservation on contrary to the unicuspid morphology. We encountered 1 patient with unicuspid valve and 2 patients with indeterminate morphology due to fusion of the commissures. Those patients had non-progressing grade I PR postoperatively and at the last echocardiographic follow up but no definite conclusion about the suitability of those valves for repair can be drawn due to the small patients' number. Hoashi et al., [14] had 66.7% bicuspid pulmonary valve in their series of 84 patients and bicuspid pulmonary valve was a significant predictor for increasing pulmonary regurgitation during the long term follow up.

Despite pulmonary regurgitation is a major cause of deterioration of the right ventricular function, several other factors can also contribute to functional deterioration following TOF repair [1, 2, 15]. Transventricular TOF repair could contribute to the progressive right ventricular dilatation. Lee et al.; found no difference in outcome between patients who had traditional versus limited right ventriculotomy [16]. In our series, all repairs were performed through trans-atrial trans-pulmonary approach with minimal resection but rather splitting of the obstructing infundibular bundles. This strategy yielded good short-term results with 1 patient had complete heart block and required a permanent pacemaker insertion and 1 patient had late operation due to persistent RVOT obstruction. No ventricular arrhythmia was reported in any of our patients.

Postoperative tricuspid regurgitation was found in other series to be a predictor of late morbidity [17]. We follow a rigorous strategy to prevent postoperative tricuspid valve regurgitation by routinely performing repair of valve with more than mild degree of regurgitation post TOF repair. 72% of our patients required tricuspid valve repair at time of primary TOF repair. This high

Table 2 Early and late clinical outcomes

Clinical outcomes	Value
ICU stay (days)	
Mean ± SD	3.1 ± 1.2
Median	3
Range	2–8
Hospital stay (days)	
Mean ± SD	8.9 ± 2.4
Median	8
Range	4–18
Hospital mortality	2 (4.35%)
Late Mortality	1/40 (2.5%)
Late reoperation	5/40 (12.5%)
Tricuspid Regurgitation (≥grade II)	1 (2.5%)
Rhythm at follow up	
Sinus	38 (95%)
Nodal	1 (2.5%)
Complete Heart block	1 (2.5%)

(Continuous variables are expressed as mean ± SD, median and range)
Categorical variables are presented as number and (percent)

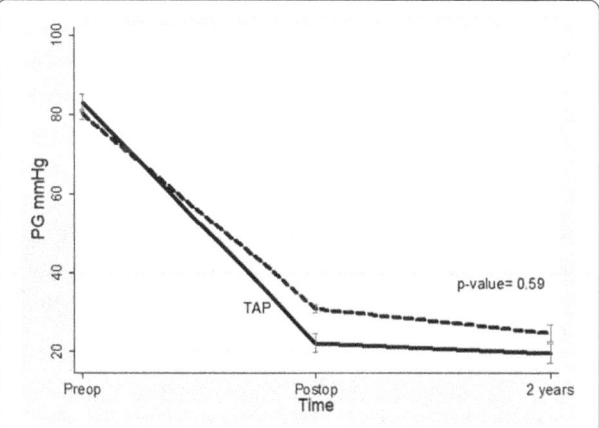

Fig. 1 Change in RVOT pressure in patients with and without transannular patch. Values are presented as preoperative, postoperative and at 2 years follow up

percentage of patients requiring concomitant tricuspid repair in our series could be attributed to the relatively older age of our patient population compared to the other published series. In older children, the right ventricle is subjected to long period of overload, with a resultant decrease in the compliance of the RV and annular dilatation. We also included repair of the regurgitation resulted from septal leaflet distortion during closure of the VSD. Tricuspid repair significantly halted the progress of tricuspid regurgitation at follow up. However long-term follow up is required to identify the effect of this procedure on right ventricular function.

Limited trans-annular pulmonary patch was required in 11 patients. We have observed no difference postoperatively and at follow up between patients with and without TAP regarding the decrease of the RVOT pressure gradient. Follow up was complete in 9 patients with TAP, 2 had progression of the degree of PR by one grade and the degree of PR remained stationary in 6 patients. On the other

hand, the degree of PR improved in patients without TAP ($n = 9$) by one grade. These results are consistent with Sen et al., [5] who found improvement in PR with valve preservation or reconstruction by biological material compared to TAP. Similar to other reports, TAP was significantly associated with postoperative PR and low weight predicts the use of the patch preoperatively [18, 19]. In contrast to our findings, Simon et al. found that limited trans-annular patch yielded similar results compared to annular sparing as regard to the degree of pulmonary regurgitation and right ventricular enlargement [20]. In summary, pulmonary leaflet sparing during TOF repair is associated with significant reduction of RVOT pressure without causing significant pulmonary regurgitation. Tricuspid valve repair halted the progression of tricuspid valve regurgitation. The use of the transannular patch is associated with increased pulmonary regurgitation compared to patients without TAP.

Study limitations

The study is retrospective in nature which bears all the drawbacks of retrospective studies. Echocardiography

Table 3 Comparison of the predischarge and last follow up RVOT pressure gradient in (mmHg) to the preoperative measurement

Timing	Mean ± SD	Standard Error	95% confidence interval	p- value
Pre-operative	80.9 ± 7.7	1.14	78.6–83.2	< 0.0001
Predischarge	28.8 ± 7.2	1.07	26.6–30.9	
Last follow up	23.6 ± 11.5	1.8	19.9–27.2	0.01

Table 4 Change in the pulmonary regurgitation (PR) grade at the last follow up compared to the predischarge grade (Numbers in the table present patients number)

Degree of predischarge PR	Degree of PR at the last follow up				
	0	1	2	3	total
0	4	1	0	0	5
1	5	18	0	0	23
2	0	5	5	1	11
3	0	0	0	1	1
Total	9	24	5	2	40

Table 5 Predictors of the use of transannular patch (TAP) in patients with moderate pulmonary annular hypoplasia

	Odds ratio	Std.Err	Z statistics	P-value	95% Confidence interval
Age	1.24	0.63	0.42	0.67	0.46–3.38
Weight	0.15	0.14	−2.06	0.03	0.26–0.9
RVOT pressure gradient	1.14	0.09	1.6	0.1	0.97–1.32

was used in follow up which is not the standard diagnostic tool for evaluation of the pulmonary valve and right ventricular function and MRI is a better tool for assessment of the right ventricular function [21]. Another drawback is the short duration of follow up and long term follow up is recommended to determine the durability of the pulmonary and tricuspid valve repair and their effect on the right ventricular function.

Conclusion

Pulmonary leaflets sparing and tricuspid repair can be safely performed at time of primary TOF repair. Pulmonary leaflets sparing doesn't result in significant pulmonary regurgitation post TOF repair and tricuspid repair protects against future development of tricuspid regurgitation. The procedure has favorable short and midterm results and low reoperation rate. Transannular patch is associated with increased postoperative pulmonary regurgitation and its progression and it should be avoided when possible.

Abbreviation
ASD: Atrial septal defect; HB: Heart block; ICU: Intensive care unit; MBT: Modified Blalock Taussig shunt; PDA: Patent ductus arteriosus; PLSVC: Persistent left superior vena cava; PR: Pulmonary regurgitation; RV: Right Ventricle; RVOT: Right ventricular outflow tract; TAP: Trans-annular patch; TEE: Transesophageal Echocardiography; TOF: Tetralogy of Fallot; TR: Tricuspid regurgitation; VSD: Ventricular septal defect

Acknowledgements
Not applicable.

Funding
This research received no specific grant from any funding agency in the public, commercial, or not-for-profit sectors.

Authors' contributions
EE, AA, MZ and AE conceived and designed the study. AAA and EE conducted the literature search. MZ, SE and NA were involved in the collection and interpretation of data. AA, AE conducted the statistical analysis and drafted the manuscript. The study was supervised by EE, AA and AE. All authors revised and approved the final manuscript.

Competing interests
The authors declare that they have no competing interests.

Author details
[1]Cardiothoracic Surgery Department, Tanta University, Al-Geish Street, Tanta 31527, Gharbya, Egypt. [2]Cardiology Department, Tanta University, Tanta, Egypt. [3]Cardiothoracic Surgery Department, Misr Children Hospital, Cairo, Egypt. [4]Cardiology Department, Misr Children Hospital, Cairo, Egypt.

References
1. Valente AM, Gauvreau K, Assenza GE, Babu-Narayan SV, Schreier J, Gatzoulis MA, et al. Contemporary predictors of death and sustained ventricular tachycardia in patients with repaired tetralogy of Fallot enrolled in the INDICATOR cohort. Heart. 2014;100(3):247–53.
2. Wijesekera VA, Raju R, Precious B, Berger AJ, Kiess MC, Leipsic JA, et al. Sequential right and left ventricular assessment in Posttetralogy of Fallot patients with significant pulmonary regurgitation. Congenit Heart Dis. 2016;11(6):606-14.
3. Kato A, Drolet C, Yoo SJ, Redington AN, Grosse-Wortmann L. Vicious circle between progressive right ventricular dilatation and pulmonary regurgitation in patients after tetralogy of Fallot repair? Right heart enlargement promotes flow reversal in the left pulmonary artery. J Cardiovasc Magn Reson. 2016;18(1):34.
4. Hiramatsu Y. Pulmonary cusp and annular extension technique for reconstruction of right ventricular outflow in tetralogy of Fallot. Ann Thorac Surg. 2014;98(5):1850–2.
5. Sen DG, Najjar M, Yimaz B, Levasseur SM, Kalessan B, Quaegebeur JM, et al. Aiming to preserve pulmonary valve function in tetralogy of Fallot repair: comparing a new approach to traditional management. Pediatr Cardiol. 2016;37(5):818–25.
6. Simon BV, Swartz MF, Egan M, Cholette JM, Gensini F, Alfieris GM. Use of a Dacron annular sparing versus limited Transannular patch with nominal pulmonary annular expansion in infants with tetralogy of Fallot. Ann Thorac Surg. 2017 Jan;103(1):186–92.
7. Vida VL, Angelini A, Guariento A, Frescura C, Fedrigo M, Padalino M, et al. Preserving the pulmonary valve during early repair of tetralogy of Fallot: Anatomic substrates and surgical strategies. J Thorac Cardiovasc Surg. 2015;149(5):1358–63. e1.
8. Roubertie F, Seguela PE, Jalal Z, Iriart X, Roques X, Kreitmann B, et al. Tricuspid valve repair and pulmonary valve replacement in adults with repaired tetralogy of Fallot. J Thorac Cardiovasc Surg. 2017;154(1):214–23.
9. Gott VL. C. Walton Lillehei and total correction of tetralogy of Fallot. Ann Thorac Surg. 1990;49(2):328–32.
10. He GW. A new technique of transannular monocusp patch-repair of the right ventricular outflow tract in repair of tetralogy of Fallot. Heart Lung Circ. 2007;16(2):107–12.
11. Brown JW, Ruzmetov M, Vijay P, Rodefeld MD, Turrentine MW. Right ventricular outflow tract reconstruction with a polytetrafluoroethylene monocusp valve: a twelve-year experience. J Thorac Cardiovasc Surg. 2007;133(5):1336–43.
12. Sasson L, Houri S, Raucher Sternfeld A, Cohen I, Lenczner O, Bove EL, et al. Right ventricular outflow tract strategies for repair of tetralogy of Fallot: effect of monocusp valve reconstruction. Eur J Cardiothorac Surg. 2013;43(4):743–51.

13. Stewart RD, Backer CL, Young L, Mavroudis C. Tetralogy of Fallot: results of a pulmonary valve-sparing strategy. Ann Thorac Surg. 2005;80(4): 1431–8. discussion 8-9.

14. Hoashi T, Kagisaki K, Meng Y, Sakaguchi H, Kurosaki K, Shiraishi I, et al. Long-term outcomes after definitive repair for tetralogy of Fallot with preservation of the pulmonary valve annulus. J Thorac Cardiovasc Surg. 2014;148(3):802–8. discussion 8-9.

15. Shin YR, Jung JW, Kim NK, Choi JY, Kim YJ, Shin HJ, et al. Factors associated with progression of right ventricular enlargement and dysfunction after repair of tetralogy of Fallot based on serial cardiac magnetic resonance imaging. Eur J Cardiothorac Surg. 2016;50(3):464–9.

16. Lee C, Lee CH, Kwak JG, Kim SH, Shim WS, Lee SY, et al. Does limited right ventriculotomy prevent right ventricular dilatation and dysfunction in patients who undergo transannular repair of tetralogy of Fallot? Matched comparison of magnetic resonance imaging parameters with conventional right ventriculotomy long-term after repair. J Thorac Cardiovasc Surg. 2014;147(3):889–95.

17. Bokma JP, Winter MM, Oosterhof T, Vliegen HW, van Dijk AP, Hazekamp MG, et al. Severe tricuspid regurgitation is predictive for adverse events in tetralogy of Fallot. Heart. 2015;101(10):794–9.

18. Cuypers JA, Menting ME, Konings EE, Opic P, Utens EM, Helbing WA, et al. Unnatural history of tetralogy of Fallot: prospective follow-up of 40 years after surgical correction. Circulation. 2014;130(22):1944–53.

19. Kim H, Sung SC, Kim S-H, Chang YH, Lee HD, Park JA, et al. Early and late outcomes of total repair of tetralogy of Fallot: risk factors for late right ventricular dilatation. Interact Cardiovasc Thorac Surg. 2013;17(6):956–62.

20. Simon BV, Swartz MF, Egan M, Cholette JM, Gensini F, Alfieris GM. Use of a Dacron annular sparing versus limited Transannular patch with nominal pulmonary annular expansion in infants with tetralogy of Fallot. Ann Thorac Surg. 2017;103(1):186–92.

21. Rudski LG, Lai WW, Afilalo J, Hua L, Handschumacher MD, Chandrasekaran K, et al. Guidelines for the echocardiographic assessment of the right heart in adults: a report from the American Society of Echocardiography endorsed by the European Association of Echocardiography, a registered branch of the European Society of Cardiology, and the Canadian Society of Echocardiography. J Am Soc Echocardiogr. 2010;23(7):685–713.

2

Effect of glycaemic control on complications following cardiac surgery

M. Navaratnarajah[*], R. Rea, R. Evans, F. Gibson, C. Antoniades, A. Keiralla, M. Demosthenous, G. Kassimis and G. Krasopoulos

Abstract

Introduction: No uniform consensus in the UK or Europe exists, for glycaemic management of patients with Diabetes or pre-diabetes undergoing cardiac surgery.

Objective: [i] Determine the relationship between glycaemic control and cardiac surgical outcomes; [ii] Compare current vs gold standard management of patients with Diabetes or pre-diabetes undergoing cardiac surgery.

Methods: Searches of MEDLINE, NHS Evidence and Web of Science databases were completed. Articles were limited to those in English, German and French. No date limit was enforced.13,232 articles were identified on initial literature review, and 50 relevant papers included in this review.

Results: No national standards for glycaemic control prior to cardiac surgery were identified. Upto 30% of cardiac surgical patients have undiagnosed Diabetes. Cardiac surgical patients without Diabetes with pre-operative hyperglycaemia have a 1 year mortality double that of patients with normoglyacemia, and equivalent to patients already diagnosed with Diabetes. Pre- and peri-operative hyperglycaemia is associated with worse outcomes. Evidence regarding tight glycaemic control vs moderate glycaemic control is conflicting. Tight control may be more effective in patients without Diabetes with pre–/peri-operative hyperglycaemia, and moderate control appears more effective in patients with pre-existing Diabetes. Patients with well controlled Diabetes may achieve comparable outcomes to patients without Diabetes with similar glycaemic control.

Conclusions: Pre / peri-operative hyperglycaemia is associated with worse outcomes in both patients with, and without Diabetes undergoing CABG. This review supports the pre-operative screening, and optimisation of glycaemic control in patients undergoing cardiac surgery. Optimal glycaemic management remains unclear and clear guidelines are needed.

Keywords: Diabetes, Cardiac surgery, CABG

Background

Diabetes is a common life-long health condition and a major risk factor for coronary artery disease. Latest estimates show a global prevalence of 382 million in 2013, with a projected rise to 592 million by 2035 [1]. Average annual increases in insulin dependent Diabetes of 3% worldwide and 4% in Europe [2] are reported. In the United Kingdom [UK] there are currently 3.2 million people diagnosed with Diabetes, while another 630,000 remain undiagnosed [1]. Approximately 26 million [8%]

people suffer from Diabetes in the United States [US] population, while an estimated additional 7 million are undiagnosed [3]. Due to the slow onset of non-insulin dependent Diabetes, and long pre-detection period, up to one-half of cases may be undiagnosed [1], and an estimated 80 million US citizens are considered to have pre-diabetes, pre-disposing them to an increased risk of developing overt Diabetes.

UK and worldwide data shows that the proportion of people with Diabetes undergoing isolated CABG surgery has increased by 33% in recent years to 25–40% [4]. These patients face increased morbidity and mortality following cardiac surgery and represent a sizeable

* Correspondence: manoraj.navaratnarajah@doctors.org.uk
Oxford Heart Centre, John Radcliffe Hospital, Headley Way, Oxfordshire OX3 9DU, UK

medico-economic predicament worldwide. Specific UK guidelines and standards exist regarding medical management of Diabetes and risk implications for cardiovascular disease [5]. In the US guidelines for the glycaemic management of patients with Diabetes, or pre-diabetes undergoing cardiac surgery have been available for nearly a decade. Surprisingly however, no uniform consensus in the UK or Europe exists for the glycaemic management of these patients.

This literature review considers the care and outcomes of patients with Diabetes and pre-diabetes undergoing cardiac surgery. The main purpose of this article is to: a] identify current standards of care of patients with Diabetes / pre-diabetes undergoing cardiac surgery and b] address the question; "what is best glycaemic management of patients with Diabetes / pre-diabetes undergoing cardiac surgery?". Based on the reviewed published literature related to the care and outcomes of patients with Diabetes and pre-diabetes undergoing cardiac surgery, it is clear that there is a lack of evidence against which institutions can benchmark their glycaemic management.

Methods
Literature review
In pursuit of clinical evidence regarding management and outcomes of patients with Diabetes or pre-diabetes undergoing cardiac surgery, an extensive search was performed using the MEDLINE, NHS Evidence and Web of Science databases. The search criteria were: ["Diabetes" OR "hyperglycaemia" OR "hypoglycaemia" OR "HbA$_{1c}$" OR "pre-diabetes" OR "glycaemic control" OR "glucose" OR "blood glucose" OR "insulin"] in title/abstract AND ["cardiac surgery" OR "surgery" OR "coronary artery bypass grafting" OR "CABG" OR "cardiovascular"] in title/abstract. Articles were limited to those in English, German and French. No date limit was enforced.

In total 13,232 articles were initially identified. Duplicates and false positives were removed. Following examination of the remaining titles and abstracts only 148 articles were regarded of relevance to the topic of review. Reference lists of these articles were also screened for any further relevant papers. Fifty papers from this search have been included in this review.

Results – Literature review
Diabetes and hyperglyacemia
Diabetes
It is established for over a decade that patients with Diabetes undergoing isolated CABG surgery are faced with a higher incidence of operation-related morbidity, mortality and post-procedural angina recurrence [6, 7]. Numerous studies show that patients with Diabetes have a significantly greater risk [up to 44%] of readmission

following discharge after CABG [6, 8–12]. This finding is also supported by most recent British national data [13]. Despite this, no specific guidance exists in the UK or Europe, as to the optimal level, or method of achieving adequate glycaemic control in patients undergoing cardiac surgery. In the US, guidelines have been available for almost a decade [12].

Hyperglycaemia
Distinct from Diabetes, isolated hyperglycaemia is a long established marker of adverse outcome and increased LOS in numerous diverse clinical settings, in both patients with, and without Diabetes. Effects appear to be "dose-dependent", as longer duration and higher levels of hyperglycaemia are both associated with increased morbidity and mortality [14]. This relationship is also apparent in patients undergoing CABG surgery [15], following acute myocardial infarction [MI] [16], severe trauma, ischaemic stroke, and in critically ill medical [17–19] and peri-operative neurosurgical patients within the ITU environment. Treatment of hyperglycaemia shows clinical outcome benefit [17, 18, 20], however the optimal range and duration of glycaemic control is unclear and remains controversial.

Pre-operative hyperglycaemia in surgical patients
At present no specific guidance exists in the UK or Europe, regarding the detection and management of pre-operative hyperglycaemia in patients undergoing cardiac surgery.

The prevalence of hyperglycaemia amongst hospitalised patients is reported as high as 38%. Newly discovered in-hospital hyperglycaemia is associated with a higher mortality rate [16%] compared with hyperglycaemia for patients with known Diabetes [21, 22], increased short-term morbidity, and also short and long-term mortality following non-cardiac surgery [23, 24].

A retrospective analysis of 60,000 patients undergoing elective non-cardiac surgery from the Cleveland Clinic showed that pre-operative hyperglycaemia [random BG ≥12 mmol/l at pre-operative assessment] in patients without an established diagnosis of Diabetes increased 1 year mortality [23]. Diabetic status significantly altered this relationship and for a given level of pre-operative hyperglycaemia; the risk of 1 year mortality was lower in the Diabetes patient group compared with non-diabetes. A similar relationship was demonstrated between pre-admission hyperglycaemia and increased in-hospital mortality in the ITU setting [25], with therapeutic glycaemic control showing benefit in only those without a diagnosis of Diabetes [18]. These findings prompted the authors to suggest that A] pre-operative hyperglycaemia should be given greater consideration in patients without Diabetes than those already diagnosed with

Diabetes, and B] the expected benefits of adequate glycaemic control may be determined by the pre-operative diagnosis of Diabetes [23]. This suggestion may be regarded as counter-intuitive, but emphasises the need to "glucose screen" all patients undergoing cardiac surgery, something that is currently not routine practice in the UK.

In another large study, over 20% of ~ 34,000 non-cardiac surgical patients were hyperglycaemic on admission [fasting BG > 6.1 mmol/l] without having a prior pre-operative diagnosis of Diabetes. In over half of these patients, a subsequent provisional diagnosis of Diabetes was made [26]. Hatzakorzian et al., in a much smaller study of non-cardiac surgical patients showed a prevalence of pre-operative hyperglycaemia of greater than 25% [27]. A study of 7310 patients by Lauruschkat et al. [28], showed that the prevalence of undiagnosed Diabetes in patients undergoing CABG to be 29.6%. This was associated with increased rate of adverse outcomes, including those of cardiac resuscitation, re-intubation and prolonged ventilation. Anderson et al., in a study of 1895 patients undergoing CABG showed that patients not known to have Diabetes, but with an elevated pre-operative fasting BG [$\geq$ 5.6 mmol/l] had double their expected 1-year mortality, and this was equivalent to patients known to have Diabetes [29]. Key studies relating to the effects of hyperglycaemia on outcomes are summarised in Table 1.

Pre-operative HbA1c
In a prospective study of 3555 CABG patients, an $HbA_{1c} \geq 8.6\%$ [70 mmol/l] was shown to be an independent risk factor for early adverse outcomes and

mortality [10]. The same group when conducting a study of 3201 patients demonstrated an $HbA_{1c} \geq 7.0\%$ [53 mmol/l] to be associated with decreased 5 year survival following CABG, compared to patients having a value < 7.0% [53 mmol/l]. More importantly, patients with well controlled Diabetes [HbA_{1c} < 7.0%], could achieve comparable outcomes to those patients without a diagnosis of Diabetes [30]. Alserius et al., also demonstrated significantly reduced 3-year survival, and elevated rates of early superficial wound infection to be associated with $HbA_{1c} \geq 6.0\%$ [42 mmol/l] following CABG [31]. However, two studies [32, 33] have failed to show a relationship between HbA_{1c} and LOS, significant early adverse outcomes, or long-term survival following CABG.

Arguably, the predictive value of pre-operative HbA_{1c} in cardiac surgical patients without Diabetes is less well studied. Hudson et al., in a retrospective observational study of 1474 elective patients showed an HbA_{1c} of $\geq 6\%$ [42 mmol/l] in almost a third of patients [31%]. This was associated with elevated intra-operative BG values, a known predictor of adverse outcomes [34], and in isolation, was shown to be an independent predictor of 30-day mortality [35]. Other studies of patients not known to have Diabetes and undergoing percutaneous coronary, vascular or cardiac [4] surgical interventions, also demonstrated a strong association between the pre-procedural elevated HbA_{1c} [30–58%], and risk of early adverse events. These findings suggest that pre-operative HbA_{1c} assessment will be useful as a screening tool in all patients undergoing cardiac surgery, both those with and without Diabetes.

Table 1 Impact of newly discovered hyperglycaemia on the outcome of patients admitted to hospital

	Aim of Study	Results
Umpierrez et al.[22] n = 2030 medical patients	To determine the prevalence of in-hospital hyperglycemia and determine the survival of patients with hyperglycemia with and without a history of Diabetes	Newly discovered hyperglycemia was associated with a higher in-hospital mortality rate compared with those patients with a prior history of Diabetes and patients with normoglycemia. Patients with hyperglycaemia had longer length of hospital stay, a higher admission rate to an intensive care unit and were less likely to be discharged home.
Abdelmalak et al.[23] n = 61,536 surgical, non-cardiac surgery patients	To study the hypothesis that pre-operative BG levels and the Diabetes diagnosis status of the patients are related to surgical outcomes	One year mortality was significantly related to pre-operative BG. Hyperglycaemic patients with diagnosed Diabetes displayed a significantly lower 1 yr. mortality than hyperglycaemic patients without Diabetes
Noordzij et al.[24] n = 108,593 surgical, non-cardiac surgery patients	To determine the relationship between pre-operative BG levels and peri-operative mortality in non-cardiac and non-vascular surgery	Pre-operative hyperglycemia was found to be associated with increased cardiovascular mortality in patients undergoing non-cardiac and non-vascular surgery
Whitcomb et al.[25] n = 2713 ITU patients	To assess the association between hyperglycemia and in-hospital mortality in different ITU departments	Higher mortality was seen in hyperglycemic patients without history of Diabetes in the cardiothoracic and neurosurgical units
Anderson et al.[29] n = 1895 cardiac surgery patients	To determine whether pre-operative fasting BG is associated with an increased mortality after CABG.	Patients not known to have Diabetes but with an elevated pre-operative fasting BG had a 30 day and a 1-year mortality twice that of patients with normal values, and equivalent to patients known to have Diabetes

Peri and post-operative hyperglycaemia

Intra-operative hyperglycaemia during cardiopulmonary bypass is an independent risk factor for mortality and morbidity in patients with and without Diabetes [34, 36]. Insulin resistance rather than impaired secretion is considered responsible for this [36]. However, it remains unclear whether hyperglycaemia per se, as opposed to increased insulin resistance, drives adverse outcomes. Furnary et al., proposed that improvement in underlying impaired myocardial glycometabolism was one of the predominant mechanisms underlying the favourable effects of insulin therapy, rather than pure achievement of euglycaemia [8, 9] and this has been subsequently supported by other studies [37, 38]. Overall, peri-operative control of hyperglycaemia via continuous insulin infusion was associated with decreased incidence of deep sternal wound infection, shortened hospital LOS, reduced rates of recurrent ischaemia, improved long-term survival and significantly decreased morbidity [8, 11], in a large number of cardiac surgical patients [> 8000]. As such, it is now a globally accepted standard practice of care, although the precise stringency of control i.e. tight vs. moderate, timing and duration of intravenous therapy remain matters of debate [7, 12].

Atrial fibrillation in patients with diabetes

The relationship between Diabetes status and post-operative AF requires clearer definition. Most studies do not show any clear association [6], however, some studies show a decreased AF incidence in patients with elevated pre-operative HbA_{1c} [10, 33, 39]. These studies reflect outcomes from a non-UK population, involving pre-dominantly off pump CABG surgery. The potential protective mechanisms of an elevated HbA_{1c} on post-operative AF are unclear. Kinoshita et al. [39], propose that one plausible explanation is that patients with elevated HbA_{1c} require more insulin for adequate glycaemic control, a therapy which is shown to reduce post-operative AF [8, 40]. In support, Lazar et al. have also demonstrated tighter glycaemic control via intravenous insulin to lower incidence of post-operative AF [11].

CABG vs non-CABG cardiac surgery

The majority of evidence reviewed in this paper relates to CABG surgery as opposed to non-CABG surgery. Studies including non-CABG cardiac surgery did not clearly delineate outcomes relating to type of surgery, with the majority of patients having undergone CABG. Therefore it is difficult to draw firm conclusions regarding the relationship between deranged glycaemic control, outcomes and precise type of surgery. It is intuitive to think that the effects of deranged glycaemic control on outcomes, would be most prominent following CABG surgery as opposed to non-CABG surgery, due to the well-recognised and established effects on lipid metabolism, endothelial cell function, coronary artery disease, as well as arterial vascular properties / function although, this remains to be proven. Future studies should focus on defining whether deranged glycaemic control has differing effects on outcomes depending on type of surgery.

Optimal glycaemic care and barriers to standardisation

A critical factor hindering the establishment of clearly defined glycaemic control guidelines is the lack of consensus on what optimal treatment actually is [7, 14]. Brief consensus was reached following 2001, when the Leuven Surgical Trial demonstrated reduced 1-year mortality among critically ill patients when BG levels were tightly controlled between 4.4–6.1 mmol/l as compared to 10.0–11.1 mmol/l [17]. This study instigated an era of tight glycaemic control for all critically ill patients including cardiac surgical patients. The aim of tight control was reinforced by further studies showing beneficial effects of intensive insulin therapy in surgical, medical [18, 20] and cardiac surgical patients [8, 38]. The Portland Diabetic Project provided strong evidence of the adverse effects of hyperglycaemia in patients with Diabetes undergoing cardiac surgery, using an 8.3 mmol/l cut off target value [8, 38].

The concept of tight glycaemic control in critically ill patients was called into question with the publication of the NICE-SUGAR Study [37]. This study of 6104 patients failed to reproduce the findings of the Leuven Surgical Trial, and in fact demonstrated increased 90-day, all-cause mortality after surgery in the tight control group [37]. In support of these findings more recent studies in CABG patients have either failed to demonstrate beneficial effects with tight control [41–44], or shown superior beneficial effects with moderate control [7.0–9.9 mmol/l] [45].

The recent randomised controlled GLUCO-CABG trial of 302 patients showed no difference in outcomes between intensive or conventional moderate glucose control in CABG patients with Diabetes [46]. However, in patients without Diabetes intensive glucose control was associated with lower complication rate. This reinforces the idea from the Portland Diabetic Project and Cleveland Clinic group of the importance of Diabetic status [pre/peri-operative hyperglycaemia in patients with and without Diabetes] [38]. Possibly a lower BG target is needed for patients without Diabetes, whereas a higher target is permissible for those with Diabetes.

The recently published American multicentre study of 4316 cardiac surgical patients by Greco et al., [47] showed that, increasing hyperglycaemia above 180 mg/dl [10 mmol/l] in patients without Diabetes was associated with worsening outcomes. However, this relationship did not hold for patients with non-insulin treated Diabetes.

Adding further complexity, this study demonstrated that in insulin treated group allowing BGs above 180 mg/dl [10 mmol/l] was beneficial, with worsening outcomes when "better" control was achieved.

Inducing unnecessary and dangerous hypoglycaemic events with insulin, historically represented another issue driving reluctance to employ stringent BG control protocols. However, these events are now recognised as being rare and avoidable [3, 46], provided BG is frequently monitored.

The lack of consensus amongst the studies we have analysed in this review may be due to the heterogeneity with regards to treatment of hyperglycaemia, glycaemic control protocols, glucose measurement protocols, the glucose metrics employed, their validity and relevance, as well as the individual population demographics. The best metric of glycaemic control remains a matter of debate, and many have been utilised. Average BG over 3 days [3-BG] is considered a good measure [38, 48]. Studies show that metrics incorporating glucose values over longer time periods have greater prognostic relevance in comparison to isolated glucose measurements from just the first 24 or 48-h of an index event e.g. surgical operation or hospitalisation [49]. Metrics of variability/complexity of the circadian glucose pattern are also proposed to be of greater importance than actual BG levels [50].

Future targeted therapies

The multiple proposed detrimental downstream pathways of hyperglycaemia / insulin resistance, and positive effects of insulin therapy following cardiac surgery are largely unknown and require further detailed definition [3]. They are not the focus of this review, but they are of importance with respect to the development of future targeted therapies. Altered free fatty acid metabolism, endothelial dysfunction, reduced nitric oxide bioavailability and accumulation of reactive oxygen species are implicated [3]. So too is protein kinase C-dependent vasoconstriction, vascular inflammation and platelet aggregation; as well as advanced glycation products [AGE] driven pro-inflammatory cascades [3]. In addition to the metabolic benefits, improved myocardial recovery following myocardial ischemia and direct improvement of contractile function are thought to occur with insulin therapy. Increasing evidence now suggests that reduction in BG variability, rather than absolute levels, to be a major determinant of the beneficial effects of insulin therapy [50]. Other proposed beneficial mechanisms include; membrane stabilization, anti-arrhythmic effects, improved glucose utilization, improved cardiac output via vasodilation and lowering of total peripheral resistance, and improved immune function [3].

Improving clinical outcomes

The detrimental effects of hyperglycaemia and Diabetes on cardiac surgery outcomes are well recognised. Despite that, clear treatment guidance is still lacking in UK and Europe and this has to be addressed. It is vital for all disciplines associated with the care of cardiac surgical patients, to engage in addressing the discrepancy in quality of outcomes observed in patients with poor glycaemic control. By looking into this discrepancy in outcomes, a decision needs to be made as to whether this discrepancy is A] acceptable, B] modifiable, and if so how, and C] is enough currently being done to minimise, or potentially abolish it. We feel that the current dogma stating that *"patients with Diabetes have worse outcomes than patients without Diabetes following cardiac surgery"* is potentially wrong, as these patients are currently not receiving best therapy, and this dogma must be challenged.

Proposal's for quality service improvement

The extensive evidence reviewed in this article provides a sufficient mandate to commence a national / international initiative to standardise and improve the quality of glycaemic control in patients undergoing cardiac surgery in UK and Europe.

In the US, a national initiative to improve post-operative glycaemic control in cardiac patients has already commenced in the form of a **S**urgical **C**are **I**mprovement **P**roject **[SCIP]** [21, 48]. This initiative involves collection and analysis of specific performance measures relating to glycaemic control in all participating cardiac centres, with subsequent public reporting of outcomes and compliance. In addition the Society of Thoracic Surgeons [STS] have published detailed US practice guidelines relating to pre-, intra- and post-operative glycaemic management of patients with and without Diabetes undergoing cardiac surgery; Table 2 [12]. The STS practice guidelines include: A] active control of BGs < 180 mg/dl[10 mmol/l] for all patients during the intra- and post-operative period B] all patients

Table 2 Summary of the US STS guidelines for glycaemic control during adult cardiac surgery (2008)

A] active control of BGs < 180 mg/dl[10 mmol/l] for all patients during the intra- and post-operative period

B] all patients with Diabetes receive an insulin infusion in the operating room and for at least 24 h postoperatively

C] pre-operative HbA$_{1c}$ measurement in all patients with Diabetes and those at high risk of post-operative hyperglycaemia, to optimise glycaemic management, and identify patients requiring more aggressive glycaemic control

D] pre-discharge in-patient education of all patients with Diabetes and

E] appropriate follow up and communication with primary care physician

with Diabetes receive an insulin infusion in the operating room and for at least 24 h postoperatively C] pre-operative HbA_{1c} measurement in all patients with Diabetes and those at high risk of post-operative hyperglycaemia, to optimise glycaemic management, and identify patients requiring more aggressive glycaemic control, D] pre-discharge in-patient education of all patients with Diabetes and E] appropriate follow up and communication with primary care physician.

It is inevitable that practice and outcomes around the UK and Europe in relation to patients with Diabetes or pre-diabetes varies between individual treatment centres. However, the formation of national guidelines, standardisation of care, centralised reporting and open sharing of glycaemic performance data is critical to improving future standards of care. Formation of this structure along with a national glycaemic SCIP would also serve to incentivise service improvement. An example of such a novel potential European SCIP is shown in Table 3. In addition the novel care pathway utilised in our unit is shown in Table 4.

Future studies

Future studies need to A] define the optimal level, duration and timing of glycaemic control of patients undergoing cardiac surgery B] quantify any potential benefit derived from pre-operative glycaemic control optimisation C] define the optimal glucose metrics for glycaemic control assessment and validate their positive predictive value for adverse events and D] mechanistically interrogate and identify potential therapeutic targets that improve outcomes in patients with Diabetes, pre-diabetes and those with peri-operative hyperglycaemia and E] aim to define the precise relationship between and deranged glycaemic control and outcomes following types of cardiac surgery; CABG vs non-CABG.

Establishing a new culture in which widespread detailed measurement, reporting and analysis of glycaemic control in relation to patient outcomes will enhance our understanding, help to identify and direct avenues for research and ultimately improve practice and outcomes in these patients.

Conclusions

The incidence of diagnosed Diabetes continues to rise, and in addition high levels of undiagnosed Diabetes and

Table 3 Potential Steps for Facilitating Service Improvement in Diabetic / Pre-diabetic Patients Undergoing Cardiac Surgery

Step 1

Publication of detailed and specific guidelines regarding:
Pre-operative screening of all patients undergoing elective cardiac surgery and therapeutic intervention for Diabetes / pre-diabetes

Pre-operative target glycaemic criteria permitting elective surgery e.g. $HbA_{1c} < 7.5\%$

Methods, triggers and duration of intra-operative and post-operative glycaemic control

Post-operative / pre-discharge target criteria of glycaemic control on ITU and ward e.g. blood glucose ≤12 mM pre-discharge

Early post-discharge follow up by family doctor / Diabetes specialist team to ensure ongoing good glycaemic control

Step 2

Establishment of a dedicated cardiac diabetic specialist team in every cardiac surgical unit to facilitate:
Pre-, peri-, post-operative and discharge glycaemic control and planning

Patient and professional education at all levels and communication with primary and community care services

Step 3

Establishment of specific national diabetic cardiac Surgical Care Improvement Project (SCIP) Europe-wide to include:
Introduction of relevant and appropriate performance quality measures e.g.:-

HbA_{1c} measurement in 100% of elective patients undergoing cardiac surgery

Pre-operative point of care fasting blood glucose of ≤8 mM in 95% of operated patients

Pre-operative HbA_{1c} value of < 7.5% in 95% of elective patients going for cardiac surgery

Median post-operative LOS of diabetic patients ≤1.0 day greater than median postoperative LOS for non-diabetic patients

Pre-discharge blood glucose range of 4–12 mM (day before discharge) in 95% of all patients going for cardiac surgery

Post-discharge review by diabetic specialist nurse or family doctor within 1 week in 95% of patients

Incidence of deep sternal wound infection for diabetic patient within the 95% CI of non-diabetic patient
A peri-operative glycaemic control multi-disciplinary working group in every cardiac surgical unit, responsible for monitoring and reporting SCIP adherence and compliance.

Table 4 Oxford Heart Centre Diabetes Care Pathway

- Routine pre-operative diabetic screening for *all* cardiac surgical elective patients (HbA_{1c}). Via *GP or part of Pre Assessment Clinic(PAC)*

- Routine diabetic screening for *all* cardiac surgical *urgent* in-patients (HbA_{1c})

- Point of care diabetic specialist team review of *all* diabetic, *OR* selectively identified *"High Glycaemic Risk"* cardiac surgical patients

- Automatic / mandatory ITU, ward, point of ITU discharge and pre-hospital discharge diabetic specialist team review of all diabetic, *OR* selectively identified *"High Glycaemic Risk"* cardiac surgical patients

- Automatic / mandatory GP or specialist nurse post-discharge follow up arrangement on agreed day e.g. day 4

- Routine pre-operative blood glucose measurement on admission of *all* surgical patients

- Establishment of a glycaemic control working group responsible for regular monitoring, auditing and presenting glycaemic control performance data

- New standardised Intravenous Insulin protocol for all patients undergoing cardiac surgery and guidelines for management of hyper and hypo-glycaemia

Table 5 The summary of the main findings of this review

- The proportion of people worldwide with Diabetes undergoing isolated CABG surgery has increased by 33% in recent years to 25–40%

- The incidence of diagnosed Diabetes continues to rise, and high levels of undiagnosed Diabetes and pre-diabetes are reported in surgical patients.

- Pre- and peri-operative hyperglycaemia is associated with worse outcomes following cardiac surgery

- Evidence suggests that pre-operative hyperglycaemia in patients without Diabetes carries greater clinical significance; than in patients already with diagnosed Diabetes.

- Cardiac surgical patients without Diabetes with pre-operative hyperglycaemia have a 1 year mortality double that of patients with normoglycaemia, and equivalent to patients already diagnosed with Diabetes.

- No uniform consensus in the UK or Europe exists, for glycaemic management of patients with Diabetes or pre-diabetes undergoing cardiac surgery.

- Patients with well controlled Diabetes *may* achieve comparable outcomes to patients without Diabetes with similar glycaemic control.

- This review supports the pre-operative screening, and optimisation of glycaemic control in patients undergoing cardiac surgery.

- The optimal glycaemic management of cardiac surgical patients remains unclear and requires definition

- Clear guidelines relating to the glycaemic management of cardiac surgical patients are needed in the UK and Europe

pre-diabetes are reported in surgical patients. Poor glycaemic control is associated with adverse outcomes following cardiac surgery, and the evidence suggests that pre-operative hyperglycaemia in patients without Diabetes carries greater clinical significance; than in patients already with diagnosed Diabetes. These results suggest that implementation of routine pre-operative glycaemic screening should be performed in all patients. There is conflicting evidence regarding the precise stringency of glycaemic control that should be employed in these patients i.e. tight vs. moderate control; and this requires clearer definition. Patients with Diabetes with good glycaemic control can achieve similar outcomes to patients without Diabetes undergoing cardiac surgery. As such, the current dogma stating that *"diabetic patients have worse outcomes than non-diabetic patients following cardiac surgery"* is potentially wrong. It is imperative that we generate national and European guidelines and standardise the care for patients with Diabetes/pre-diabetes undergoing cardiac surgery.

The main findings from this review are summarised in Table 5.

Acknowledgements
None

Funding
Not applicable

Authors' contributions
MN and RR were specifically involved in performing a through literature review and both made significant contributions to the writing of the paper. RE and FG were specifically involved in the vetting of the quality of the papers subject to review in this article and made significant contributions to the formatting and structure of this paper. CA was involved in the literature review and assessment of the quality of papers included in this paper and also made significant contributions to the writing of this paper. AK and MD performed the initial literature search and selection of relevant papers. GK and GK were responsible for the editing of the final submitted paper. All authors read and approved the final manuscript.

Competing interests
The authors declare that they have no competing interests.

References
1. Forouhi NG, Wareham NJ. Epidemiology of diabetes. Medicine [Abingdon]. 2014;42(12):698–702.
2. Patterson CC, Dahlquist GG, Gyurus E, Green A, Soltesz G. Incidence trends for childhood type 1 diabetes in Europe during 1989-2003 and predicted new cases 2005-20: a multicentre prospective registration study. Lancet. 2009;373(9680):2027–33.
3. Reddy P, Duggar B, Butterworth J. Blood glucose management in the patient undergoing cardiac surgery: a review. World J Cardiol. 2014;6(11): 1209–17.
4. JT MG Jr, Shariff MA, Bhat TM, Azab B, Molloy WJ, Quattrocchi E, Farid M, Eichorn AM, Dlugacz YD, Silverman RA. Prevalence of dysglycemia among coronary artery bypass surgery patients with no previous diabetic history. J Cardiothorac Surg. 2011;6:104.
5. Ryden L, Grant PJ, Anker SD, Berne C, Cosentino F, Danchin N, Deaton C, Escaned J, Hammes HP, Huikuri H, Marre M, Marx N, Mellbin L, Ostergren J, Patrono C, Seferovic P, Uva MS, Taskinen MR, Tendera M, Tuomilehto J, Valensi P, Zamorano JL. ESC guidelines on diabetes, pre-diabetes, and cardiovascular diseases developed in collaboration with the E. Diab Vasc Dis Res. 2014;11(3):133–73.
6. Thourani VH, Weintraub WS, Stein B, Gebhart SS, Craver JM, Jones EL, Guyton RA. Influence of diabetes mellitus on early and late outcome after coronary artery bypass grafting. Ann Thorac Surg. 1999;67(4):1045–52.
7. Tsai LL, Jensen HA, Thourani VH. Intensive Glycemic control in cardiac surgery. Curr Diab Rep. 2016;16(4):25.
8. Furnary AP, Zerr KJ, Grunkemeier GL, Starr A. Continuous intravenous insulin infusion reduces the incidence of deep sternal wound infection in diabetic patients after cardiac surgical procedures. Ann Thorac Surg. 1999;67(2):352–60.
9. Furnary AP, Gao G, Grunkemeier GL, Wu Y, Zerr KJ, Bookin SO, Floten HS, Starr A. Continuous insulin infusion reduces mortality in patients with diabetes undergoing coronary artery bypass grafting. J Thorac Cardiovasc Surg. 2003;125(5):1007–21.
10. Halkos ME, Puskas JD, Lattouf OM, Kilgo P, Kerendi F, Song HK, Guyton RA, Thourani VH. Elevated preoperative hemoglobin A1c level is predictive of adverse events after coronary artery bypass surgery. J Thorac Cardiovasc Surg. 2008;136(3):631–40.
11. Lazar HL, Chipkin SR, Fitzgerald CA, Bao Y, Cabral H, Apstein CS. Tight glycemic control in diabetic coronary artery bypass graft patients improves perioperative outcomes and decreases recurrent ischemic events. Circulation. 2004;109(12):1497–502.
12. Lazar HL, McDonnell M, Chipkin SR, Furnary AP, Engelman RM, Sadhu AR, Bridges CR, Haan CK, Svedjeholm R, Taegtmeyer H, Shemin RJ. The Society of Thoracic Surgeons practice guideline series: blood glucose management during adult cardiac surgery. Ann Thorac Surg. 2009;87(2):663–9.
13. National Adult Cardiac Surgical Database Report. 2008. Available http://www.scts.org/_userfiles/resources/SixthNACSDreport 2008.
14. Girish G, Agarwal S, Satsangi DK, Tempe D, Dutta N, Pratap H. Glycemic control in cardiac surgery: rationale and current evidence. Ann Card Anaesth. 2014;17(3):222–8.

15. Fish LH, Weaver TW, Moore AL, Steel LG. Value of postoperative blood glucose in predicting complications and length of stay after coronary artery bypass grafting. Am J Cardiol. 2003;92(1):74–6.

16. Capes SE, Hunt D, Malmberg K, Pathak P, Gerstein HC. Stress hyperglycemia and prognosis of stroke in nondiabetic and diabetic patients: a systematic overview. Stroke. 2001;32(10):2426–32.

17. Van den Berghe G, Wouters P, Weekers F, Verwaest C, Bruyninckx F, Schetz M, Vlasselaers D, Ferdinande P, Lauwers P, Bouillon R. Intensive insulin therapy in critically ill patients. N Engl J Med. 2001;345(19):1359–67.

18. Van den Berghe G, Wilmer A, Milants I, Wouters PJ, Bouckaert B, Bruyninckx F, Bouillon R, Schetz M. Intensive insulin therapy in mixed medical/surgical intensive care units: benefit versus harm. Diabetes. 2006;55(11):3151–9.

19. Van den Berghe G. Intensive insulin therapy in the ICU–reconciling the evidence. Nat Rev Endocrinol. 2012;8(6):374–8.

20. Van den Berghe G, Wilmer A, Hermans G, Meersseman W, Wouters PJ, Milants I, Van WE, Bobbaers H, Bouillon R. Intensive insulin therapy in the medical ICU. N Engl J Med. 2006;354(5):449–61.

21. Stoodley L, Wung SF. Hyperglycemia after cardiac surgery: improving a quality measure. AACN Adv Crit Care. 2014;25(3):221–7.

22. Umpierrez GE, Isaacs SD, Bazargan N, You X, Thaler LM, Kitabchi AE. Hyperglycemia: an independent marker of in-hospital mortality in patients with undiagnosed diabetes. J Clin Endocrinol Metab. 2002;87(3):978–82.

23. Abdelmalak BB, Knittel J, Abdelmalak JB, Dalton JE, Christiansen E, Foss J, Argalious M, Zimmerman R, Van den Berghe G. Preoperative blood glucose concentrations and postoperative outcomes after elective non-cardiac surgery: an observational study. Br J Anaesth. 2014;112(1):79–88.

24. Noordzij PG, Boersma E, Schreiner F, Kertai MD, Feringa HH, Dunkelgrun M, Bax JJ, Klein J, Poldermans D. Increased preoperative glucose levels are associated with perioperative mortality in patients undergoing noncardiac, nonvascular surgery. Eur J Endocrinol. 2007;156(1):137–42.

25. Whitcomb BW, Pradhan EK, Pittas AG, Roghmann MC, Perencevich EN. Impact of admission hyperglycemia on hospital mortality in various intensive care unit populations. Crit Care Med. 2005;33(12):2772–7.

26. Abdelmalak B, Abdelmalak JB, Knittel J, Christiansen E, Mascha E, Zimmerman R, Argalious M, Foss J. The prevalence of undiagnosed diabetes in non-cardiac surgery patients, an observational study. Can J Anaesth. 2010;57(12):1058–64.

27. Hatzakorzian R, Bui H, Carvalho G, Shan WL, Sidhu S, Schricker T. Fasting blood glucose levels in patients presenting for elective surgery. Nutrition. 2011;27(3):298–301.

28. Lauruschkat AH, Arnrich B, Albert AA, Walter JA, Amann B, Rosendahl UP, Alexander T, Ennker J. Prevalence and risks of undiagnosed diabetes mellitus in patients undergoing coronary artery bypass grafting. Circulation. 2005;112(16):2397–402.

29. Anderson RE, Klerdal K, Ivert T, Hammar N, Barr G, Owall A. Are even impaired fasting blood glucose levels preoperatively associated with increased mortality after CABG surgery? Eur Heart J. 2005;26(15):1513–8.

30. Halkos ME, Lattouf OM, Puskas JD, Kilgo P, Cooper WA, Morris CD, Guyton RA, Thourani VH. Elevated preoperative hemoglobin A1c level is associated with reduced long-term survival after coronary artery bypass surgery. Ann Thorac Surg. 2008;86(5):1431–7.

31. Alserius T, Anderson RE, Hammar N, Nordqvist T, Ivert T. Elevated glycosylated haemoglobin [HbA1c] is a risk marker in coronary artery bypass surgery. Scand Cardiovasc J. 2008;42(6):392–8.

32. Knapik P, Ciesla D, Filipiak K, Knapik M, Zembala M. Prevalence and clinical significance of elevated preoperative glycosylated hemoglobin in diabetic patients scheduled for coronary artery surgery. Eur J Cardiothorac Surg. 2011;39(4):484–9.

33. Matsuura K, Imamaki M, Ishida A, Shimura H, Niitsuma Y, Miyazaki M. Off-pump coronary artery bypass grafting for poorly controlled diabetic patients. Ann Thorac Cardiovasc Surg. 2009;15(1):18–22.

34. Gandhi GY, Nuttall GA, Abel MD, Mullany CJ, Schaff HV, Williams BA, Schrader LM, Rizza RA, McMahon MM. Intraoperative hyperglycemia and perioperative outcomes in cardiac surgery patients. Mayo Clin Proc. 2005; 80(7):862–6.

35. Hudson CC, Welsby IJ, Phillips-Bute B, Mathew JP, Lutz A, Chad HG, Stafford-Smith M. Glycosylated hemoglobin levels and outcome in non-diabetic cardiac surgery patients. Can J Anaesth. 2010;57(6):565–72.

36. Doenst T, Wijeysundera D, Karkouti K, Zechner C, Maganti M, Rao V, Borger MA. Hyperglycemia during cardiopulmonary bypass is an independent risk factor for mortality in patients undergoing cardiac surgery. J Thorac Cardiovasc Surg. 2005;130(4):1144.

37. Finfer S, Chittock DR, Su SY, Blair D, Foster D, Dhingra V, Bellomo R, Cook D, Dodek P, Henderson WR, Hebert PC, Heritier S, Heyland DK, McArthur C, McDonald E, Mitchell I, Myburgh JA, Norton R, Potter J, Robinson BG, Ronco JJ. Intensive versus conventional glucose control in critically ill patients. N Engl J Med. 2009;360(13):1283–97.

38. Furnary AP, Wu Y, Bookin SO. Effect of hyperglycemia and continuous intravenous insulin infusions on outcomes of cardiac surgical procedures: the Portland diabetic project. Endocr Pract. 2004;10(Suppl 2):21–33.

39. Kinoshita T, Asai T, Suzuki T, Kambara A, Matsubayashi K. Preoperative hemoglobin A1c predicts atrial fibrillation after off-pump coronary bypass surgery. Eur J Cardiothorac Surg. 2012;41(1):102–7.

40. Lazar HL, Chipkin S, Philippides G, Bao Y, Apstein C. Glucose-insulin-potassium solutions improve outcomes in diabetics who have coronary artery operations. Ann Thorac Surg. 2000;70(1):145–50.

41. Desai SP, Henry LL, Holmes SD, Hunt SL, Martin CT, Hebsur S, Ad N. Strict versus liberal target range for perioperative glucose in patients undergoing coronary artery bypass grafting: a prospective randomized controlled trial. J Thorac Cardiovasc Surg. 2012;143(2):318–25.

42. Mulla I, Schmidt K, Cashy J, Wallia A, Andrei AC, Johnson OD, Aleppo G, Li C, Grady KL, McGee E, Molitch ME. Comparison of glycemic and surgical outcomes after change in glycemic targets in cardiac surgery patients. Diabetes Care. 2014;37(11):2960–5.

43. Pezzella AT, Holmes SD, Pritchard G, Speir AM, Ad N. Impact of perioperative glycemic control strategy on patient survival after coronary bypass surgery. Ann Thorac Surg. 2014;98(4):1281–5.

44. Lazar HL, McDonnell MM, Chipkin S, Fitzgerald C, Bliss C, Cabral H. Effects of aggressive versus moderate glycemic control on clinical outcomes in diabetic coronary artery bypass graft patients. Ann Surg. 2011;254(3):458–63.

45. Bhamidipati CM, LaPar DJ, Stukenborg GJ, Morrison CC, Kern JA, Kron IL, Ailawadi G. Superiority of moderate control of hyperglycemia to tight control in patients undergoing coronary artery bypass grafting. J Thorac Cardiovasc Surg. 2011;141(2):543–51.

46. Umpierrez G, Cardona S, Pasquel F, Jacobs S, Peng L, Unigwe M, Newton CA, Smiley-Byrd D, Vellanki P, Halkos M, Puskas JD, Guyton RA, Thourani VH. Randomized controlled trial of intensive versus conservative glucose control in patients undergoing coronary artery bypass graft surgery: GLUCO-CABG trial. Diabetes Care. 2015;38(9):1665–72.

47. Greco G, Ferket BS, D'Alessandro DA, Shi W, Horvath KA, Rosen A, Welsh S, Bagiella E, Neill AE, Williams DL, Greenberg A, Browndyke JN, Gillinov AM, Mayer ML, Keim-Malpass J, Gupta LS, Hohmann SF, Gelijns AC, O'Gara PT, Moskowitz AJ. Diabetes and the Association of Postoperative Hyperglycemia with Clinical and Economic Outcomes in cardiac surgery. Diabetes Care. 2016;

48. McDonnell ME, Alexanian SM, Junqueira A, Cabral H, Lazar HL. Relevance of the surgical care improvement project on glycemic control in patients undergoing cardiac surgery who receive continuous insulin infusions. J Thorac Cardiovasc Surg. 2013;145(2):590–4.

49. Kosiborod M, Inzucchi SE, Krumholz HM, Xiao L, Jones PG, Fiske S, Masoudi FA, Marso SP, Spertus JA. Glucometrics in patients hospitalized with acute myocardial infarction: defining the optimal outcomes-based measure of risk. Circulation. 2008;117(8):1018–27.

50. Ogawa S, Okawa Y, Sawada K, Goto Y, Yamamoto M, Koyama Y, Baba H, Suzuki T. Continuous postoperative insulin infusion reduces deep sternal wound infection in patients with diabetes undergoing coronary artery bypass grafting using bilateral internal mammary artery grafts: a propensity-matched analysis. Eur J Cardiothorac Surg. 2016;49(2):420–6.

3

The wearable cardioverter defibrillator as a bridge to reimplantation in patients with ICD or CRT-D-related infections

L. Castro[1][*][†] (iD), S. Pecha[1][†], M. Linder[1], J. Vogler[2], N. Gosau[2], C. Meyer[2], S. Willems[2], H. Reichenspurner[1] and S. Hakmi[1]

Abstract

Background: The approach to treat device infection in patients with implantable cardioverter defibrillator (ICD) or cardiac resynchronization therapy defibrillator (CRT-D) is a challenging procedure. Optimal treatment is complete extraction of the infected device. To protect these patients from sudden cardiac arrest while waiting for reimplantation and to avoid recurrent infection, a wearable cardioverter defibrillator (WCD) seems to be a valuable solution. Therefore, we investigated the management and outcome of patients with ICD or CRT-D infections using the WCD as a bridge to re-implantation after lead extraction procedures.

Methods: We conducted a retrospective study on consecutive patients who underwent ICD or CRT-D removal due to device-related local or systemic infections. All patients were prescribed a WCD at our center between 01/2012 and 10/2015. All patients returned to our outpatient clinic for regular ICD or CRT-D monitoring initially 1 and 3 months after reimplantation followed by 6-months intervals.

Results: Twenty-one patients (mean age 65.0 ± 8.0 years, male 76.2%) were included in the study. Complete lead extraction was achieved in all patients. While waiting for reimplantation one patient experienced a symptomatic episode of sustained ventricular tachycardia. This episode was converted successfully into sinus rhythm by a single 150 J shock. Mean follow-up time 392 ± 206 days, showing survival rate of 100% and freedom from reinfection in all patients.

Conclusion: The WCD seems to be a valuable bridging option for patients with ICD or CRT-D infections, showing no recurrent device infection.

Keywords: Wearable cardioverter defibrillator, CIED-infection, ICD infection, Sudden cardiac arrest, Lead/ device extraction, Ventricular tachycardia

Background

Due to the increasing indications for cardiac resynchronization-therapy devices (CRT-D) and implantable cardioverter defibrillator devices (ICD) for heart failure therapy and prevention of sudden cardiac arrest (SCA), the implantation rates for cardiovascular implantable electronic devices (CIEDs) have increased over time [1, 2]. In this context, there is also a rising number of devices that have to be extracted due to local or systemic device-related infections.

The choice of treatment strategy for the prevention of sudden cardiac arrest (SCA) among patients after removal of an infected implantable cardioverter-defibrillator (ICD) system is still an important clinical challenge. The underlying pathologies – such as, structural heart disease, previous myocardial infarction or genetic abnormality – pose a constant and ongoing risk for ventricular tachycardia. Current guidelines recommend complete removal of the infected device and parenteral antibiotic treatment, followed by two-stage contralateral reimplantation [3]. Care of patients in this period is critical. On one hand, implanting the device too early may result in recurrent infection. On the other hand, patients still remain at risk for SCA.

Using a wearable cardioverter defibrillator (WCD) seems to be a valuable approach to protect patients from

---
* Correspondence: l.castro@uke.de
†Equal contributors
[1]Department of Cardiovascular Surgery, University Heart Center Hamburg, Hamburg, Germany
Full list of author information is available at the end of the article

SCA while waiting for reimplantation and to avoid too early reimplantation leading to recurrent infection.

We here investigated the management and outcomes of patients with ICD or CRT-D infections using the WCD as a bridge to reimplantation after device extraction procedures.

Methods

Patient characteristics

Patient characteristics are shown in Table 1. We conducted a retrospective study on consecutive patients who underwent ICD or CRT-D removal due to local or systemic infection at our center between January 2012 and October 2015. Patient information was de-identified in all cases and all patients were prescribed a WCD (LifeVest, ZOLL, Pittsburgh, PA, USA). We discussed all cases in an interdisciplinary heart team, including a cardiothoracic surgeon and a cardiologist/ electrophysiologist.

Removal techniques

All procedures were performed in a hybrid operating room with patients under general anesthesia. For monitoring during lead extraction we used continuous arterial blood pressure measurement via an arterial line placed in the radial artery and 3D transoesophageal echocardiography.

After removal of the generator we did extensive wound debridement and collected specimens from the pocket. Leads were dissected from the scar tissue and the sleeves were removed.

Leads implanted less than 24 months ago were extracted under fluoroscopic guidance with use of a lead locking device (Spectranetics Corporation, Colorado Springs, CO, USA) making the traction procedure more efficient.

Table 1 Baseline and clinical characteristics

Patients	(n = 21)
Demographics	
Age, years	65 ± 8
Male gender, n (%)	16 (76.2)
Medical history	
Renal failure, n (%)	7 (33.3)
Diabetes mellitus, n (%)	9 (42.85)
Coronary artery disease, n (%)	11 (52.4)
Symptoms	
Pocket infection, n (%)	14 (66.7)
Systemic infection, n (%)	7 (33.3)
Laboratory	
Leucocytes billion/l	8.7 ± 2.2
C-reactive protein mg/l	66.0 ± 61

Continuous variables are expressed as mean ± standard deviation and categorical are expressed by values and percentages

When the attempt to remove leads was not successful because of aggressive adhesions, a Spectranetics laser sheath (Spectranetics Corporation, Colorado Springs, CO, USA) was applied in 12 cases. Lead tips were collected for microbiological work up.

Postoperative management

According to antibiotic sensitivity testing we initiated an antibiotic treatment. All patients were prescribed a WCD and were trained in handling the WCD 1–2 days after explantation. Very thoroughly programming was required due to unavailable antitachycardia pacing in WCD. The recommended programming is 170–220 beats/min for rate detection with VT shock delay programmed from 60 to 180 s. Depending on former device programming and ECG recordings from the explanted device, rate and treatment criteria of the WCD were adjusted and programmed. Although the VT detection can be programmed to as low as 120 beats/min, we avoided to program lower rates than 160 beats/min to prevent inappropriate shocks.

Before discharge appointments were made for every patient to return to our outpatient clinic for first follow-up four weeks after the respective device explantation. A new device was implanted on contralateral side when C-reactive protein (CRP) value and leucocyte counts were within normal ranges and blood culture samples showed negative results.

Follow-up and endpoints

Patients returned to our outpatient clinic for regular ICD or CRT-D monitoring initially 1 and 3 months after re-implantation followed by 6-months intervals. The primary endpoints of the study were absence of serious arrhythmic complications and freedom from reinfection.

Definitions

Local infection was defined as the presence of local inflammation-signs (pocket abscess, skin adherence, chronic draining sinus) at the generator pocket or erosion of a lead or device through the skin without clinically evident involvement of the intravenous portion of the lead system [3, 4].

Systemic infection was defined as valvular endocarditis with or without definite involvement of the leads and/or device, occult gram-positive bacteremia (not contaminant) or sepsis. Freedom from reinfection was defined as the absence of such detection during the observational period [3, 4].

Complete procedural success was defined as removal of all infected device elements (generator, leads, sleeves) without any complications or procedure related death.

Statistical analysis

All data were recorded prospectively into a database and analyzed retrospectively with SPSS statistical software version 23 (IBM SPSS Statistics for Windows, Version 23.0). All continuous variables are expressed as mean ± standard deviation and categorical variables are displayed as numbers and percentages.

Results
Patients
Twenty-one patients with a mean age of 65.0 ± 8.0 years were included in the study. The indication for initial device implantation was primary prevention in 10 (47.6%) patients and secondary prevention in 11 (52.4%) patients.

Infection was local in 14 patients (66.7%; 6 ICD; 8 CRT-D) and systemic in 7 patients (33.3%; 4 ICD; 3 CRT-D). In all patients serological infection parameters were elevated, mean leucocytes counts were 8.7 ± 2.2 billion/l (range 4.8–16.2) and mean CRP values were 66 ± 61 mg/dl (range 5–343).

Laser lead extraction had to be performed in 12 (57.1%) patients. Mean procedural time was 74 ± 30 (range 15–150) minutes with a mean fluoroscopic time of 215 ± 164 (range 20–390) seconds. During extraction, one major adverse event occurred. This was a tear at the coronary sinus (CS) during the extraction procedure of a StarFix™ (Medtronic Inc., Minneapolis, MN, USA) active fixation CS lead in a 57-years old male with subsequent need for sternotomy. Under the use of cardiopulmonary bypass the tear was successfully patched and the patient made an uneventful recovery thereafter.

Microbiology and antibiotic treatment
Antibiotic treatment had been initiated prior to surgery in 8 (38.1%) patients. If necessary, the antibiotic treatment was escalated or adapted following accomplished antibiotic sensitivity testing. After microbiological work up of the pocket specimen and lead tips, *Staphylococcus epidermidis* was the predominant infectious organisms (38.1%) found in swab and on the lead-tips. Mean postoperative duration of antibiotic treatment was 15.0 ± 5.0 (range 7–28) days.

Reimplantation
When CRP- and leucocyte values were in normal range and 3 blood culture samples showed negative results, a new CIED was successfully implanted on the contralateral side. Before reimplantation we reviewed the initial indication for CIED-implantation and if necessary a different CIED - adapted to the current diagnostic findings - was implanted as show in Table 2. Nine (42.85%) patients were re-implanted with an ICD, 9 (42.85%) patients with CRT-D and 3 (14.3%) patients with subcutaneous-ICD. The mean time to reimplantation was 51.6 ± 16.9 (range 28–108) days.

Table 2 Device characteristics

Devices	($n = 21$)
Indication for implantation	
Ischemic cardiomyopathy, n (%)	7 (33.3)
Non-ischemic cardiomyopathy, n (%)	14 (66.7)
Long QT syndrome, n (%)	1 (4.8)
ARVC, n (%)	2 (9.5)
Secondary prophylaxis, n (%)	11 (52.4)
Explanted	
VVI-ICD, n (%)	5 (23.8)
DDD-ICD, n (%)	6 (28.6)
CRT-D, n (%)	10 (47.6)
Reimplanted	
VVI-ICD, n (%)	6 (28.6)
DDD-ICD, n (%)	3 (14.3)
CRT-D, n (%)	9 (42.8)
S-ICD, n (%)	3 (14.3)
Time to re-implantation, days	51.6 ± 16.9

ARVC Arrhythmogenic right ventricular cardiomyopathy
Continuous variables are expressed as mean ± standard deviation and categorical are expressed by values and percentages

Follow-up
While waiting for reimplantation 1 (4.8%) patient experienced an episode of sustained (> 30 s) ventricular tachycardia 6 weeks after explantation. This episode was converted into sinus rhythm by a single 150 J shock of the WCD (Fig. 1). The patient was admitted to our emergency department for further monitoring and treatment. He did not show any local or systemic infection signs, thus it was decided to implant a new CRT-D.

All patients returned to our outpatient clinic for CIED monitoring after 1 and 3 months and none of the patients showed recurrent infection. The follow up was continued by regular ICD monitoring every 6 months. Mean follow-up time was 454 ± 263 (range 114–1068) days, showing survival rate of 100% and freedom from reinfection in all patients.

All patients were comfortable with wearing WCD and compliance with device use was 100% showing a mean daily wear time of 22.0 (15–24) hours per day.

Discussion
In this study we have shown that the use of WCD is a safe and efficient solution to protect patients from SCA while waiting for re-implantation of a new ICD/CRT-D device. During the period of WCD treatment, one patient experienced a symptomatic sustained ventricular tachycardia, which has been successfully treated by a single 150 J WCD shock. No inappropriate shocks were delivered. The WCD bridging concept, with the possibility to delay reimplantation until freedom from infection

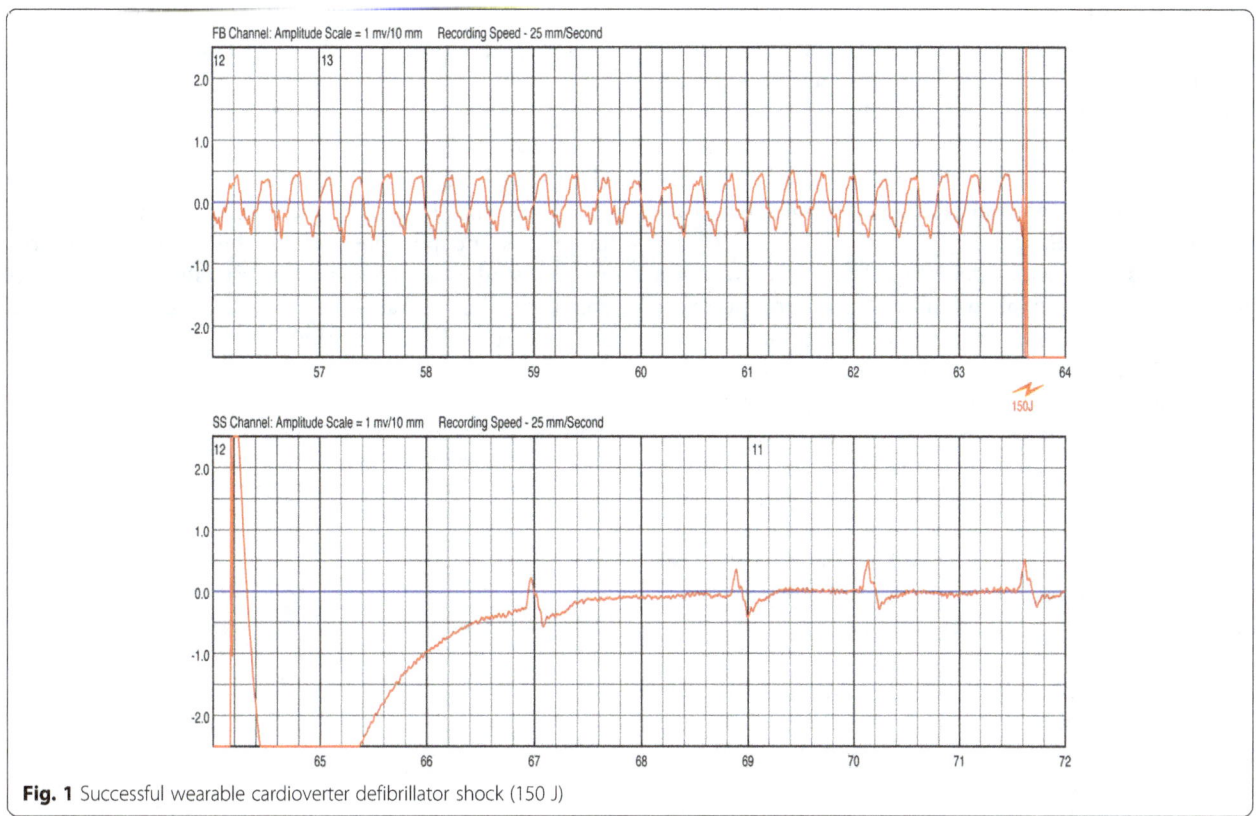

Fig. 1 Successful wearable cardioverter defibrillator shock (150 J)

is achieved, enabled for the absence of recurrent infection observed in this study.

For patients with systemic device infection, the complete removal of the device and all leads is a class I recommendation in 2010 AHA/HRS Scientific Statement (AHA) [4]. Conservative treatment of those patients is associated with high mortality and the complete device removal has been shown to significantly reduce morbidity and mortality in those patients.

Furthermore, a two-step approach with an extended period of antibiotic treatment before re-implantation is recommended [4]. In several studies it has been proven that this two-step re-implantation strategy is associated with reduced re-infection rates. The ideal timing for re-implantation is still discussed controversially in literature. However, treatment regimen should be individualized for each patient and clinical situation [4]. In patients with systemic infection and positive blood cultures, antibiotic treatment should be performed for an extended period of time, and blood cultures should be negative for at least 72 h before a re-implantation is conducted [4]. In patients with positive blood cultures and evidence for valvular involvement, implantation of a new transvenous system should even be delayed for at least 14 days, after first negative blood cultures are drawn.

These data underline the importance of a suitable bridging concept after device removal, especially in patients with

pacemaker dependency or risk for sudden cardiac arrest after ICD explantation. In patients with pacemaker dependency, as a bridging concept, a temporary RV lead can be implanted, tunneled subcutaneously and connected to an externalized pacemaker device [5].

In ICD/CRT-D patients with device removal due to infection and ongoing risk for SCA, hospitalization of the patient and continuous rhythm monitoring has been the only safe and reasonable treatment option for a long time. However, continuous inpatient monitoring is cost-effective and undesirable to the patient from a quality-of-life standpoint [6]. Furthermore this situation might lead to too early re-implantation of a new ICD/CRT-D device in some cases, carrying a high risk for recurrent infection.

Using a WCD allows extension of the period of antibiotic treatment until re-implantation up to several weeks, if necessary. During this time the patient can be discharged home safely until re-implantation is scheduled [6].

Safety and efficacy of WCD has been proven in clinical studies [7–9]. In a large prospective clinical registry, the WEARIT-II registry, 2000 patients with WCD were included. In this registry, 120 sustained ventricular tachycardia (VT)/ ventricular fibrillation (VF) episodes occurred in 41 patients. Importantly, most of the sustained VTs were not treated by the WCD, while patients used the response button to delay therapy and the VT episodes self-terminated. However, 30 events in 22 patients needed shock delivery due to hemodynamic instability [8]. All patients requiring shock delivery had their VT/VF episode terminated successfully with the first shock, showing the high efficacy of WCD therapy. In the largest WCD registry including 3569 patients, Chung et al. demonstrated a first shock efficacy of 99% [10]. Although a smaller study, our experience of one appropriate and successful shock demonstrated a shock efficacy of 100%.

In contrast to previous published data by Tanawuttiwat et al. and Chung et al. we observed no inappropriate shocks in our study. In the study by Wuttiwat et al. one patient (1.0%) received an inappropriate shock due to oversensitivity of a signal artifact. Regarding inappropriate shocks, across studies with WCDs, the rate is with 0.67–1.4% per month of use, similar to those of ICDs [8, 11, 12]. Reasons that account for inappropriate shocks are noise, supraventricular tachycardia above the preset rate criteria or device malfunction. In contrast to an ICD, the WCD enables the patient to press a response button while awake and abort shock delivery. This tool might help to reduce the rate of inappropriate shock delivery.

Patients being prescribed a WCD need detailed teaching and instructions. On the one hand the patient needs to know all important device functions, like e.g. the response button and on the other hand needs to understand the importance of wearing the WCD to prevent SCA, ensuring a good compliance and high daily wear time.

In our study a mean daily wear time of 22.0 (15–24) hours shows that the WCD is a practical solution, which is easy to handle. Daily wear time, in studies by Tanawuttiwat 2014, Kutyifa et al. was with 20–22.5 h per day comparable. WCD discontinuation rates of up to 22%, which have been described by Feldman et al. were not observed in our series [9]. Another important aspect of the WCD therapy is cost-effectiveness. By avoiding expensive and uncomfortable inpatient monitoring, Healy et al. have shown that use of WCD and discharging patients home is associated with reduced costs and improvement in quality-adjusted-life-year (QALY) analysis, when compared with inpatient monitoring [6].

The protection from SCA with WCD, allowing for an appropriate time of antibiotic therapy with mean duration of 15.0 days was surely one of the reasons for the favourable outcome of our patients, showing no mortality and no recurrence of infection during mean follow-up time of 392 days. Another important factor was the successful lead extraction with complete removal rate of 100%. The combination of these two therapy aspects seems to be the ideal treatment option in patients with ICD/CRT device infection.

Conclusion

The WCD is a safe, comfortable and cost-effective bridging solution for these patients, showing survival rate of 100% and no recurrent device infection after a mean follow-up time of 454 ± 263 (range 114–1068) days.

Limitations

The major limitation of this study is the small number of patients and the retrospective design with its inherent limitations and possible bias. In the future, larger prospective studies are needed to investigate safety and efficiency of the wearable cardioverter defibrillator as a bridge to reimplantation solution.

Abbreviations

CIED: Cardiovascular Implantable Electronic Device; CRT: Cardiac Resynchronization Therapy; ICD: Implantable Cardioverter Defibrillator; SCA: Sudden Cardiac Arrest; VF: Ventricular Fibrillation; VT: Ventricular Tachycardia; WCD: Wearable Cardioverter Defibrillator

Acknowledgements

Not applicable

Funding

No funding was received for this study.

Authors' contributions

LC: conceived of the study, participated in its design and coordination, recorded data, performed the statistical analysis. SP: conceived of the study, participated in its design and coordination, helped to draft the manuscript. ML: helped to record the data. JV: helped to record the data. NG: participated in the design of the study, helped to draft the manuscript. CM: helped to draft the manuscript. SW: helped to draft the manuscript. HR: helped to draft the manuscript. SH: conceived of the study, and participated in its design and coordination. All authors read and approved the final manuscript.

Competing interests

The authors declare that they have no competing interests.

Author details

[1]Department of Cardiovascular Surgery, University Heart Center Hamburg, Hamburg, Germany. [2]Department of Cardiology, Electrophysiology, University Heart Center Hamburg, Hamburg, Germany.

References

1. Klug D, Balde M, Pavin D, Hidden-Lucet F, Clementy J, Sadoul N, Rey JL, Lande G, Lazarus A, Victor J, et al. Risk factors related to infections of implanted pacemakers and cardioverter-defibrillators: results of a large prospective study. Circulation. 2007;116:1349–55.
2. Voigt A, Shalaby A, Saba S. Continued rise in rates of cardiovascular implantable electronic device infections in the United States: temporal trends and causative insights. Pacing Clin Electrophysiol. 2010;33:414–9.
3. Wilkoff BL, Love CJ, Byrd CL, Bongiorni MG, Carrillo RG, Crossley GH 3rd, Epstein LM, Friedman RA, Kennergren CE, Mitkowski P, et al. Transvenous lead extraction: Heart Rhythm Society expert consensus on facilities,

training, indications, and patient management: this document was endorsed by the American Heart Association (AHA). Heart Rhythm. 2009;6:1085–104.

4. Baddour LM, Epstein AE, Erickson CC, Knight BP, Levison ME, Lockhart PB, Masoudi FA, Okum EJ, Wilson WR, Beerman LB, et al. Update on cardiovascular implantable electronic device infections and their management: a scientific statement from the American Heart Association. Circulation. 2010;121:458–77.

5. Pecha S, Aydin MA, Yildirim Y, Sill B, Reiter B, Wilke I, Reichenspurner H, Treede H. Transcutaneous lead implantation connected to an externalized pacemaker in patients with implantable cardiac defibrillator/pacemaker infection and pacemaker dependency. Europace. 2013;15:1205–9.

6. Healy CA, Carrillo RG. Wearable cardioverter-defibrillator for prevention of sudden cardiac death after infected implantable cardioverter-defibrillator removal: a cost-effectiveness evaluation. Heart Rhythm. 2015;12:1565–73.

7. Tanawuttiwat T, Garisto JD, Salow A, Glad JM, Szymkiewicz S, Saltzman HE, Kutalek SP, Carrillo RG. Protection from outpatient sudden cardiac death following ICD removal using a wearable cardioverter defibrillator. Pacing Clin Electrophysiol. 2014;37:562–8.

8. Kutyifa V, Moss AJ, Klein H, Biton Y, McNitt S, MacKecknie B, Zareba W, Goldenberg I. Use of the wearable cardioverter defibrillator in high-risk cardiac patients: data from the prospective registry of patients using the wearable cardioverter defibrillator (WEARIT-II registry). Circulation. 2015;132:1613–9.

9. Feldman AM, Klein H, Tchou P, Murali S, Hall WJ, Mancini D, Boehmer J, Harvey M, Heilman MS, Szymkiewicz SJ, et al. Use of a wearable defibrillator in terminating tachyarrhythmias in patients at high risk for sudden death: results of the WEARIT/BIROAD. Pacing Clin Electrophysiol. 2004;27:4–9.

10. Chung MK, Szymkiewicz SJ, Shao M, Zishiri E, Niebauer MJ, Lindsay BD, Tchou PJ. Aggregate national experience with the wearable cardioverter-defibrillator: event rates, compliance, and survival. J Am Coll Cardiol. 2010;56:194–203.

11. Sohail MR, Uslan DZ, Khan AH, Friedman PA, Hayes DL, Wilson WR, Steckelberg JM, Stoner S, Baddour LM. Management and outcome of permanent pacemaker and implantable cardioverter-defibrillator infections. J Am Coll Cardiol. 2007;49:1851–9.

12. Tarakji KG, Chan EJ, Cantillon DJ, Doonan AL, Hu T, Schmitt S, Fraser TG, Kim A, Gordon SM, Wilkoff BL. Cardiac implantable electronic device infections: presentation, management, and patient outcomes. Heart Rhythm. 2010;7:1043–7.

4

Quantifying the learning curve for pulmonary thromboendarterectomy

Smita Sihag[1,4]*(iD), Bao Le[1], Alison S. Witkin[2], Josanna M. Rodriguez-Lopez[2], Mauricio A. Villavicencio[3], Gus J. Vlahakes[3], Richard N. Channick[2] and Cameron D. Wright[1]

Abstract

Background: Pulmonary thromboendarterectomy (PTE) is an effective treatment for chronic thromboembolic pulmonary hypertension (CTEPH), but is a technically challenging operation for cardiothoracic surgeons. Starting a new program allows an opportunity to define a learning curve for PTE.

Methods: A retrospective case review was performed of 134 consecutive PTEs performed from 1998 to 2016 at a single institution. Outcomes were compared using either a two-tailed t-test for continuous variables or a chi-squared test for categorical variables according to experience of the program by terciles (T).

Results: The 30-day mortality was 3.7%. The mean length of hospital stay, length of ICU stay, and duration on a ventilator were 12.6 days, 4.6 days, and 2.0 days, respectively. The mean decrease in systolic pulmonary artery pressure (sPAP) was 41.3 mmHg. Patients with Jamieson type 2 disease had a greater change in mean sPAP than those with type 3 disease ($p = 0.039$). The mean cardiopulmonary bypass time was 180 min (T1–198 min, T3–159 min, $p = <0.001$), and the mean circulatory arrest time was 37 min (T1-44 min, T3-31 min, $p < 0.001$). Plotting circulatory arrest times as a running sum compared to the mean demonstrated 2 inflection points, the first at 22 cases and the second at 95 cases.

Conclusions: PTE is a challenging procedure to learn, and good outcomes are a result of a multi-disciplinary effort to optimize case selection, operative performance, and postoperative care. Approximately 20 cases are needed to become proficient in PTE, and nearly 100 cases are required for more efficient clearing of obstructed pulmonary arteries.

Keywords: Pulmonary thromboendarterectomy, Outcomes, Learning curve

Background

Chronic thromboembolic pulmonary hypertension (CTEPH) is a relatively rare disease affecting less than 5% of patients subsequent to an acute pulmonary embolism [1]. It is characterized by pulmonary hypertension resulting from pulmonary vascular obstruction which leads to progressive right ventricular dysfunction. Riedel et al. reported that patients with mean pulmonary artery pressures greater than 30 mmHg have only a 30% 5-year survival, and in patients with mean PAPs greater than 50 mmHg, 5-year survival further decreases to as low as 10% [2]. Medical therapy is palliative and can mitigate symptoms in the short-term, while only surgical treatment via pulmonary thromboendarterectomy (PTE) offers the potential for cure [3].

PTE is a technically challenging operation that involves complete removal of organized fibrotic and thrombotic material from bilateral pulmonary arteries extending to segmental branches under intermittent deep hypothermic circulatory arrest [4]. The effectiveness of the operation is directly related to the location and accessibility of pulmonary arterial occlusive disease and the extent to which it is cleared by the surgeon [5]. It is performed predominantly at a few experienced centers across the country, and these centers have been able to demonstrate excellent outcomes in appropriately selected patients. Thus far, the group at University of California San Diego Medical Center (UCSD) has reported the largest experience with PTE with an overall mortality rate of 4.9% and a mean decrease in pulmonary artery systolic pressures of 28 mmHg correlating

* Correspondence: sihags@mskcc.org
[1]Division of Thoracic Surgery, Massachusetts General Hospital, 55 Fruit Street, Founders 7, Boston, Massachusetts 02114, USA
[4]Thoracic Surgery Service, Memorial Sloan Kettering Cancer Center, 12 75 York Avenue, C-881, New York, NY 10065, USA
Full list of author information is available at the end of the article

with a mean increase in cardiac output of 1.6 L/min. Reperfusion pulmonary edema was the most frequent postoperative complication at 10.9% [6]. In their more recent experience after completing 2700 cases, they reported a similarly substantial improvement in hemodynamics and cardiac function with an even lower mortality rate of 2.2% [7].

Our center initiated a program to surgically treat patients with CTEPH in 1998 as a product of a multi-disciplinary collaboration between experts in pulmonary hypertension and cardiothoracic surgery. Since then, we have performed a total of 134 cases, and we have averaged 31 cases per year over the past 3 years, thereby becoming the only high volume center in PTE in our region. All patients were selected by a multi-disciplinary team led by an experienced pulmonologist in CTEPH, and all PTEs were performed jointly by a cardiac and thoracic attending surgeon. Here, we report our experience with building a CTEPH program and define a learning curve for surgeons interested in achieving proficiency in PTE.

Methods

All patients who underwent PTE from 1998 to 2016 at Massachusetts General Hospital in Boston, MA were retrospectively analyzed with the approval of the Partners Institutional Review Board Committee. A total of 134 patients were included in our study. Patients were selected for operation based on preoperative findings on pulmonary angiography, echocardiography, and nuclear ventilation-perfusion scans [8]. All cases were reviewed by a multi-disciplinary team of pulmonologists and cardiothoracic surgeons at our institution. PTE was performed jointly by a senior-level cardiac and thoracic attending surgeon in a manner similar to that described at UCSD [9]. A thoracic surgeon (CDW) performed or directly supervised all endarterectomies, and one of two cardiac surgeons assisted with cardiopulmonary bypass (GJV or MAV). Median sternotomy, cardiopulmonary bypass, aortic cross-clamping, hypothermia to 18 degrees °C, and periods of circulatory arrest of up to 20 min for each side were all essential components of operative conduct for optimal exposure and clearance of pulmonary vasculature. Additional cardiac procedures were performed during the re-warming period if indicated. Preoperative hemodynamics were assessed during right heart catheterization, while postoperative hemodynamics were monitored via Swan-Ganz catheter (Edwards Life Sciences, Irvine, CA) in the operating room and intensive care unit. Of note, pulmonary capillary wedge pressures (PCWP) were not measured routinely in our intensive care unit postoperatively. All surgical, hemodynamic, and 30-day postoperative outcomes were recorded in our database.

For data review, patients were divided into 3 evenly distributed groups or terciles by case number. The first tercile (T1) ($n = 44$) spanned from October 1998 to September 2012 and represented a more sporadic experience that began ramping up in 2010. The second tercile (T2) ($n = 45$) extended from November 2012 to February 2015, and the third tercile (T3) ($n = 45$) from February 2015 to August 2016. Statistical comparisons between T1 and T3 were carried out using a two-tailed unpaired student's t test for continuous variables, and a Chi-squared test for categorical variables. Significance was set at a threshold of $p < 0.05$. We utilized STATA statistical software package, release 14 (StataCorp LP, College Station, TX) for all analyses.

To compute a learning curve, we plotted the cumulative running sum (CUSUM) of the difference of each value from the mean deep hypothermic circulatory arrest time across 134 consecutive cases, as this parameter improved dramatically with increasing surgeon experience. This methodology has been previously validated in the surgical literature for defining a learning curve for complex procedures [10, 11].

Results

We included all consecutive patients who underwent PTE since the inception of our institution's CTEPH program in 1998 ($n = 134$) and divided them into terciles (T1 – T3) to evaluate surgical, hemodynamic, and postoperative outcomes over time as our experience increased. Preoperative characteristics of all patients in our study are summarized in Table 1. Patients had an average age of 54 years, and 60% were male. The degree of pulmonary hypertension in these patients was severe with an average systolic pulmonary artery pressure (sPAP) of 78 mmHg and diastolic pulmonary artery pressure (dPAP) of 28 mmHg. Mean pulmonary vascular resistance (PVR) was calculated at 639 dynes-sec-cm^{-5}. Preoperatively, 87.3% of patients were classified as New York Heart Association (NYHA) Heart Failure Class II or III, and nearly all patients had either Jamieson type 2 or 3 disease (none had type 4 disease) [5]. These preoperative parameters did not vary significantly by tercile.

Postoperatively, we observed a mean decrease in sPAP of 41 mmHg and a mean decrease in right atrial pressure (RAP) of 6 mmHg overall (Table 2). The mPAP decreased from 49 mmHg to 22 mmHg overall, and there was no difference in the number of patients with residual pulmonary hypertension (mPAP >30 mmHg) across terciles. These favorable hemodynamic results following PTE were achieved consistently across all 3 terciles of patients, and therefore increased surgeon experience did not appear to influence the degree of improvement in pulmonary artery pressures. Rather, patients with Jamieson type 2 disease had a significantly

Table 1 Preoperative patient characteristics

| Variable | Overall (n = 134) | Tercile (T) | | | P value |
		T1 (n = 44)	T2 (n = 45)	T3 (n = 45)	T1 vs. T3
Age (y)	54 ± 15	54 ± 14	54 ± 14	53 ± 16	0.757
Male Sex (%)	81 (60.4)	22 (50.0)	32 (71.1)	27 (60.0)	0.343
PAP (mm Hg)					
Systolic	78 ± 20	77 ± 19	78 ± 21	78 ± 20	0.778
Diastolic	28 ± 9	26 ± 10	30 ± 8	27 ± 9	0.882
PVR (dynes-sec-cm^{-5})	639 ± 373	695 ± 442	618 ± 371	602 ± 292	0.243
CO (L/min)	4.7 ± 1.5	4.5 ± 1.5	4.8 ± 1.4	4.7 ± 1.5	0.531
DLCO (% predicted)	64 ± 19	66 ± 17	67 ± 20	56 ± 18	0.011
NYHA class					
I	1 (0.7)	0 (0)	1 (2.2)	0 (0)	0.218
II	43 (32.1)	17 (38.6)	14 (31.1)	12 (26.7)	
III	74 (55.2)	21 (47.7)	26 (57.8)	27 (60.0)	
IV	15 (11.2)	6 (13.6)	3 (6.7)	6 (13.3)	
Jamieson classification					
Type 1	1 (0.7)	0 (0)	1 (2.2)	0 (0)	0.226
Type 2	64 (47.8)	24 (54.5)	20 (44.4)	20 (44.4)	
Type 3	61 (45.5)	20 (45.5)	17 (37.8)	24 (53.3)	
Type 4	0 (0)	0 (0)	0 (0)	0 (0)	

Data are shown as mean ± standard deviation or numbers (percentages)
PAP pulmonary artery pressure, *PVR* pulmonary vascular resistance, *CO* cardiac output, *DLCO* diffusing capacity of carbon monoxide, *NYHA* New York Heart Association

greater mean decrease in sPAP than patients with Jamieson type 3 disease (45 vs. 37, $p = 0.039$), further validating that anatomic and pathological classification of thromboembolic disease in the pulmonary arteries is a major predictor of outcome after PTE [5].

Similarly, mortality and other postoperative outcomes remained relatively consistent across our experience (Table 3). The 30-day mortality rate following PTE was 3.7% overall, which is on par with other high volume centers [12, 13]. In the postoperative setting, 44.4% of patients experienced at least one complication, 20.8% of patients experienced a major complication, and 16.4% of patients experienced at least one pulmonary complication (Table 3). By far, the most common complication was atrial fibrillation at 29.7%, and major complications included acute respiratory distress syndrome, pneumonia, or respiratory failure requiring re-intubation, sepsis, and return to the operating room for any reason. Though the

Table 2 Comparison of perioperative hemodynamic and surgical parameters

| Variable | Overall (n = 134) | Tercile (T) | | | P value |
		T1 (n = 44)	T2 (n = 45)	T3 (n = 45)	T1 vs. T3
Postoperative					
sPAP (mm Hg)	37 ± 13	38 ± 13	35 ± 13	40 ± 14	0.468
mPAP (mm Hg)	22 ± 7	21 ± 6	20 ± 7	23 ± 8	0.183
RAP (mm Hg)	5 ± 4	5 ± 3	5 ± 4	5 ± 3	1.000
Mean Δ sPAP (mm Hg)	41 ± 21	40 ± 19	43 ± 22	41 ± 21	0.908
Mean Δ mPAP (mm Hg)	24 ± 13	25 ± 11	24 ± 13	24 ± 14	0.570
Mean Δ RAP (mm Hg)	6 ± 8	7 ± 11	6 ± 6	5 ± 6	0.287
CPB time (min)	180 ± 41	198 ± 42	182 ± 42	159 ± 28	<0.001
Aortic cross-clamp time (min)	132 ± 31	140 ± 35	134 ± 28	123 ± 28	0.018
DHCA time (min)	37 ± 15	44 ± 17	35 ± 13	31 ± 10	<0.001

Data are shown as mean ± standard deviation
sPAP systolic pulmonary artery pressure, *mPAP* mean pulmonary artery pressure, *RAP* right atrial pressure, *CPB* cardiopulmonary bypass, *DHCA* deep hypothermic circulatory arrest

Table 3 Comparison of postoperative outcomes

Variable	Overall (n = 134)	Tercile			P value T1 vs. T3
		T1 (n = 44)	T2 (n = 45)	T3 (n = 45)	
30-day mortality	5 (3.7)	0 (0)	3 (6.6)	2 (4.4)	0.159
At least one complication	72 (44.4)	28 (63.6)	17 (37.8)	27 (60.0)	0.724
At least one pulmonary complication	19 (14.8)	5 (11.4)	7 (15.6)	7 (15.6)	0.563
At least one major complication	26 (20.3)	11 (25.0)	9 (20.0)	6 (13.3)	0.162
Residual mPAP >30 mmHg	11 (8.2)	4 (9.1)	4 (8.9)	3 (6.7)	0.671
30-day readmission rate	7 (5.2)	3 (6.8)	0 (0)	4 (8.9)	0.713
Length of hospital stay (d)	12.6 ± 9.0	12.8 ± 7.8	13.0 ± 11.7	11.8 ± 6.7	0.517
Length of ICU stay (d)	4.6 ± 4.7	4.5 ± 3.4	4.7 ± 5.6	4.6 ± 4.8	0.910
Duration on ventilator (d)	2.0 ± 3.0	1.6 ± 1.5	2.6 ± 4.5	1.8 ± 2.2	0.618

Data are shown as mean ± standard deviation or numbers (percentages)
ICU intensive care unit, *mPAP* mean pulmonary artery pressure

rate of major complications trended downward across terciles, this was not statistically significant. A total of 4 patients in our series had massive hemoptysis postoperatively, and there was no correlation with surgeon experience. The average length of hospital stay was 12.6 days, with an average of 4.6 days in the intensive care unit and 2.0 days on the ventilator. After undergoing PTE, 74.6% of patients had marked relief of their symptoms and were reclassified as NYHA class I from class II-IV, and 65% of patients in T1 were NYHA class I in comparison to 80% in T3 (p = 0.15).

We did, however, detect a significant improvement in operative parameters with increased surgeon experience. Total cardiopulmonary bypass, aortic cross-clamp, and deep hypothermic circulatory arrest times steadily shortened from T1 to T3, and these differences were statistically significant (Table 2). Total cardiopulmonary bypass time decreased from a mean of 198 min to 159 min (p < 0.001) from T1 to T3, and total deep hypothermic circulatory arrest time decreased from a mean of 44 min to 31 min (p < 0.001). In order to further illustrate a learning curve of PTE, Fig. 1 depicts a CUSUM plot of deep hypothermic circulatory arrest times over 134 cases as compared to the mean value. Interestingly, two inflection points are seen in this curve at 22 and 95 cases. The first inflection point at 22 cases suggests a threshold of transitioning from novice to intermediate with PTE, as arrest times begin to trend downward thereafter. After the second inflection point at 95 cases, arrest times plummet even more steeply, indicating a threshold of attaining advanced expertise in clearing obstructed pulmonary arteries.

Discussion

All complex procedures are associated with a learning curve for surgeons, and PTE is among one of the more technically demanding operations in cardiothoracic surgery. It is undoubtedly a challenging procedure to learn, and our experience demonstrates that favorable outcomes can be achieved in the setting of a dedicated multi-disciplinary team of pulmonologists, surgeons, and intensivists working in concert to select appropriate patients, improve operative efficiency, and provide meticulous postoperative care. Accurate diagnosis of

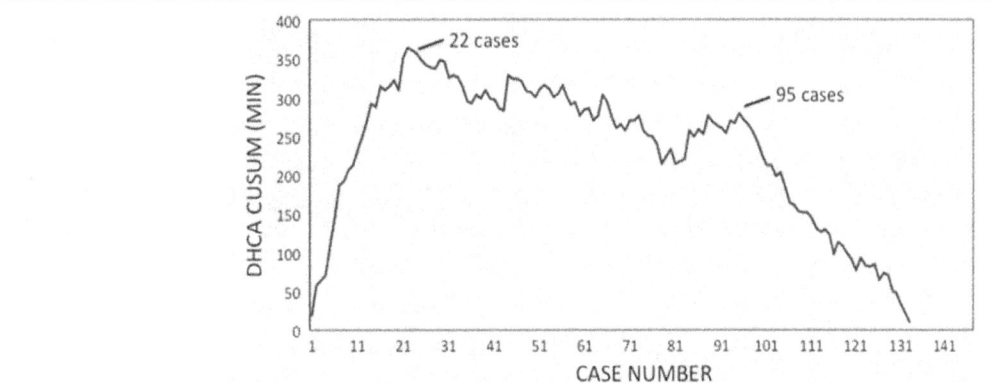

Fig. 1 CUSUM plot depicts learning curve for PTE. Cumulative running sum (CUSUM) of the difference in DHCA (deep hypothermic circulatory arrest) time from the mean value is plotted on the vertical axis vs. case number on the horizontal axis. Two inflection points are seen at 22 and 95 cases

CTEPH and recognition of patients with disease amenable to surgical intervention are the first steps, and having the benefit of an expert pulmonologist in CTEPH as part of our team has greatly facilitated evaluation and subsequent referral of excellent surgical candidates. The other key components included the involvement of two senior-level cardiothoracic surgeons on each case, and 24-h coverage of our cardiothoracic surgery ICU by a certified intensivist. Even early in our program's existence, we were able to obtain adequate clearance of obstructed pulmonary arteries with significant postoperative hemodynamic improvements, despite much longer operative and circulatory arrest times. However, overall morbidity and mortality were not adversely affected during the initial phases of building our program, as there were no early deaths in our first 44 cases.

As we would expect, our learning curve suggests that operative efficiency is greatly enhanced with increasing case numbers. According to Fig. 1, approximately 20 cases are needed for a surgeon to become proficient at reliably recognizing and dissecting the thromboendarterectomy plane during circulatory arrest, while nearly 100 cases are needed to demonstrate mastery. To our knowledge, no other high volume center has described a learning curve for this procedure. The main limitation of our study is the fact that we have described the learning curve of a single team of providers at a single institution based on a retrospective analysis. We believe that the fundamental tenets that allowed us to successfully build our program, however, can be generalized and may prove useful to other programs early on in their trajectory. Surgical treatment of patients with CTEPH remains largely focused at regional centers of excellence at this time. As of 2013, only approximately 30 centers worldwide offered PTE surgery, and over half of cases were performed at the highest volume program at UCSD [14]. As CTEPH appears to be gaining prevalence in the U.S. and the limits of surgically curable disease are expanding [15–17], the need for more widespread access to PTE surgery is surely to arise in the future.

Conclusions

In summary, our experience offers other centers which aspire to build a multi-disciplinary program to treat CTEPH a road-map on how to achieve this goal. We conclude that adopting a team-based approach with an emphasis on proper patient selection and adequate surgical clearance of obstructed pulmonary arteries can lead to favorable outcomes from the outset. Operative expediency is largely a function of case volume, and may be less critical with respect to influencing surgical and hemodynamic outcomes.

Abbreviations
CTEPH: Chronic thromboembolic pulmonary hypertension; CUSUM: Cumulative running sum; DHCA: Deep hypothermic circulatory arrest; dPAP: Diastolic pulmonary artery pressure; ICU: Intensive care unit; mPAP: Mean pulmonary artery pressure; NYHA: New York Heart Association; PAP: Pulmonary artery pressure; PCWP: Pulmonary capillary wedge pressure; PTE: Pulmonary thromboendarterectomy; PVR: Pulmonary vascular resistance; RAP: Right atrial pressure; sPAP: Systolic pulmonary artery pressure; T: Tercile

Acknowledgements
None

Funding
The authors have no sources of funding to disclose for this study.

Authors' contributions
SS contributed to data analysis and wrote the bulk of the manuscript. BL contributed to cumulative running sum learning curve analysis. AW contributed to data collection and interpretation related to classification of pulmonary hypertension. JR contributed to data collection and interpretation related to classification of pulmonary hypertension. MV contributed to data collection and interpretation related to surgical outcomes. GV contributed to data collection and interpretation related to surgical outcomes. RC contributed to data interpretation and manuscript preparation. CW contributed to data collection, interpretation, and manuscript preparation. All authors have read and approved the final manuscript.

Competing interests
The authors declare that they have no competing interests.

Author details
[1]Division of Thoracic Surgery, Massachusetts General Hospital, 55 Fruit Street, Founders 7, Boston, Massachusetts 02114, USA. [2]Division of Pulmonary and Critical Care Medicine, Massachusetts General Hospital, 55 Fruit Street, Boston, Massachusetts 02114, USA. [3]Division of Cardiac Surgery, Massachusetts General Hospital, 55 Fruit Street, Cox 6, Boston, Massachusetts 02114, USA. [4]Thoracic Surgery Service, Memorial Sloan Kettering Cancer Center, 12 75 York Avenue, C-881, New York, NY 10065, USA.

References
1. Pengo V, Lensing AW, Prins MH, Marchiori A, Davidson BL, Tiozzo F, Albanese P, Biasiolo A, Pegoraro C, Iliceto S, et al. Incidence of chronic thromboembolic pulmonary hypertension after pulmonary embolism. N Engl J Med. 2004;350:2257–64.
2. Riedel M, Stanek V, Widimsky J, Prerovsky I. Longterm follow-up of patients with pulmonary thromboembolism. Late prognosis and evolution of hemodynamic and respiratory data. Chest. 1982;81:151–8.
3. Ishida K, Masuda M, Tanabe N, Matsumiya G, Tatsumi K, Nakajima N. Long-term outcome after pulmonary endarterectomy for chronic thromboembolic pulmonary hypertension. J Thorac Cardiovasc Surg. 2012;144:321–6.
4. Thistlethwaite PA, Kaneko K, Madani MM, Jamieson SW. Technique and outcomes of pulmonary endarterectomy surgery. Ann Thorac Cardiovasc Surg. 2008;14:274–82.
5. Thistlethwaite PA, Mo M, Madani MM, Deutsch R, Blanchard D, Kapelanski DP, Jamieson SW. Operative classification of thromboembolic disease determines outcome after pulmonary endarterectomy. J Thorac Cardiovasc Surg. 2002;124:1203–11.
6. Thistlethwaite PA, Madani M, Jamieson SW. Outcomes of pulmonary endarterectomy surgery. Semin Thorac Cardiovasc Surg. 2006;18:257–64.
7. Madani MM, Auger WR, Pretorius V, Sakakibara N, Kerr KM, Kim NH, Fedullo PF, Jamieson SW. Pulmonary endarterectomy: recent changes in a single

institution's experience of more than 2,700 patients. Ann Thorac Surg. 2012;94:97–103. discussion 103

8. Witkin AS, Channick RN. Chronic Thromboembolic pulmonary hypertension: the end result of pulmonary embolism. Curr Cardiol Rep. 2015;17:63.

9. Jamieson SW, Kapelanski DP. Pulmonary endarterectomy. Curr Probl Surg. 2000;37:165–252.

10. Tapias LF, Morse CR. Minimally invasive Ivor Lewis esophagectomy: description of a learning curve. J Am Coll Surg. 2014;218:1130–40.

11. Chen PD, Wu CY, Hu RH, Chen CN, Yuan RH, Liang JT, Lai HS, Wu YM. Robotic major hepatectomy: Is there a learning curve? Surgery. 2017;161:642–9.

12. Mayer E, Jenkins D, Lindner J, D'Armini A, Kloek J, Meyns B, Ilkjaer LB, Klepetko W, Delcroix M, Lang I, et al. Surgical management and outcome of patients with chronic thromboembolic pulmonary hypertension: results from an international prospective registry. J Thorac Cardiovasc Surg. 2011;141:702–10.

13. Jamieson SW, Kapelanski DP, Sakakibara N, Manecke GR, Thistlethwaite PA, Kerr KM, Channick RN, Fedullo PF, Auger WR. Pulmonary endarterectomy: experience and lessons learned in 1,500 cases. Ann Thorac Surg. 2003;76: 1457–62. discussion 1462-1454.

14. Ryan JJ, Rich S, Archer SL. Pulmonary endarterectomy surgery–a technically demanding cure for WHO Group IV Pulmonary Hypertension: requirements for centres of excellence and availability in Canada. Can J Cardiol. 2011;27:671–4.

15. Madani M, Mayer E, Fadel E, Jenkins DP. Pulmonary Endarterectomy. Patient selection, technical challenges, and outcomes. Ann Am Thorac Soc. 2016;13 Suppl 3:S240-7.

16. D'Armini AM, Morsolini M, Mattiucci G, Grazioli V, Pin M, Valentini A, Silvaggio G, Klersy C, Dore R. Pulmonary endarterectomy for distal chronic thromboembolic pulmonary hypertension. J Thorac Cardiovasc Surg. 2014;148:1005–11.

17. Jenkins DP, Biederman A, D'Armini AM, Dartevelle PG, Gan HL, Klepetko W, Lindner J, Mayer E, Madani MM. Operability assessment in CTEPH: lessons from the CHEST-1 study. J Thorac Cardiovasc Surg. 2016;152:669–674 e663.

5

Chest-wall reconstruction with a customized titanium-alloy prosthesis fabricated by 3D printing and rapid prototyping

Xiaopeng Wen[†], Shan Gao[†], Jinteng Feng, Shuo Li, Rui Gao and Guangjian Zhang[*]

Abstract

Background: As 3D printing technology emerge, there is increasing demand for a more customizable implant in the repair of chest-wall bony defects. This article aims to present a custom design and fabrication method for repairing bony defects of the chest wall following tumour resection, which utilizes three-dimensional (3D) printing and rapid-prototyping technology.

Methods: A 3D model of the bony defect was generated after acquiring helical CT data. A customized prosthesis was then designed using computer-aided design (CAD) and mirroring technology, and fabricated using titanium-alloy powder. The mechanical properties of the printed prosthesis were investigated using ANSYS software.

Results: The yield strength of the titanium-alloy prosthesis was 950 ± 14 MPa (mean $\pm$ SD), and its ultimate strength was 1005 ± 26 MPa. The 3D finite element analyses revealed that the equivalent stress distribution of each prosthesis was unifrom. The symmetry and reconstruction quality contour of the repaired chest wall was satisfactory. No rejection or infection occurred during the 6-month follow-up period.

Conclusion: Chest-wall reconstruction with a customized titanium-alloy prosthesis is a reliable technique for repairing bony defects.

Keywords: 3D printing, Titanium-alloy prosthesis, Chest-wall bony defect, Rapid prototyping

Background

Customized chest implants are widely used in the repair of chest-wall bony defects. The fixing plate is the most important and complicated component, and an inappropriate prosthesis might eventually lead to repair failure. Compared with prostheses manufactured by traditional methods, customized implants have the significant advantages of accurately restoring the appearance and normal function of the missing part. Optimizing the design and fabricating process of a customized implant markedly influences the strength of the prosthesis and the final outcome, and

such techniques have been widely used by orthodontic and maxillofacial surgeons [1, 2].

This article presents two case reports on the utilization of three-dimensional (3D) image reconstruction technology, computer-aided design (CAD), and reverse-engineering mirroring to optimize the design of prostheses. Laser rapid-prototyping technology was used to produce titanium-alloy prostheses. The clinical results obtained in these two cases confirm the high quality of the chest-wall repairs.

Methods

Patient information

Case 1

A 62-year-old male was admitted for an anterior chest-wall mass. Chest CT revealed a right lung mass with right anterior chest-wall invasion. The tumor protruded

* Correspondence: michael8039@163.com
[†]Equal contributors
Department of Thoracic Surgery, First Affiliated Hospital of Xi'an Jiaotong University, #277 West Yanta Road, Xi'an, Shaanxi Province 710061, People's Republic of China

from the chest wall with destruction of the second and third ribs, and invaded the upper edge of the fourth rib (Fig. 1a). The pathological diagnosis of a biopsy specimen was squamous cell carcinoma. A PET/CT evaluation showed no metastasis in the hilar or mediastinal lymph nodes, and no distant metastases were revealed. The patient was planned for surgery including resection of the tumor and ribs. The patient signed an informed-consent form and the surgery was approved by the appropriate ethics committee. Resection of the second and third ribs would lead to a large bone defect of the chest wall, and so an implantable rib prosthesis was designed for repairing the chest wall.

Case 2

A 64-year-old male was admitted for a chest-wall mass. Chest CT revealed a $5 \times 5 \times 5$ cm^3 mass in the middle of the chest wall. The tumor had destroyed sternal body and was considered to be a chondrosarcoma (Fig. 1b). No obvious contraindication or distant metastasis was revealed, and so the patient was assigned for surgery. The planned surgery included resection of the affected sternum, bilateral cartilage from the third to seventh ribs, and the related soft tissue. A sternum–rib prosthesis implantation was designed for reconstructing the chest wall.

Design of the prosthesis

A helical CT scan was acquired using a General Electric CT scanner at The First Affiliated Hospital of Xi'an Jiaotong University in Xi'an, China. This scan acquisition was performed with a 1.3-mm slice thickness, a slice reconstruction interval of 0.6 mm, and a 512×512 imaging matrix. The two-dimensional image slices obtained from the CT scans were imported into commercial Materialise Interactive Medical Image Control System (MIMICS) software (Materialise, Leuven, Belgium). After removing the soft tissue, the skeleton was visualized using a 3D display for diagnosing and evaluating the chest defect. Figure 2a and c show 3D images of the sternum–rib defects in cases 1 and 2, respectively.

Digisurf (3D–Family Corporation, Taiwan) software was used to design the surface shape of the prosthesis. MIMICS cannot directly interface the CT scanner with Digisurf software since the software can read only data obtained from a 3D laser scanner. Software called Point-Data-Processing was therefore developed in the Institute of Advanced Manufacturing Technology (Xi'an Jiaotong University) to convert the output from MIMICS in IGS format into the format readable by the Digisurf software for surface reconstruction. The CAD data for the prosthesis with corresponding resection templates were translated into the STL file format and imported into the prototyping machine to fabricate the physical prostheses (Fig. 2b and d). Alternatively, the stereolithographic apparatus (SLA) model prosthesis could be fitted on the 3D chest model to evaluate characteristics such as the symmetry and the accuracy of the surface fitting. Finally, the SLA prosthesis pattern was directly used in investment casting performed using Quick-Cast to produce the titanium-alloy prosthesis. Holes were made in the implant body after completing the CAD/CAM (computer-aided manufacturing) process in order to facilitate soft-tissue integration.

Since surgeries utilizes prefabricated titanium-alloy implants require a negative tumor margin, or ideally include more safety margin for some type of pathology, we estimate the resection margin and the dimensions of the implants based on preoperative 3D reconstruction. To ensure there is enough healthy bone to attach the implants, we also include a 2 cm redundant fixing area to accommodate the intraoperative alteration of surgical plan when designing the

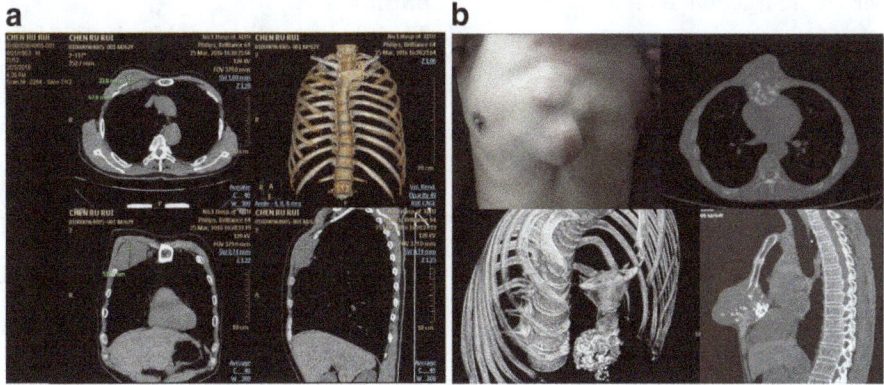

Fig. 1 Preoperative images of the patients. **a** In case 1, the tumor protruded from the chest wall with destruction of the second and third ribs, and invaded the upper edge of the fourth rib. **b** In case 2, the tumor had destroyed infrasternal bone and protruded from the chest wall

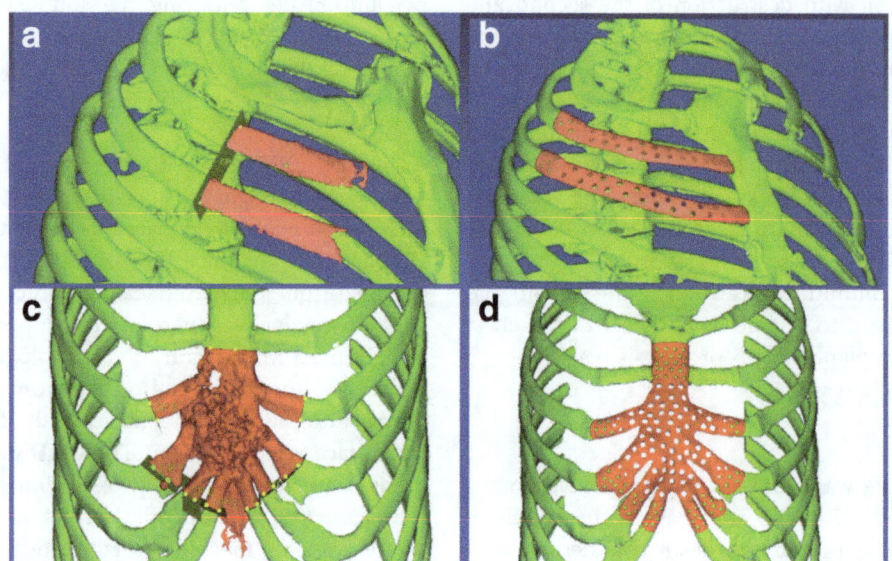

Fig. 2 a, **c** The sternum and rib defects in the 3D reconstruction model for cases 1 and 2, respectively. **b**, **d** The corresponding customized prostheses designed by CAD and mirroring technology

implants. This redundancy of fixing area greatly improves the safety of the surgery on both oncological and mechanical aspects.

3D finite element analysis

The CAD-generated virtual implants were positioned along the bony orbit according to surgical convention and prosthesis design considerations. The implants were virtually placed in the 3D viewing window, and then ANSYS (version 5.7, ANSYS, Pittsburgh, USA) finite element analysis software was used to analyze the stress distribution. The available bone at selected locations was evaluated in coronal, axial, and sagittal views, and implant positions were adjusted as needed while taking into account the prosthesis design requirements.

In this study we assumed that all of the materials were continuous, homogeneous, and isotropic linearly elastic. The material properties are listed in Table 1.

Manufacturing the prosthesis

The 3D model of the patient's chest was printed from the STL data of the patient's skeletal anatomy (ZPrinter® 310 Plus, Z Corporation, Cambridge, MA, USA). The model was printed using high-performance composite

Table 1 Elastic modulus and Poisson's ratio of the study materials

Material	Elastic modulus (MPa)	Poisson's ratio
Cortical bone	13,800	0.26
Cancellous bone	345	0.31
Titanium-alloy	110,000	0.3

powder and binder with a layer thickness of 0.102 mm. The surgical guide was test fitted on the 3D–printed model conforming to the patient's anatomy to ensure a precise fit in the area in which the implant was to be placed surgically (Fig. 3a and c). The locations of the drilling sites were assessed by clinicians to ensure that they adequately represented the surgical plan before proceeding to surgery. Finally, the 3D data of the prosthesis was imported into the printing device to produce the titanium-alloy prosthesis, this step usually takes 3 work days. After mechanical polishing and sandblasting, the titanium-alloy prosthesis appeared silver white with a rough granular surface. No microscale defects such as scratches, cracks, burrs, or spiral edges were found in the inspection (Fig. 3b and d).

Mechanical properties of the 3D–printed titanium-alloy prosthesis

The titanium-alloy prosthesis was fabricated by a laser rapid-prototyping system (EOS, Munich, Germany) from the raw material of spherical particles of titanium alloy with a diameter of 20–65 μm (Ti6Al4V, UNS R56400). The entire process was carried out in an environment protected using 99.999% argon to prevent the oxidation of titanium-alloy powder. In order to test the mechanical properties of titanium-alloy materials obtained by laser rapid prototyping, standard tensile specimens and three-point-bending specimens were prepared by the EOS system. The yield strength and ultimate strength of the formed titanium alloy were measured by SANS material testing machine (MTS Shenzhen, China) according to the

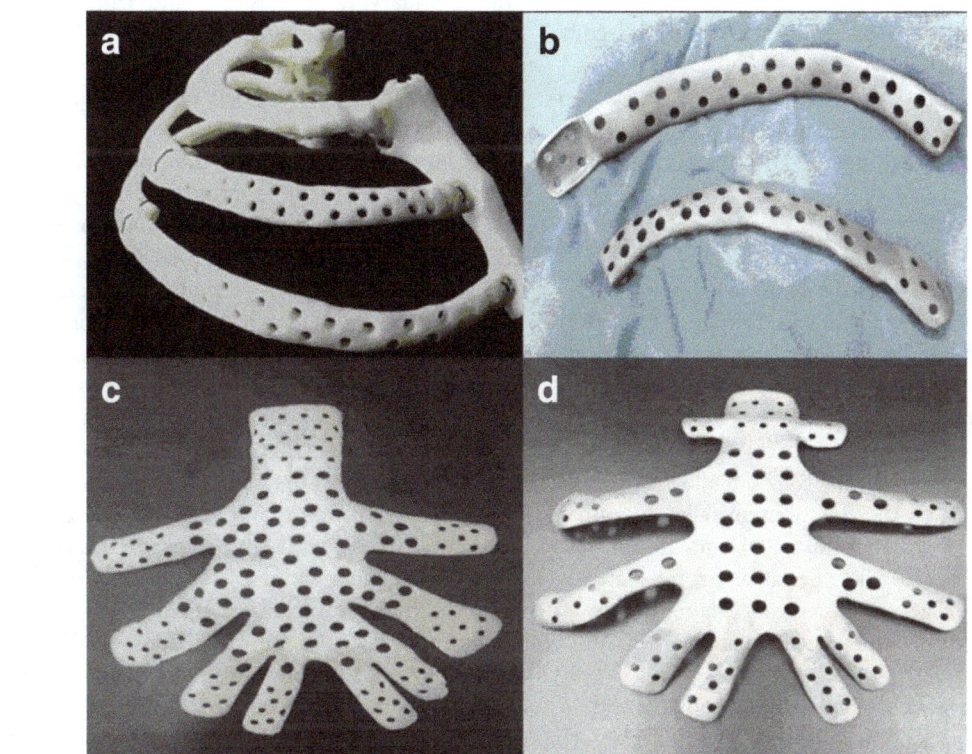

Fig. 3 a, **c** Chest reference models for cases 1 and 2, respectively. **b**, **d** The corresponding 3D printed titanium-alloy prostheses

test standard and environment temperature designated by the Ministry of Industry and Information Technology (GB 6892). The mechanical properties of the titanium-alloy prosthesis is listed in Table 2.

Titanium-alloy rib prosthesis implantation and postoperative follow-up

Case 1

In the first case, the second to fourth ribs were resected along with the upper lobe of the right lung. The seventh and tenth groups of lymph nodes were also dissected to allow pathology analysis. After en-bloc resection of the tumor-bearing area, the measured defect area was 14×20 cm^2. After disinfection and sterilization, the rib prosthesis was fixed with steel wire. Frozen section pathology of the resected edge is sent and came back negative. The skin incision was closed after the prosthesis was covered with a flap of the pectoralis major muscle. A chest

drainage tube was routinely placed, and an elastic bandage was fixed with pressure. The operating time was 120 min and involved a minimal amount of blood loss. The postoperative pathology analysis showed squamous cell carcinoma of the right upper lung infiltrating the ribs. No lymph node metastasis was detected.

Case 2

In the second case, the prosthesis is designed to include a 2 cm error margin above the line of bone destruction. The sternum was resected below the 3rd sternal costal joints, the lateral border contains 3–7 costal cartilages, and a 1 cm margin above the intended resection line is also included due to unsatisfactory gross margin. The sternal prosthesis was fixed with the broken ends of the ribs and the rest of the sternum using screws. A flap of the rectus abdominis muscle was created and transferred to cover the prosthesis before closing the skin incision.

Table 2 Mechanical properties of the titanium-alloy prosthesis compared with industry standards

	Tensile strength (MPa)	Specified nonproportional extension strength, $RP_{0.2}$ (MPa)	Elongation rate (%)
3D printed titanium-alloy prosthesis	1002	819	13.3
Pharmaceutical industry standards from YY0117.1–2005	≥860	≥780	≥10

Note: The YY0117.1–2005 pharmaceutical industry standards are entitled "Surgical implants: bone prosthesis forging, casting -Ti6Al4V titanium alloy forgings"

Two drainage tubes were placed. The postoperative pathology analysis showed grade II chondrosarcoma with negative margins.

The integrity of the fixation was examined on postoperative day 1 in a chest x-ray, and a CT 3D reconstruction of the chest was reviewed 1 month after the surgery.

Results
3D finite element analysis of the customized prosthesis
A rapid biomechanical analysis was carried out to evaluate the stress distribution of each prosthesis. As shown in Fig. 4, the equivalent stress distribution of each prosthesis was uniform.

Mechanical properties of the 3D titanium-alloy prosthesis
The yield strength of the 3D titanium-alloy rib prosthesis was 950 ± 14 MPa (mean $\pm$ SD), and its ultimate strength was 1005 ± 26 MPa. Sandblasting was applied to increase the surface roughness and thereby improve the connection between the prosthesis and soft tissue.

Recovery and follow-up of rib prosthesis implantation
The radiological and clinical results obtained after reconstruction of the chest defects were ideal in the two patients. The customized prefabricated prostheses fit the chest defects well in both patients, and no adjustments were needed during the surgery. These features shortened the operating time. Rigid fixation of both implants was achieved using screws. Complications were not observed during the 6-month follow-up period. X-ray examinations showed no loosening of the prosthesis and no deformity of the chest (Fig. 5a and c). The 3D reconstruction of CT data showed that each prosthesis was well fixed and surrounded by fibrous tissue around the periosteum (Fig. 5b and d).

Discussion
Large chest-wall defects can be caused by sternum or rib dysplasia, congenital malformation, trauma, and primary or secondary tumor lesions, and can have devastating functional and cosmetic consequences [3, 4]. Several reconstruction techniques such as autologous tissue transfers and alloplastic materials have been applied for many years, but reconstructing extensive defects with autologous bone is restricted by the amount of available donor bone, difficulty in 3D contouring, poor tissue tolerance and acceptance, and risk of long-term pain syndrome or discomfort [5]. Most thoracic surgeons agree that total or subtotal sternum resection or resecting more than three or four ribs increases the likelihood of chest-wall instability, and therefore is the typical indication for chest-wall reconstruction and the use of synthetic materials [6]. The use of alloplastic materials such as Marlex® mesh, bone cement, Prolene® mesh, Prolene® mesh composite bone cement, a sandwich complex, stainless steel net, titanium mesh, titanium plate, or plexiglass is more widely adopted [7], although commercially available materials are generally more cost-efficient but this is associated with risks including plate exposure, plate-screw fracture, screw loosening, infection, and poor cosmetic and functional restoration. It is also worth to point out that the cost of the custom prosthesis is not that high: $1200 for two ribs and $1300 for the sternum, depending on the weight of the prosthesis (how much alloys used) and complexity of the design.

Creating a 3D model of bone structures extracted from CT image data allows not only for precise prosthesis design but also provides adequate visualization of the defect for preoperative surgical evaluation and thorough planning of the repair. Few studies have focused on applying this technique to repairing chest defects. The two cases we report here have demonstrated the efficacy and accuracy of using combined technologies of 3D CT data and a stereolithography produced model for tumor resection guidance and defect reconstruction. The implantation of a titanium-alloy prosthesis covered with a flap of the pectoralis major muscle completely restored the normal chest appearance. The preoperative preparation, symmetry, and precise fit obtained during implant evaluation were greatly facilitated by using a

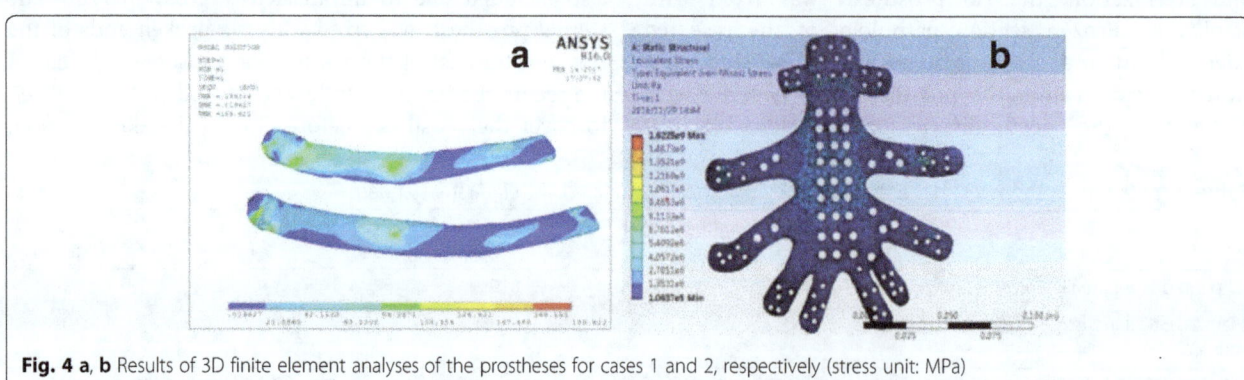

Fig. 4 a, b Results of 3D finite element analyses of the prostheses for cases 1 and 2, respectively (stress unit: MPa)

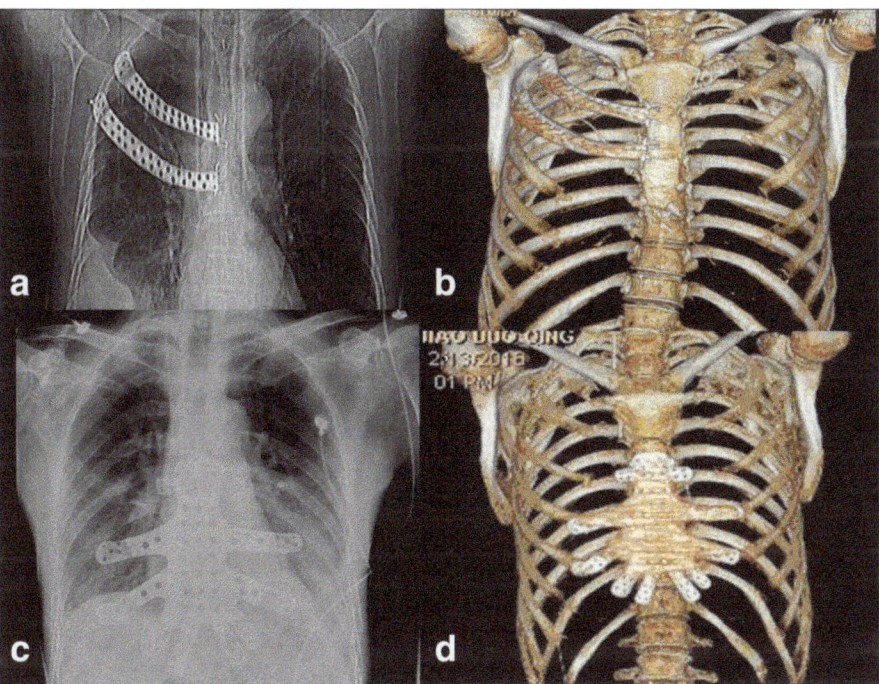

Fig. 5 a, c Postoperative X-ray images showing that the prostheses fit well in the chest. **b, d** 3D reconstructions of CT data showing that the prostheses were well fixed in the chest

physical model generated by rapid prototyping. This approach shortened the operating time and allowed for potential intraoperative errors to be modified preoperatively and thus avoided having to address them during the actual surgery. No complications occurred during the early postoperative period, other than slight chest-wall floating in case 2.

Until now most implants have been manually shaped intraoperatively at the surgical site [8]. However, modifying an implant intraoperatively is difficult. Furthermore, intraoperative modeling is time-consuming and is associated with unsatisfactory accuracy, sometimes even leading to more-invasive surgery or repair failure [9]. The intraoperative adaptation of the prosthesis can be avoided when using prefabricated customized titanium-alloy implants, and a CAD/CAM system can be used to design and fabricate prostheses with very complex 3D shapes. Moreover, CAD-based prosthesis modeling can avoid indirect manual manipulation on a life-size model. The application of prefabricated titanium-alloy implants in the two patients reported here has demonstrated that the prosthesis accuracy and the symmetry of the chest contour can be greatly improved.

Conclusion

This study has shown that using a computer-generated model makes it possible to fabricate a custom implant that very accurately represents an anatomical defect. In addition to eliminating intraoperative errors and achieving a precise fit and high stability after screw fixation, the use of these techniques also leads to (i) better titanium-alloy bone and joint fixation with the use of titanium alloy, (ii) reduced occurrence of postoperative chest-wall floating and paroxysmal breathing, (iii) better tissue compatibility, fewer foreign-body reactions, and lower susceptible to infection, and (iv) overall better physiological and morphological contour of the chest. From the experience gained in the two present cases we can safely conclude that rapid-prototyping and CAD modeling can dramatically improved the presurgical planning workflow, with the subsequent fabrication process achieving sufficient precision after immediate reconstruction.

Abbreviations
3D: Three-dimensional; CAD: Computer-aided design; CAM: Computer-aided manufacturing; MIMICS: Materialise interactive medical image control system; SLA: Stereolithographic apparatus

Acknowledgements
Not applicable.

Funding
This study was funded by the departmental budget.

Authors' contributions

XW performed the surgery and researched the mechanical properties, SG analyzed the patient and prosthesis data and was responsible for writing the manuscript, JF and SL were responsible for collecting the patient data and fabricating the models, RG critically revised the manuscript and prepared the figures and tables, and GZ conceived and designed the study. All of the authors have read and approved the final version of the manuscript.

Competing interests

The authors declare that they have no competing interests.

References

1. Nayar S, Bhuminathan S, Bhat WM. Rapid prototyping and stereolithography in dentistry. J Pharm Bioallied Sci. 2015;7(Suppl 1):S216–9.
2. Peng Q, Tang Z, Liu O, Peng Z. Rapid prototyping-assisted maxillofacial reconstruction. Ann Med. 2015;47(3):186–208.
3. Bennett DT, Weyant MJ. Extended chest wall resection and reconstruction in the setting of lung cancer. Thorac Surg Clin. 2014;24(4):383–90.
4. Yang H, Tantai J, Zhao H. Clinical experience with titanium mesh in reconstruction of massive chest wall defects following oncological resection. J Thorac Dis. 2015;7(7):1227–34.
5. Jakoi A, Iorio J, Cahill PJ. Autologous bone graft harvesting: a review of grafts and surgical techniques. Musculoskelet Surg. 2015;99(3):171–8.
6. Tukiainen E. Chest wall reconstruction after oncological resections. Scand J Surg. 2013;102(1):9–13.
7. Hameed A, Akhtar S, Naqvi A, Pervaiz Z. Reconstruction of complex chest wall defects by using polypropylene mesh and a pedicled latissimus dorsi flap: a 6-year experience. J Plast Reconstr Aesthet Surg. 2008;61(6):628–35.
8. Rocco G. Chest wall resection and reconstruction according to the principles of biomimesis. Semin Thorac Cardiovasc Surg. 2011;23(4):307–13.
9. McCormack PM. Use of prosthetic materials in chest-wall reconstruction. Assets and liabilities. Surg Clin N Am. 1989;69(5):965–76.

6

Suture fixation of tracheal stents for the treatment of upper trachea stenosis: a retrospective study

Jingtao Huang[*], Zhongwei Zhang and Tao Zhang

Abstract

Background: Stent migration is a common complication in treating trachea stenosis. There is no report concerning suture fixation of tracheal stent. The aim of this study was to investigate whether suture fixation of tracheal stent could avoid stent migration in patients with upper trachea stenosis. The complications were further investigated.

Methods: The patients with upper trachea stenosis who underwent tracheal stent placement for benign/malignant conditions in our hospital between May 2016 and April 2018 were retrospectively reviewed. Clinical data were collected for each patient, including age, gender, co-morbid diseases, site of tracheal obstruction, degree of tracheal obstruction, success of stent placement, impact on patient's symptoms, complications, etc.

Results: Eleven patients (8 males and 3 females; range of age: 17–85, and average age of 63) were enrolled into this study. Six silicone stents and five membrane-covered metal stents were used. The surgery was successfully performed in all the cases. The postoperative recovery was uneventful. All symptoms of the patients were relieved. No complications occurred. The average follow-up for patients was 5 months (range of 1–13 months). During the follow-up, no stent migration was observed according to CT and bronchoscope.

Conclusion: The results suggested that suture fixation of stents could avoid stent migration in treating upper trachea stenosis with metal stent or silicone stent. This method seemed to be effective without operation complications.

Keywords: Tracheal stenosis, Tracheal stent, Stent migration, Suture fixation, Complication

Background

Tracheal stenosis refers to abnormal narrowing of the central air passageways, [1] which can occur at the larynx, trachea, carina or main bronchi [2]. The causes for tracheal stenosis are various and the optimal therapy is not well defined, depending largely on the type of the stenosis [3]. Generally, in some very experienced surgery centers, tracheal resection and reconstruction might be considered as the best treatment to completely cure the stenosis and allows to obtain good results [4]. For example, it is available in tracheal stenosis resulting from prolonged endotracheal intubation or tracheostomy [5]. Nowadays tracheal stenting is a preferred alternative, which can be used for patients with malignant stenosis and benign stenosis [6]. Airway stents are the most common tracheobronchial prosthesis and can be inserted into the trachea. They can rapidly relieve the narrowing air passageway and breathing difficulty [7, 8].

With improved design of stents and advanced technology to aid in the stent insertion, more patients are being treated with tracheal stents. However, numerous complications associated with the use of stents have been reported, including partial or complete trachea obstruction, stent migration and infections [9]. Among those complications, migration of the stent is very common [10]. Martinez-Ballarin et al. reported the rate of migration of stents as 17.5%, [11] and Park et al. found migration of stents in 34% patients [9]. Migration of silicone stents is reported to be 16.6–24%, [12, 13] and migration of metal stent is reported as 2.2–6.4% [12, 14]. Stent migration brings a lot of pain to the patient and increase therapy cost. Silicone Y-stents can be used

* Correspondence: huangjingtaot@163.com
Department of Thoracic Surgery, Tianjin Nankai Hospital, No. 6 Changjiang Road, Nankai District, Tianjin 300100, China

to inhibit the stent migration, however they are only reserved for the patients with stenosis around the area of tracheal carina [7]. Therefore, it is a critical issue to avoid tracheal stent migration.

Although there are many reports on the efficacy and complications of stents for the treatment of trachea stenosis, as far as we know, there is no report concerning suture fixation of tracheal stent in treating upper trachea stenosis. Since May 2016, our institution has been using suture fixation of stent to treat patient with upper trachea stenosis. Our clinical experience suggested that it seemed to be an effective method. Therefore, we retrospectively reviewed the patients who underwent suture fixation of tracheal stent in order to see if it could avoid stent migration. The complications were also investigated.

Methods

Patients

This study was approved by the ethic committee of our hospital. The patients with upper trachea stenosis who underwent tracheal stent placement for benign/malignant conditions in our hospital between May 2016 and April 2018 were retrospectively reviewed. The inclusion criteria were patients with upper trachea stenosis and patient who underwent suture fixation of the stent.

As for diagnosis of trachea stenosis, it was evaluated with computed tomography and bronchoscopy. According to CT images, the cross section area of the narrowest part of the trachea (ANWT) and the cross section area of the normal part of the trachea (ANT) were evaluated. The stenosis degree was defined as ANWT/ANT. Each patient underwent a standard assessment, including physical examination, routine laboratory tests, chest radiography and chest computed tomography prior to the stenting operation. In our institute, the indications for stent placement were trachea stenosis > 50% and dyspnea above grade III. The grade of dyspnea was assessed in reference to World Health Organization (WHO). The indications for suture fixation in this study were patients with upper tracheal stent migration and the patient who needs upper tracheal stenting.

Surgery procedures

After general anesthesia, the patients were placed in trendelenburg position. A rigid bronchoscope was inserted into the trachea under the guidance of a flexible bronchoscope. Ventilation was assured by using a ventilator. After tracheal stenosis was treated with cryoresection, acusection, argon plasma coagulation, balloon dilatation properly, the membrane-covered metal stents (Micro-Tech Co. Ltd., Nanjing, China) or Dumon stent (Novatech, La Ciotat, France) were placed during a rigid bronchoscopy procedure. Under endoscope, a double-needle gastropexy device of PEG kit (Create Medic Co., Ltd., Yokohama, Japan) was applied. The puncture was performed at the part between the inferior margin of the cricoid cartilage and the suprasternal notch. After the position of stent was adjusted satisfactory, the anterior of the stent was fixed onto the antetheca of the trachea and its front tissue under endoscopic monitoring. To prevent surgical suture from cutting the skin, a silicon pad (width of 1–1.5 cm and length of 3-4 cm) was placed on the skin at the puncture site (Fig. 1). A suture fixation about 1–3 stitches were done. Postoperatively, phone call following-up was done every month to see if there's any complication.

In the patients with benign stenosis, the suture was removed under the following conditions. Silicon stent was inserted for more than 3 months; the uncovered part of metal stent was covered by granulation scar; the patient asked for suture removal.

Data collection

Demographic and clinical data were collected for each patient, including age, gender, co-morbid diseases, site of trachea obstruction, degree of trachea obstruction, previous interventional bronchoscopic procedures (including or not including trachea stenting), duration of procedure, success of stent placement, impact on patient's symptoms, procedure- and stent-related complications, duration of follow-up, and the final outcomes.

Results

Basic information of the patients

Eleven patients (8 males and 3 females; range of age: 17–85, and average age of 63) met the inclusion criteria and were enrolled into this study. The upper margins of the stenosis were at 2–5 cm below the glottis. The main symptoms of those patients were dyspnea of grade V. Stent migration occurred in two patients at 1 day and 46 days after the first stent implantation respectively. Those two patients were treated with stent implantation again and suture fixation was performed. The characteristics of the patients were listed in Table 1.

Surgery profile and results

The surgery was successfully performed in the 11 cases. The suture fixation of the stent took about 5-15 min. During the operation, oxyhemoglobin saturation was stable and no haemorrhage was observed. The patients were managed in the post-anesthesia care unit and they were then sent to the ward after the vital parameters were normal. The postoperative recovery was uneventful, and the patient was discharged from hospital after 4–18 days (average: 8 days) of observation (Table 2). The patients who only had treatment for tracheal stenosis

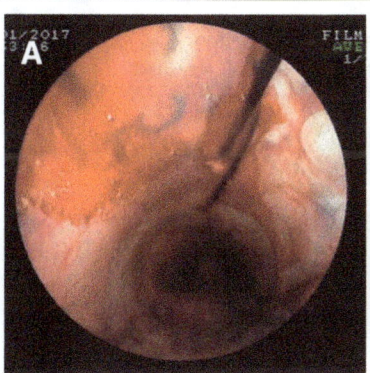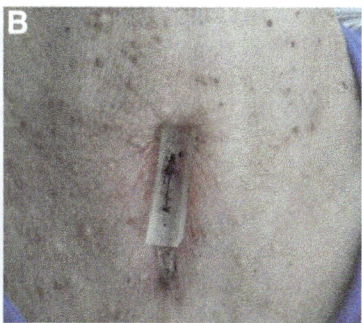

Fig. 1 Images of the operation procedures. **a**: Suture fixation method for the tracheal stent. **b**: Postoperative CT showing the silicon pad on the skin at the puncture site (as the arrow indicates)

were discharged within 5 days postoperatively; those having other treatments had longer hospital stay. Post operatively, the patients' symptoms were relieved.

The suture was successfully removed in the patients with benign stenosis at 4 months, 6 months and 12 months after stent placement respectively. The stents didn't migrate after the suture removal.

Complications

Postoperatively, there was slight hyperemia around the silicon pad due to the pressure from the suture in four patients. Regarding this, the patients had mild discomfortable feeling in the suture site, which didn't affect coughing or deglutition. The discomfortableness was relieved within 3–5 days. As for pain evaluation, Visual Analogue Scale (VAS) was used; the results were detailed in Table 2. All patients were satisfactory with the results. No other complications were observed.

Follow-up results

The average follow-up for patients was 5 months (range of 1–13 months). During the follow-up, no stent migration was observed according to CT and bronchoscope (Figs. 2 and 3). The patients' symptoms disappeared.

Discussion

Migration of stent is still a serious clinical issue, with a reported migration rate of 16.6–24% in silicone stents [12, 13] and 2.2–6.4% in metal stent [12, 14]. Thus, it calls for effective measures to prevent the tracheal stents from migrating. In this study, we mainly found that suture fixation of stents avoided stent migration in patients with upper trachea stenosis. The patients' symptoms were successfully relieved without stent migration.

To prevent tracheal stent from migrating, the studs are particularly designed in the silicon stent. Still it can't completely avoid stent migration. In fact, there are several factors that may contribute to migration of stent.

Table 1 General information of the patients

Case No.	Age	Gender	B/M	Medical History (month)	Location of the stenosis/ degree of stenosis (90%)	Length of the stenosis (mm)	Previous interventional procedures
1	85	F	M	10	Middle&Upper/95	30	Yes
2	74	M	B	3	Upper/90	20	No
3	84	F	M	3	Middle&upper/90	20	No
4	75	M	B	11	Upper/90	25	Yes
5	28	F	B	6	Upper/90	20	no
6	54	M	M	2	Upper/95	40	No
7	81	M	M	1	Upper/90	40	No
8	17	M	B	2	Upper/95	50	No
9	75	M	M	3	Upper/90	30	No
10	66	M	M	2	Middle&upper/95	20	No
11	55	M	M	6	Upper/95	30	No

F female, *M* male, *B* benign, *M* malignant

Table 2 Intraoperative and postoperative information of the patients

Case No.	Stenosis treatment	Stent Type/stent diameter (mm)/ stent length (mm)	VAS	Suture removal after the stent replacement (month)	Postoperative hospital stay (day)	Postoperative survival time (month)	Follow-up (month)
1	Cryoresection, APC	Silicone/16/50	2	/	5	5	5
2	Acusection, balloon dilatation	Silicone/16/50	3	4	4	/	8
3	Cryoresection, APC	MCMS /18/40	1	/	17	7	7
4	Acusection, balloon dilatation	Silicone/16/50	2	6	5	/	6
5	Acusection, balloon dilatation	Silicone/16/50	1	12	12	/	13
6	Cryoresection, APC	MCMS /20/60	1	/	14	6	6
7	Balloon dilatation	MCMS /20/60	1	/	4	4	4
8	Acusection, balloon dilatation	Silicone/16/60	2	/	5	/	3
9	/	MCMS /20/60	2	/	18	1	1
10	Balloon dilatation	MCMS /18/60	1	/	5	Under radiotherapy	1
11	Balloon dilatation	Silicone/16/60	3	/	4	Under chemotherapy	1

VAS Visual Analogue Scale, *MCMS* membrane-covered metal stents, *APC* argon plasma coagulation

Firstly, we found that the middle and lower trachea appeared wider than upper trachea according to CT 3D reconstructions in those patients, which might be attributed to the migration of the upper tracheal stent. Besides, with the rather narrow lumen in the stenosis site, the stenosed segment may exert more compression to the stent. Secondly, patients with tracheal disease usually suffer cough which may contribute to stent migrating. Thirdly, the gravity of the stent is also a contributing factor. Fourthly, another cause is the higher pressure in the superior of the glottis than in the inferior part. In the past, we would use a longer stent or a stent with larger-diameter when there's stent migration, which however might still failed to avoiding stent migration. Besides, a longer stent might result in sputum drainage disorder in some patients and then the stent

had to be removed. It brought a lot of pain and risk to the patients.

In fact, there are some researches concerning the methods for external fixation of tracheal stents [15–18]. For example, Colt et al. described a technique of external fixation of subglottic stents, which appeared to be applicable to some carefully-selected patients with subglottic stenosis who have failed indwelling stent placement because of stent migration [15]. Miwa et al. reported a method utilizing an external fixation apparatus for silicone stents in the subglottic trachea [17]. Majid et al. suggested a technique of securing endoluminal stents using an Endo Close suturing device (Coviden, Boston, MA) and an external silicone button. And their method was proved to be effective in nine patients [16]. Considering the efficacy and

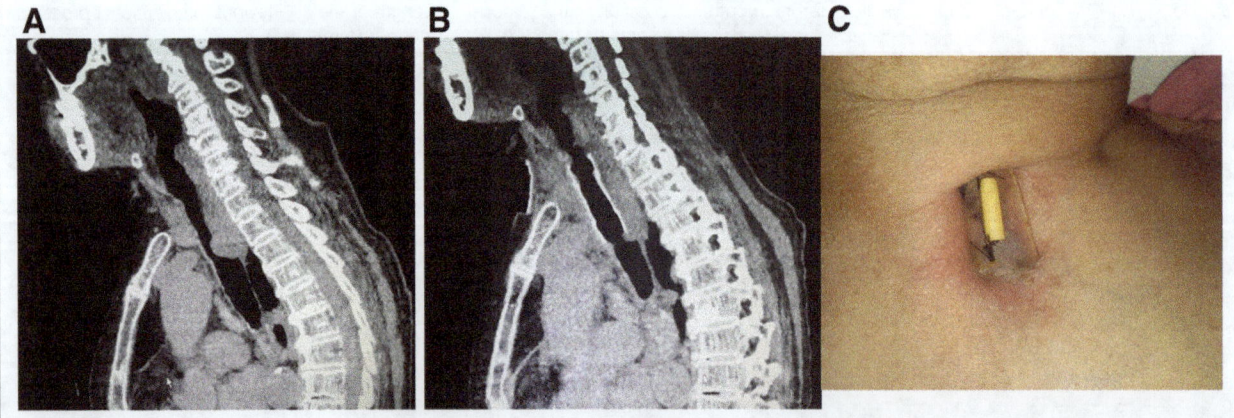

Fig. 2 Preoperative and postoperative images of one patient (Case No. 1). **a**: Preoperative sagittal CT showing the upper tracheal stenosis. **b**: Postoperative sagittal CT showing the normal trachea. **c**: The appearance of the suture fixation on the neck

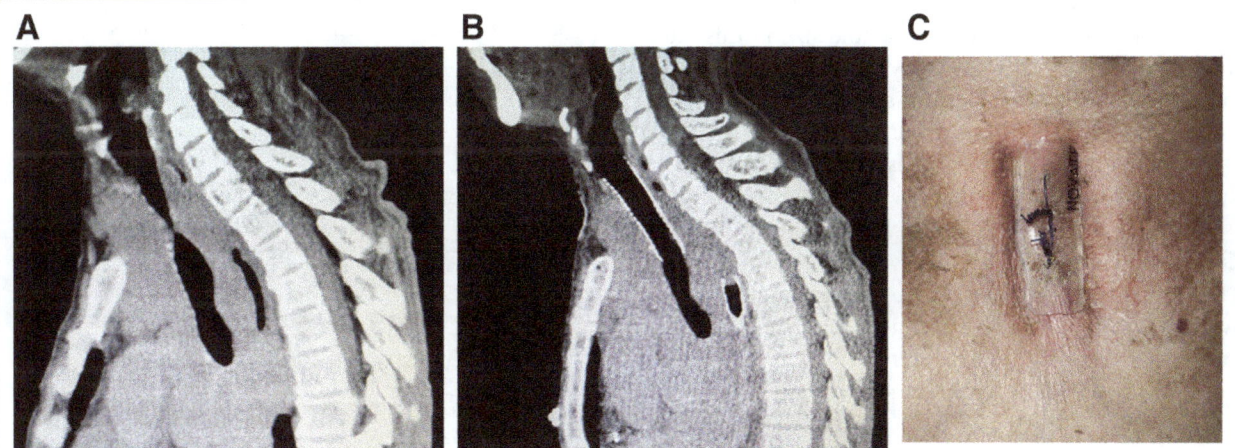

Fig. 3 Preoperative and postoperative images of one patient (Case No. 9). **a**: Sagittal preoperative CT showing the upper tracheal stenosis. **b**: Postoperative sagittal CT showing the normal trachea. **c**: The appearance of the suture on the neck

surgical complications, we have been using suture fixation of the stent in recent years. According to our clinical experience, it seemed that the present method was effective and could avoid stent migration without any complication. There are some points requiring careful attention when perform this method. To gain a better suture fixation, the acupuncture should be perpendicular to the course of the upper trachea. Besides, the patients were placed in trendelenburg position when implanting the stent, in which condition the neck skin was tracked slightly to the head. Therefore, the shoulder pad should be removed before acupuncture to guarantee satisfactory suture fixation.

The suture in the neck would produce certain tension with patients' swallowing and coughing. Besides, the suture would have a long retention in the neck. Thus, it cut the neck skin easily and may even cut into the subcutaneous part. To reduce the stress of the suture on the neck skin, a silicon pad was place on the skin at the fixation site in this study. Postoperatively, there was only slight hyperemia around the silicon pad in four patients. Although it gave the patients some mild discomfortable feelings in the suture part, it didn't affect normal function of coughing or deglutition. The discomfortableness was relieved within 3–5 days. All patients were satisfactory with the results. As for removing the suture, it was done in the patient with benign stenosis in this study. On the contrast, in the patients with malignant stenosis, it's difficult to well fix the stent without the suture because of the softness of the malignant tumor. Besides, considering the short lifetime of those patients, the suture were not removed in the present patients with malignant stenosis. As for the patients with benign stenosis, silicone stents were used in the present study. After the suture fixation for a proper period, the trachea and stent could remain stable even if the suture fixation was removed. In this study, the suture was removed at 4 months, 6 months and 12 months after stent placement respectively. The stents didn't migrate after the suture removal. However, it's uncertain when to remove the sure. It's far from drawing a solid conclusion due to the very small sample size. According to our clinical experience, we suggested the following three criteria. Firstly, silicon stent was inserted for more than 3 months; the uncovered part of metal stent was covered by granulation scar; the patient asked for suture removal. It still needs close attention in further clinical practice to determine the proper criteria for suture removal.

As for complications following the stent placement, Martinez-Ballarin et al. found migration of stents in 17.5%, granulation tissue formation in 6.3%, and trachea obstruction due to mucostasis in 6.3% of cases [11]. Park et al. found restenosis in 40%, granulation tissue formation in 38%, migration of stents in 34%, and mucostasis in 31% of cases [9]. The formation of tracheoesophageal fistula (TEF) has been reported after placement of esophageal stent for stricture esophagus and metallic tracheal stent for tracheal stenosis [19]. The probable cause of fistula formation may be due to the injury at the time of stent deployment or erosion of the tracheal/bronchial wall by proximal/distal margin of a malpositioned stent for prolonged time. In present study, no complications occurred except for slight hyperemia around the silicon pad which was relieved within 3–5 days.

Besides, this suture fixation procedure is relatively easy to perform and usually take short operation time, that is several minutes. Thus, during our clinical experience, this method was used to the patients with upper tracheal stent migration and the patient who needs upper tracheal stenting, in order to avoid stent migration. There are several limitations in this study. Except for the nature of retrospective study, the sample size in this study was too small to draw a highly valid conclusion. The follow-up is not very long in some cases at present; those patients are still under our observation. A further study with a larger sample size is needed to further verify the efficacy of this method.

Conclusion

The results suggested that suture fixation of stents could avoid stent migration in treating upper trachea stenosis with metal stent and silicone stent. This method seemed to be effective without operation complications.

Abbreviations

ANT: The cross section area of the normal part of the trachea; ANWT: The cross section area of the narrowest part of the trachea; APC: Argon plasma coagulation; MCMS: Membrane-covered metal stents; VAS: Visual Analogue Scale; WHO: World Health Organization

Authors' contributions

JH carried out the study design, analyzed the data and wrote the manuscript. ZZ participated in the study design, data collecting and data analysis. TZ participated in the study design, data collecting and helped to draft the manuscript. All authors read and approved the final manuscript.

Competing interests

The authors declare that they have no competing interests.

References

1. Gelbard A, Francis DO, Sandulache VC, Simmons JC, Donovan DT, Ongkasuwan J. Causes and consequences of adult laryngotracheal stenosis. Laryngoscope. 2015;125:1137–43.
2. Burdett E, Mitchell V. Anatomy of the larynx, trachea and bronchi. Anaesthesia Intensive Care Med. 2011;12:335–9.
3. Brichet A, Verkindre C, Dupont J, Carlier ML, Darras J, Wurtz A, et al. Multidisciplinary approach to management of postintubation tracheal stenoses. Eur Respir J. 1999;13:888–93.
4. Gómezcaro A, Morcillo A, Wins R, Molins L, Galan G, Tarrazona V. Surgical management of benign tracheal stenosis. Multimed Manual Cardiothorac Surg 2011;2011:mmcts.2010.004945.
5. Kumar B, Munirathinam GK, Puri GD, Mishra AK, Arya VK. Silicone tracheobronchial stent: a rare cause for bronchoesophageal fistula and distortion of airway anatomy. Ann Card Anaesth. 2017;20:355–8.
6. Puma F, Ragusa M, Avenia N, Urbani M, Droghetti A, Daddi N, et al. The role of silicone stents in the treatment of cicatricial tracheal stenoses. J Thorac Cardiovasc Surg. 2000;120:1064.
7. Chin CS, Litle V, Yun J, Weiser T, Swanson SJ. Airway stents. Ann Thorac Surg. 2008;85:S792–6.
8. Wood DE, Liu YH, Vallières E, Karmy-Jones R, Mulligan MS. Airway stenting for malignant and benign tracheobronchial stenosis. Ann Thorac Surg. 2003; 76:167–74.
9. Park HY, Kim H, Koh WJ, Suh GY, Chung MP, Kwon OJ. Natural stent in the management of post-intubation tracheal stenosis. Respirology. 2009; 14:583–8.
10. Bolliger CT, Probst R, Tschopp K, Solèr M, Perruchoud AP. Silicone stents in the Management of Inoperable Tracheobronchial Stenoses : indications and limitations. Chest. 1993;104:1653–9.
11. Martinezballarin JI, Diazjimenez JP, Castro MJ, Moya JA. Silicone stents in the management of benign tracheobronchial stenoses. Tolerance and early results in 63 patients. Chest. 1996;109:626–9.
12. Noppen M, Meysman M, Claes I, D'Haese J, Vincken W. Screw-thread vs Dumon Endoprosthesis in the Management of Tracheal Stenosis. Chest. 1999;115:532.
13. Olze H, Dörffel W, Kaschke O. Endotracheal silicon stents in therapy management of benign tracheal stenoses. HNO. 2001;49:895.
14. Lemaire A, Burfeind WR, Toloza E, Balderson S, Petersen RP, Jr HD, et al. Outcomes of tracheobronchial stents in patients with malignant airway disease. Ann Thorac Surg. 2005;80:434–7.
15. Colt HG, Harrell J, Neuman TR, Robbins T. External fixation of subglottic tracheal stents. Chest. 1994;105:1653–7.
16. Majid A, Fernandez-Bussy S, Kent M, Folch E, Fernandez L, Cheng G, et al. External fixation of proximal tracheal airway stents: a modified technique. Ann Thorac Surg. 2012;93:e167–e9.
17. Miwa K, Takamori S, Hayashi A, Fukunaga M, Shirouzu K. Fixation of silicone stents in the subglottic trachea: preventing stent migration using a fixation apparatus. Ann Thorac Surg. 2004;78:2188–90.
18. Spelsberg FW, Wollenberg B, Weidenhagen R, Lang RA, Winter H, Jauch KW, et al. Trachealstents wegen ösophagotrachealer Fistel beim Laryngektomierten. HNO. 2009;57:1065–70.
19. Madan K, Venuthurimilli A, Ahuja V, Hadda V, Mohan A, Guleria R. Tracheal penetration and tracheoesophageal fistula caused by an esophageal self-expanding metallic stent. Case Rep Pulmonol. 2014;2014:567582.

7

Is there a difference in bleeding after left ventricular assist device implant: centrifugal versus axial?

Ann C. Gaffey[1*], Carol W. Chen[1], Jennifer J. Chung[1], Jason Han[1], Christian A. Bermudez[1], Joyce Wald[2] and Pavan Atluri[1]

Abstract

Background: Continuous-flow left ventricular assist devices (CF-LVAD) have become the standard of care for patients with end stage heart failure. Device reliability has increased, bringing the potential for VAD, compared to transplant, into debate. However, complications continue to limit VADs as first line therapy. Bleeding is a major morbidity. A debate exists as to the difference in bleeding profile between the major centrifugal and axial flow devices. We hypothesized that there would be similar adverse bleeding event profiles between the 2 major CF-LVADs.

Methods: We retrospectively investigated isolated CF LVADs performed at our institution between July 2010 and July 2015: HeartMateII (HMII, $n = 105$) and HeartWare (HVAD, $n = 34$). We reviewed demographic, perioperative and short- and long-term outcomes.

Results: There was no significant difference in demographics or comorbidities. There was a low incidence of gastrointestinal (GI) bleed 3.9% in HMII and 2.9% in HVAD ($p = 0.78$). Preoperatively, the cohorts did not differ in coagulation measures ($p = 0.95$). Within the post-operative period, there was no difference in product transfusion: red blood cells ($p = 0.10$), fresh frozen plasma ($p = 0.19$), and platelets ($p = 0.89$). Post-operatively, a higher but not significantly different number of HMII patients returned to the operating room for bleeding ($n = 27$) compared to HVAD ($n = 6$, $p = 0.35$). There was no difference in rates of stroke ($p = 0.65$), re-intubation ($p = 0.60$), driveline infection ($p = 0.05$), and GI bleeding ($p = 0.31$). The patients had equivalent ICU LOS ($p = 0.86$) and index hospitalization LOS ($p = 0.59$).

Conclusion: We found no difference in the rate of bleeding complications between the current commercially available axial and centrifugal flow devices.

Keywords: Left ventricular assist device, Gastrointestinal bleeding

Background

During the past several decades, left ventricular assist devices (LVADs) have become a valuable and indispensable therapeutic option in the management of end stage heart failure. Recent data suggest that one of the most common adverse events within the first 30 days after LVAD implantation is bleeding in particular bleeding not requiring a return to the operating room [1–5]. Data from the Interagency Registry for Mechanically Assisted Circulatory Support (INTERMACS) have shown that the most frequent location of the first bleeding episode after implantation to be mediastinal (45%), thoracic-pleural space (12%), lower gastrointestinal (GI) tract (10%), chest wall (8%), and upper GI tract (8%) with no difference in the overall bleeding rates between axial- and pulsatile flow devices [6].

The etiology of the greater rate of non-surgical bleeding is due to the relatively high non-physiological stress imparted on the blood components as they move through the device. Stress coupled with the reduced pulse pressure may result in the unanticipated

* Correspondence: Ann.gaffey@uphs.upenn.edu
[1]Division of Cardiovascular Surgery, Department of Surgery, Perelman School of Medicine, University of Pennsylvania, Silverstein 6, 3400 Spruce St, Philadelphia, PA 19104, USA
Full list of author information is available at the end of the article

increases in nonsurgical bleeding related to arteriovenous malformations (AVMs) in the GI tract. Bleeding specifically from the GI tract has been identified as the most common adverse event in implantation and is a major cause of morbidity in patients supported with LVAD therapy [7–10]. One of the proposed mechanisms for GI bleeding following implantation of an LVAD is acquired von Willebrand syndrome. Von Willebrand factor (vWF) is a protein expressed by vascular endothelial cells that is essential in preventing coagulopathy or bleeding; however, excessive cleavage of large vWF results in bleeding syndrome in the acquired syndrome as seen in patients with LVADs [11]. This paper aims to compare outcomes between axial (HeartMate II) and centrifugal (HeartWare) flow LVADs with respect to bleeding outcomes at a single institution.

Methods
Study design
All patients who underwent implantation of a CF-LVAD from July 2010 to July 2015 (n = 139) at the University of Pennsylvania were retrospectively reviewed. After initial data accrual, all patient identifiers were removed from the database. The University of Pennsylvania Institutional Review Board (IRB 7) approved this study for investigation.

Device selection was based on patient characteristics and surgeons' preference. Patients were initially not anti-coagulated on post-operative day zero. On post-operative day one, the patients were started on a heparin drip with a goal partial thromboplastin time of 45–50 s. Ultimately, all patients were anticoagulated with 325 mg of aspirin and Coumadin to a target International Normalized Ratio (INR) of 2.0–3.0. No additional anti-platelet agents were used in either cohort.

Patient demographics, co-morbidities, laboratory values, and complications were retrospectively analyzed using our institutional database. Baseline information was collected the day before LVAD implantation. Patient demographic information and co-morbidities included age, sex, diabetes, etiology of cardiomyopathy, indication for LVAD, and INTERMACS patient profile risk score. Height and weight were collected in order to calculate body mass index (BMI). We also collected cardiopulmonary bypass time, days of mechanical ventilation, duration of hospital stay, and ICU length of stay.

Patients were followed on LVAD support for complications and intraoperative outcomes out to 36 months. Potential device related complications included: GI bleeding, infection, right ventricular failure, stroke, VAD malfunction, and wound infection. We defined GI bleeding by hematemesis, melena, or active bleeding at the time of endoscopy or colonoscopy. All complications were recorded during ICU stay except for device malfunction, GI bleeding, and death, which were also followed after discharge.

Outcomes analysis
The primary outcomes were post-operative bleeding events. Secondary outcomes included postoperative complications and length of stay outcomes. Normally distributed variables were presented as mean value ± standard deviation; non-normally distributed were presented as median value with interquartile range. Normality of all data variables was tested. Non-parametric data was analyzed using Kruskal-Wallis one way analysis of variance and parametric data was analyzed by a two-sample t-test. Significance was set at α = 0.05. All statistical analyses were performed using commercially available software (STATA 13.1; Statacorp LP, College Station, Texas).

Results
Patient characteristics
During the study time frame, 105 HMII implants and 34 HVAD implants were performed at our institution. Between the two cohorts, no difference existed with regard to age (p = 0.83) and gender with the majority of patients being male (p = 0.73, Table 1). The most common indication for LVAD implantation in both groups was destination therapy with 59.1% in the HMII cohort and 52.9% in the HVAD cohort (p = 0.89). The second indication for LVAD implantation was bridge to transplantation in 26.7% of the HMII cohort and 35.3% in the HVAD cohort. There was no difference in INTERMACS classification between the two cohorts (p = 0.19) with the greatest percentage in both being class 2 with 37.1% in HMII and 41.2% in HVAD.

In terms of past medical history, there was a low frequency of GI bleeding in both cohorts at less than 4%

Table 1 Baseline characteristics of patients implanted with the HeartMate II (HMII) and HeartWare (HVAD)

	HMII (n = 105)	HVAD (n = 34)	p-value
Age	56.5 + 13.9	57.2 + 14.6	0.82
Sex male, n (%)	83 (79.1)	27 (81.8)	0.73
Body mass index	29.2 + 6.8	29.5 + 6.2	
LVAD Indication, n (%)			0.89
Bridge to transplantation	28 (26.7)	12 (35.3)	
Destination therapy	62 (59.1)	18 (52.9)	
Bridge to decision	13 (12.4)	1 (2.9)	
Bridge to recovery	2 (1.9)	3 (8.8)	
INTERMACS Classification			0.19
1	12 (14.3)	5 (14.7)	
2	39 (37.1)	14 (41.2)	
3	36 (34.3)	15 (44.1)	
4	14 (13.3)		
5	1 (0.9)		
Heart failure duration, months	2.2 + 1.1	2.3 + 0.8	0.59

($p = 0.78$). For all other past medical history, there was no difference with regards to coronary artery disease ($p = 0.53$), hypertension ($p = 0.76$), atrial fibrillation ($p = 0.82$) and chronic renal insufficiency ($p = 0.60$). The etiology of heart failure was similar between the groups, with ischemic and idiopathic being the two most common causes ($p = 0.59$) (Table 2).

Intraoperative outcomes

For the HMII cohorts, 21% of the patients were redo-sternotomy compared to 30% in the HVAD ($p = 0.31$). The cardiopulmonary bypass time (85.1 ± 37.7 vs. 81.8 ± 47.9 min, $p = 0.72$) was low and similar in the cohorts. Additionally, there was no difference in blood product transfusion between the two groups (Table 3).

Post-operative outcomes

Within the HVAD cohort, there was a higher requirement for temporary RVAD at 29% compared to 15% in HMII ($p = 0.02$). There was no difference in immediate

Table 2 Pre-implantation past medical history, heart failure, etiology, and laboratory values of patients implanted with the HeartMate II (HMII) and HeartWare (HVAD)

	HMII ($n = 105$)	HVAD ($n = 34$)	p-value
Past medical history, n (%)			
History of gastrointestinal bleeding	4 (3.9)	1 (2.9)	0.78
Coronary artery disease	49 (46.7)	18 (53.0)	0.53
Diabetes mellitus	48 (45.7)	14 (41.2)	0.65
Smoking	38 (36.2)	22 (66.7)	0.002
Hypertension	55 (52.9)	19 (55.9)	0.76
Atrial fibrillation	44 (41.9)	15 (44.1)	0.82
Cerebral vascular accident	13 (12.4)	3 (8.8)	0.55
Chronic renal insufficiency	37 (35.2)	10 (30.3)	0.60
Heart failure etiology, n (%)			0.59
Ischemic	47 (45.2)	12 (55.2)	
Idiopathic	45 (43.3)	10 (34.5)	
Viral	1 (1.0)	–	
Peripartum	4 (3.9)	1 (3.5)	
Alcoholic	1 (1.0)	–	
Myocarditis	1 (1.0)	2 (6.9)	
Chemotherapy Induced cardiomyopathy	2 (1.9)	–	
Vavlular	3 (2.9)	–	
Lab values			
White blood cell (THO/uL)	8.9 + 4.9	7.9 _ 2.5	0.15
Hemoglobin (g/dL)	12.0 + 0.9	10.8 + 0.4	0.23
Platelet (THO/uL)	184.9 + 69.8	191.9 + 83.4	0.66
Prothrombin Time (seconds)	52.6 + 2.5	52.3 + 3.9	0.95

Table 3 Intraoperative outcomes and product utilization of patients implanted with the HeartMate II (HMII) and HeartWare (HVAD)

	HMII ($n = 105$)	HVAD ($n = 34$)	p-value
Redo sternotomy, n (%)	22 (21)	10 (30)	0.31
Cardiopulmonary bypass time, minutes	85.1 + 37.7	81.8 + 47.9	0.72
Product Transfusion, peri-operative (72 h)			
Red blood cells, units	8.2 + 1.0	4.9 + 1.6	0.10
Fresh frozen plasma, units	3.3 + 0.5	2.0 + 0.6	0.19
Platelets, units	1.1 + 0.2	1.2 + 0.5	0.89

post-operative day one laboratory values with regards to hemoglobin (9.9 ± 1.5 vs. 9.7 ± 1.8 d/dL, $p = 0.63$) and international normalized ratio (1.4 ± 0.3 vs. 1.3 ± 0.1, $p = 0.06$); however, partial thromboplastin time was greater in the HVAD compared to HMII (34.7 ± 9.3 vs. 40.1 ± 8.4 s, $p = 0.003$).

Prior to return to possible return the operating room, hemodynamics were measured as included in Table 4. Mean arterial pressure was equivalent between the two cohorts (72 ± 11 vs. 68 ± 9 mmHg, $p = 0.29$). As surrogate marker of right ventricular function, central venous pressure was noted to be elevated within the HVAD compared to the HMII cohort (10 ± 3 vs. 13 ± 2 mmHg, $p = 0.05$). Additionally, the cardiac index was reduced in the HVAD cohort compared to HMII (2.5 ± 1.1 vs. $2.2 + 1.3$ L/min/m^2, $p = 0.04$).

Within the index hospitalization, there was a higher but not significantly different incidence of intra-thoracic bleeding requiring operative exploration within the HMII compared to the HVAD cohort (25.7% vs. 18.2%, $p = 0.35$). The rate of GI bleeding within the index hospitalization was similar between the two groups (11.5% vs. 5.9%, $p = 0.28$). Throughout follow-up, there was no difference between GI bleeding at 3, 12, 24, and 36 months ($p = 0.35$, 0.45, 0.48, and 0.23, respectively).

As shown in Fig. 1, there was no difference in post-VAD implantation survival between the two cohorts (log rank $p = 0.0769$).

Discussion

Balancing bleeding and thrombotic complications has become a difficult clinical dilemma, made more challenging by the poorly understood difference in risk factors. This study showed that overall, patients had similar outcomes with regards to bleeding, irrespective of whether they received a HMII or HVAD and there was no difference in associated mortality.

Overall, the patient cohorts were similar with regard to pre-operative conditions. The only significant difference between the two cohorts was nearly a one third greater incidence of smoking within the HVAD cohort

Table 4 Postoperative outcomes for patients implanted with the HeartMate II (HMII) and HeartWare (HVAD)

	HMII (n = 105)	HVAD (n = 34)	p-value
Temporary RVAD Requirement, n (%)	16 (15)	10 (29)	0.02
Time to extubation, days	1.5 (1,5)	2 (1.5)	0.63
ICU length of stay, days	7 (4,14)	8 (6,15)	0.86
Hospital length of stay, days	20 (14,32)	20 (15, 27)	0.59
Post-operative day one lab values			
White blood cells (THO/uL)	15.6 + 6.7	15.5 + 5.7	0.96
Hemoglobin (d/dL)	9.9 + 1.5	9.7 + 1.8	0.63
Platelet (THO/uL)	138.1 + 52.6	147.7 + 57.9	0.39
International normalized ratio	1.4 + 0.3	1.3 + 0.1	0.06
Prothrombin time (seconds)	34.7 + 9.3	40.1 + 8.4	0.003
Lactic acid dehydrogenase (U/L)	499.8 + 228.1	411.6 + 96.1	0.14
Hemodynamics			
Mean Arterial Pressure (mmHg)	72 + 11	68 + 9	0.29
Central Venous Pressure (mmHg)	10 + 3	13 + 2	0.05
Systolic Pulmonary Artery Pressure (mmHg)	28 + 4	26 + 6	0.07
Cardic Index (L/min/m²)	2.5 + 1.1	2.2 + 1.3	0.04
Complications- index hospitalization, n (%)			
Intra-thoracic bleeding	27 (25.7)	6 (18.2)	0.35
Stroke	4 (3.8)	2 (5.9)	0.65
Re-intubation	20 (19.1)	5 (15.2)	0.6
Drive line infection	2 (3.9)	0 (0.0)	0.05
Gastrointestinal bleeding, n (%)			
Index hospitalization	12 (11.5)	2 (5.9)	0.28
3 months	17 (19.5)	3 (11.5)	0.35
12 months	8 (16.33)	0 (0.0)	0.54
24 months	3 (15.0)	0 (0.0)	0.48
36 months	3 (15.0)	0 (0.0)	0.23

compared the HMII; however, this pre-operative difference did not translate into a difference in post-operative outcomes. Both groups had a low incidence of prior GI bleeding and with no significant difference in pre-implant coagulation factors. During the operation, and within 30 days post-operatively, there was a low blood product requirement without any difference between the two cohorts.

Post-operatively, a greater percentage of the HVAD cohort required temporary RVAD support. This finding is supported by the reduced right ventricular function within the HVAD cohort immediately prior to RVAD implantation. The CVP was noted to be significantly elevated within the HVAD cohort suggesting right heart strain. The incidence of right ventricular support was

higher than that reported in the ADVANCE trial at 2.1% requiring mechanical support and 12.1% on inotropic support [12]. Given that there are no significant differences pre-operatively and intra-operatively between the two groups, it seems as though this difference is likely attributed to small numbers in both cohorts. Overall, both the HMII and HVAD patients had nearly equivalent time to extubation, ICU length of stay, and hospital length of stay.

Furthermore, the incidence of post-operative complications was low between both groups. Examining the implantation technique between the devices, the HMII requires creation and tunneling of subcutaneous pocket while the HVAD has a smaller dissection for the intrapericardial implantation. Despite the differences in technique, no difference existed in overall bleeding events. This similar outcome between the two groups suggests that a meticulous dissection of the pump pocket, as well as hemostasis, is essential to keep bleeding events low for those patients receiving HMII. Additionally, the rate of intra-thoracic bleeding requiring a return to the operating room for a washout was similarly low between the groups. These low rates are further supported by those of the ADVANCE trial with risk of 0.26/patient-year in the HVAD and 0.45/patient-year for the HMII [12].

Furthermore, numerous studies have been published showing that the incidence of GI bleeding after LVAD implantation to vary between 18 and 40% [13–15]. GI bleeding after implantation is classified as upper GI bleeding (proximal to the ligament of Trietz) or lower GI bleeding (distal to the ligament of Trietz). Most common causes are vascular malformations like AVMs and Dieulafoy lesions, which account for 30–40% and 15–20%, respectively [16]. Within our study, the rates of GI bleeding we reported in both cohorts are similar to past studies which reported rates between 11% and 13% [17–19] in the HVAD cohort and 22% in HMII patients [20]. During the index hospitalization only 11.5% of HMII and 5.9% HVAD experienced GI bleeding in our cohort of patients. Throughout follow up there was no difference in the occurrence of a GI bleed between the cohorts out to 36 months of follow-up.

The etiology of the GI bleeding following LVAD implantation is multifactorial given the need for chronic anticoagulation as well as the changes in systemic immunologic and thrombostatic functions [21]. One proposed mechanism of GI bleeding is acquired von Willebrand syndrome due to the fragmentation of high molecular weight multimers of vWF. A study by Meyer et al. [22] demonstrated a reduction in high molecular weight vWF in HVAD patients. This finding suggest that although HVAD shear forces are low due to the contact free design and lower revolutions per minute in the HVAD, the shear force still reaches a

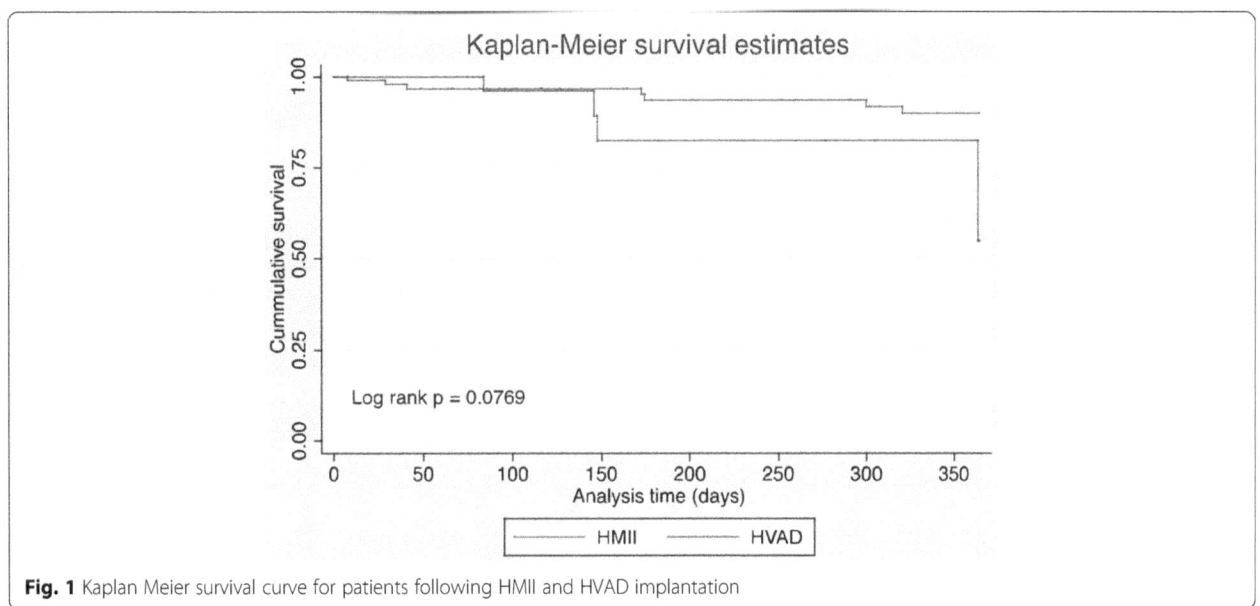

Fig. 1 Kaplan Meier survival curve for patients following HMII and HVAD implantation

sufficient threshold to induce vWF unfolding [23]. As result, that both HMII and HVAD patients develop acquired von Willebrand syndrome, it is anticipated that they would have similar rates of GI bleeding.

For management of an LVAD patient with GI bleeding, a multidisciplinary approach is needed involving possible reversal of anticoagulation, holding of anticoagulants, and possible medical and surgical interventions. Overall, the main goals are to locate the bleeding source and the severity by holding anti-coagulation and resuscitation to maintain stable hemodynamics.

Conclusions
Overall, balancing bleeding and thrombosis risks continues to be a critical component of LVAD patient management moving forward, especially with the advent of novel anticoagulant agents. Our study further adds to the literature that the rate of bleeding between axial and centrifugal pumps is low without significant difference between the two.

Limitations
Limitations of this study include its retrospective nature. Due to sample size restrictions, we were unable to perform adjusted analysis. Furthermore, the small sample sized may have limited the study's ability to detect statistically significant differences in some of the variables compared. The value of transthoracic echocardiogram within the immediate postoperative period is difficult to gain value given the obscure windows, as a result, cardiac index provides a better measurement of function. Additionally, although we did not observe high INR before GI bleeding events, some of the incidences may have been precipitated by high INR in patients.

Abbreviations
AVMS: Arteriovenous malformations; CF-LVAD: Continuous-flow left ventricular assist devices; GI: Gastrointestinal; HMII: HeartMate II; HVAD: HeartWare; INR: International normalized ratio; INTERMACS: Interagency Registry for Mechanically Assisted Circulatory Support; LVAD: Left ventricular assist device; vWF: Von Willebrand factor (vWF)

Acknowledgments
Not applicable

Authors' contributions
AG conceived of the study, and participated in its design, coordination, and drafted the manuscript. CC participated in the design of the study and performed the statistical analysis. JC and JH performed statistical analysis and assisted with drafting of the manuscript. CB, JW, and PA conceived of the study, and participated in its design and coordination and helped to draft the manuscript. All authors read and approved the final manuscript.

Competing interests
The authors declare that they have no competing interests.

Author details
[1]Division of Cardiovascular Surgery, Department of Surgery, Perelman School of Medicine, University of Pennsylvania, Silverstein 6, 3400 Spruce St, Philadelphia, PA 19104, USA. [2]Division of Cardiology, Department of Medicine, Perelman School of Medicine, University of Pennsylvania, Philadelphia, USA.

References

1. Slaughter MS, Rogers JG, Milano CA, et al. Advanced heart failure treated with continuous-flow left ventricular assist device. N Engl J Med. 2009; 361(23):2241–51. https://doi.org/10.1056/NEJMoa0909938.
2. Genovese EA, Dew MA, Teuteberg JJ, et al. Incidence and patterns of adverse event onset during the first 60 days after ventricular assist device implantation. Ann Thorac Surg. 2009;88(4):1162–70. https://doi.org/10.1016/j.athoracsur.2009.06.028.
3. Pagani FD, Miller LW, Russell SD, et al. Extended mechanical circulatory support with a continuous-flow rotary left ventricular assist device. J Am Coll Cardiol. 2009;54(4):312–21. https://doi.org/10.1016/j.jacc.2009.03.055.
4. Uriel N, Pak S-W, Jorde UP, et al. Acquired von Willebrand syndrome after continuous-flow mechanical device support contributes to a high prevalence of bleeding during long-term support and at the time of transplantation. J Am Coll Cardiol. 2010;56(15):1207–13. https://doi.org/10.1016/j.jacc.2010.05.016.
5. Pal JD, Piacentino V, Cuevas AD, et al. Impact of left ventricular assist device bridging on posttransplant outcomes. Ann Thorac Surg. 2009;88(5):1457–61; discussion 1461. https://doi.org/10.1016/j.athoracsur.2009.07.021.
6. Jessup ML, Goldstein D, Ascheim DD, et al. 5 risk for bleeding after MCSD implant: an analysis of 2358 patients in INTERMACS. J Hear Lung Transplant. 2011;30(4) https://doi.org/10.1016/j.healun.2011.01.012.
7. Stern DR, Kazam J, Edwards P, et al. Increased incidence of gastrointestinal bleeding following implantation of the HeartMate II LVAD. J Card Surg. 2010;25(3):352–6. https://doi.org/10.1111/j.1540-8191.2010.01025.x.
8. Stulak JM, Mehta V, Schirger JA, et al. Temporal Differences in Causes of Mortality After Left Ventricular Assist Device Implantation. Ann Thorac Surg. 2015;99(6):1969-74. https://doi.org/10.1016/j.athoracsur.2015.01.036.
9. Geisen U, Heilmann C, Beyersdorf F, et al. Non-surgical bleeding in patients with ventricular assist devices could be explained by acquired von Willebrand disease. Eur J Cardiothorac Surg. 2008;33(4):679–84. https://doi.org/10.1016/j.ejcts.2007.12.047.
10. Crow S, John R, Boyle A, et al. Gastrointestinal bleeding rates in recipients of nonpulsatile and pulsatile left ventricular assist devices. J Thorac Cardiovasc Surg. 2009;137(1):208–15. https://doi.org/10.1016/j.jtcvs.2008.07.032.
11. Suarez J, Patel CB, Felker GM, Becker R, Hernandez AF, Rogers JG. Mechanisms of bleeding and approach to patients with axial-flow left ventricular assist devices. Circ Heart Fail. 2011;4(6):779–84. https://doi.org/10.1161/CIRCHEARTFAILURE.111.962613.
12. Aaronson KD, Slaughter MS, Miller LW, et al. Use of an intrapericardial, continuous-flow, centrifugal pump in patients awaiting heart transplantation. Circulation. 2012;125(25):3191-200. https://doi.org/10.1161/CIRCULATIONAHA.111.058412.
13. John R, Kamdar F, Eckman P, et al. Lessons learned from experience with over 100 consecutive HeartMate II left ventricular assist devices. Ann Thorac Surg. 2011;92(5):1593–9; discussion 1599–1600. https://doi.org/10.1016/j.athoracsur.2011.06.081.
14. Morgan JA, Paone G, Nemeh HW, et al. Gastrointestinal bleeding with the HeartMate II left ventricular assist device. J Heart Lung Transplant. 2012; 31(7):715–8. https://doi.org/10.1016/j.healun.2012.02.015.
15. Aggarwal A, Pant R, Kumar S, et al. Incidence and management of gastrointestinal bleeding with continuous flow assist devices. Ann Thorac Surg. 2012;93(5):1534–40. https://doi.org/10.1016/j.athoracsur.2012.02.035.
16. Demirozu ZT, Radovancevic R, Hochman LF, et al. Arteriovenous malformation and gastrointestinal bleeding in patients with the HeartMate II left ventricular assist device. J Heart Lung Transplant. 2011;30(8):849–53. https://doi.org/10.1016/j.healun.2011.03.008.
17. Wieselthaler GM, Gerry O, Jansz P, Khaghani A, Strueber M. Initial clinical experience with a novel left ventricular assist device with a magnetically levitated rotor in a multi-institutional trial. J Heart Lung Transplant. 2010; 29(11):1218–25. https://doi.org/10.1016/j.healun.2010.05.016.
18. Miller LW, Pagani FD, Russell SD, et al. Use of a Continuous-Flow Device in Patients Awaiting Heart Transplantation. N Engl J Med. 2007;357(9):885-96. https://doi.org/10.1056/NEJMoa067758.
19. Popov AF, Hosseini MT, Zych B, et al. Clinical experience with HeartWare left ventricular assist device in patients with end-stage heart failure. Ann Thorac Surg. 2012;93(3):810–5. https://doi.org/10.1016/j.athoracsur.2011.11.076.
20. Demirozu ZT, Radovancevic R, Hochman LF, et al. Arteriovenous malformation and gastrointestinal bleeding in patients with the HeartMate II left ventricular assist device. J Hear Lung Transplant. 2011;30(8):849-53. https://doi.org/10.1016/j.healun.2011.03.008.
21. John R, Lee S. The biological basis of thrombosis and bleeding in patients with ventricular assist devices. J Cardiovasc Transl Res. 2009;2(1):63–70. https://doi.org/10.1007/s12265-008-9072-7.
22. Meyer AL, Malehsa D, Budde U, Bara C, Haverich A, Strueber M. Acquired von Willebrand syndrome in patients with a centrifugal or axial continuous flow left ventricular assist device. JACC Heart Fail. 2014;2(2):141–5. https://doi.org/10.1016/j.jchf.2013.10.008.
23. Crow SS, Joyce DD. Are centrifugal ventricular assist devices the answer to reducing post-implantation gastrointestinal bleeding? JACC Heart Fail. 2014; 2(2):146–7. https://doi.org/10.1016/j.jchf.2013.11.008.

8

The correlation between the coaptation height of mitral valve and mitral regurgitation after mitral valve repair

Dan Wei, Jie Han, Haibo Zhang, Yan Li, Chunlei Xu and Xu Meng[*]

Abstract

Background: To investigate the association between the coaptation height of mitral valve and mitral regurgitation after mitral valve repair.

Methods: From Sep 2014 to Jun 2015, 20 patients underwent mitral valve valvuloplasty for mitral regurgitation were included. Ring annuloplasty was performed in all cases. Mitral valve short-axis dimension (MVd), coaptation height (CH), Left ventricular ejection fraction (LVEF) were measured by the transesophageal echocardiography before the operation in operation room and 3 months and 12 months after the operation by the transthoracic echocardiography. A degree from 0 to 4 was used to measure the degree of mitral regurgitation.

Results: There were 14 patients with 0, 3 patients with 1, 3 patients with 2 of mitral regurgitation 12 months after the operation. CH (3.53 ± 1.91 mm) increased significantly at 3 months (5.05 ± 1.09 mm) and 12 months after operation (5.22 ± 1.15 mm) ($p < 0.05$). MVd and LVEF were not significantly changed after mitral valve repair. Furthermore, CH after resuscitation have a statistically significant negative correlation with the degree of mitral regurgitation 12 months after operation.

Conclusion: The mitral valve repair with mitral valve ring induce the morphologic change of the mitral valve structure. The increase of CH after mitral valve repair may be one of the main factors in regulation of mitral regurgitation.

Keywords: Coaptation Height of mitral valve, Mitral regurgitation, Mitral valve repair

Background

Mitral valve repair is a surgical procedure that has continuously developed through decades. Since 1968, Carpentier has developed the concept of prosthetic ring annuloplasty which aimed to restore the shape of the deformed annulus fibrosus of the MV [1]. With the development of the comprehension and evaluation of the pathology, standardization of the surgical techniques, the long term results from this surgery have gained a great progress. The remodeling of mitral annular provide the predictability and stability which has made MVP the most attractive approach on the treatment of mitral regurgitation in the United States [2, 3]. Nowadays, mitral valve repair (MVR) is the gold standard for severe degenerative mitral regurgitation (MR). Resection of the prolapsed leaflet has been widely performed and has shown excellent outcomes for posterior leaflet prolapse. The concept of leaflet preservation has become increasingly appreciated. In mitral valve repair, the greater the mitral valve coaptation area is, the lighter the mitral regurgitation is. Falk et al. found that chordal placement with minimal or no leaflet resection may contribute to better durability of MVR compared with leaflet resection, because of a longer zone of coaptation [4]. Post-repair coaptation length (CL) has been shown to be related to durability of MVR in patients with ischemic MR. [5] However, the association between post-repair CL and durability of MVR in degenerative MR has not been investigated. However, the exact value of the mitral valve coaptation area is not easy to obtain.

Doppler echocardiography was used to detect the functional information of transvalvular flow velocity, which could be used to measure the pressure gradient across valve and regurgitant flow [6]. Mitral valve area (MVA), a

* Correspondence: caiyan951@yeah.net
Department of cardiac surgery, Capital medical university affiliated Beijing anzhen hospital, Chaoyang District Anzhen Road No. 2, Beijing 100029, China

important functional index, can be detected by either 2-D echocardiography or Doppler pressure half-time [7]. In additional, transesophageal echocardiography (TEE) was also used to evaluate situation of the patients who has underwent percutaneous mitral BV in whom left atrial thrombus (LAT) is suspected [8] and for the intraoperative monitoring of the valvuloplasty procedure [9]. More recently, three-dimensional (3D) transoesophageal (TEE) echocardiography has provided accurate measurement of mitral valve morphology [10].

Therefore, in this study we used above methods to investigated whether it is possible to measure the degree of mitral regurgitation by measuring the mitral coaptation height. Accordingly, the present study aimed to evaluate the correlation between the height of mitral valve coaptation and mitral regurgitation after mitral valve repair.

Methods

This was a retrospective study with the prospective follow-up of mitral valve regurgitation patients who underwent mitral regurgitation using a annuloplasty strip for mitral valve repair. This study was approved by Capital medical university affiliated Beijing anzhen hospital.

Patients

A total of 20 patients were treated with the MV at Capital medical university affiliated Beijing anzhen hospital between Sep 2014 and Jun 2015. Transesophageal echocardiography (TEE) assessment assessment were routinely performed before the intervention to assess LVEF, mitral valve morphology and mitral regurgitation grade, and evaluation of factors that may contraindicate the procedure. Transthoracic echocardiographic (TTE) examination was performed after the operation. This study was approved by the ethics committee of Capital medical university affiliated Beijing Anzhen hospital. The informed consent was obtained form all the included patients.

Operative procedure

All operations included in this study were performed via a median sternotomy approach. Cardiopulmonary bypass was established by ascending aortic and bicaval cannulation. The aorta was cross-clamped and cardiac asystole was achieved using intermittent antegrade and retrograde cardioplegia. Posterior leaflet prolapse was primarily repaired by leaflet resection. The resection size and shape were determined by a surgeon in charge of each case. Neochordal placement was added if necessary. Ring annuloplasty was performed in all cases. The type of ring was chosen based on surgeon's preference. The size of ring was determined by sizing the area of anterior leaflet using prosthetic sizers made by each manufacturer.

The surgical procedures with prosthetic ring annuloplasty were performed in all patients. Prosthetic ring annuloplasty was performed in 5 cases with 30-mm prosthetic ring (Edwards physio 2), 8 cases with 32-mm prosthetic ring (Edwards 5200), 5 cases with 34-mm prosthetic ring (Edwards physio 2) and 2 cases with 36-mm prosthetic ring (Edwards physio 4450).

Echocardiographic measurements

TTE was performed using commercially available ultrasound systems (E33; Philips, Netherlands) equipped with an S5–1 transducer, and 2D, M-mode and Doppler data were acquired with the patient in the left lateral decubitus position. Transthoracic echocardiography was performed at 3 months and 12 months postoperatively. TEE with X7-2 t transducer was applied. The TEE view for the measurement was 3-chamber view and the middle square of mitral apparatus in short axis (Fig. 1). Mitral valve short-axis dimension (MVd) and Coaptation height (CH) at endsystole were measured (Fig. 1). The coaptation height was defined as the length between the free edge of the leaflet and the anterior and posterior lobes to left atrial surface level at end-systole stage. Carpentier typing was used to unify the mitral leaflet partition. The posterior lobe is divided into three leaves, the lateral fan as P1, the middle fan leaf as P2 and the medial fan leaf as P3. The corresponding anterior lobe was also divided into three parts, the lateral 1/3 part as A1, the middle 1/3 as A2, the medial 1/3 as A3. 20 cases in the operation room under anesthesia were examined by TEE.The Height of the corresponding section were set. The A2P2 was measured by four chamber view of the middle esophagus. The A1P1 was measured by five chamber view of the middle esophagus. The A3P3 was measured by deep esophageal short four chamber view showing coronary sinus. Three cardiac cycles were selected to measure the corresponding height. The mitral regurgitation grade was determined according to the following scale: 0, no or trivial mitral regurgitation; 1+, mild; 2+, mild to moderate mitral regurgitation; 3+, moderate to severe mitral regurgitation; and 4+, severe mitral regurgitation. The coaptation height (the longest coaptation height of the anterior and posterior leaflets) was measured in early systole.

Statistical analysis

The values obtained were analyzed with Student's T test. Linear regression analysis was determined using the least squares method. A p value <0.05 was considered as indicative of significant significance. Data are presented as the means ± standard deviation (SD).

Results
Baseline characteristics

The mean age of all patients was 52.45 ± 14.26 years and 11 patients (55%) were women. In the 20 cases studied, mitral regurgitation was degree 1 in 2 patients, degree 2 in 4 cases, and degree 3 in 14 cases before the operation. All

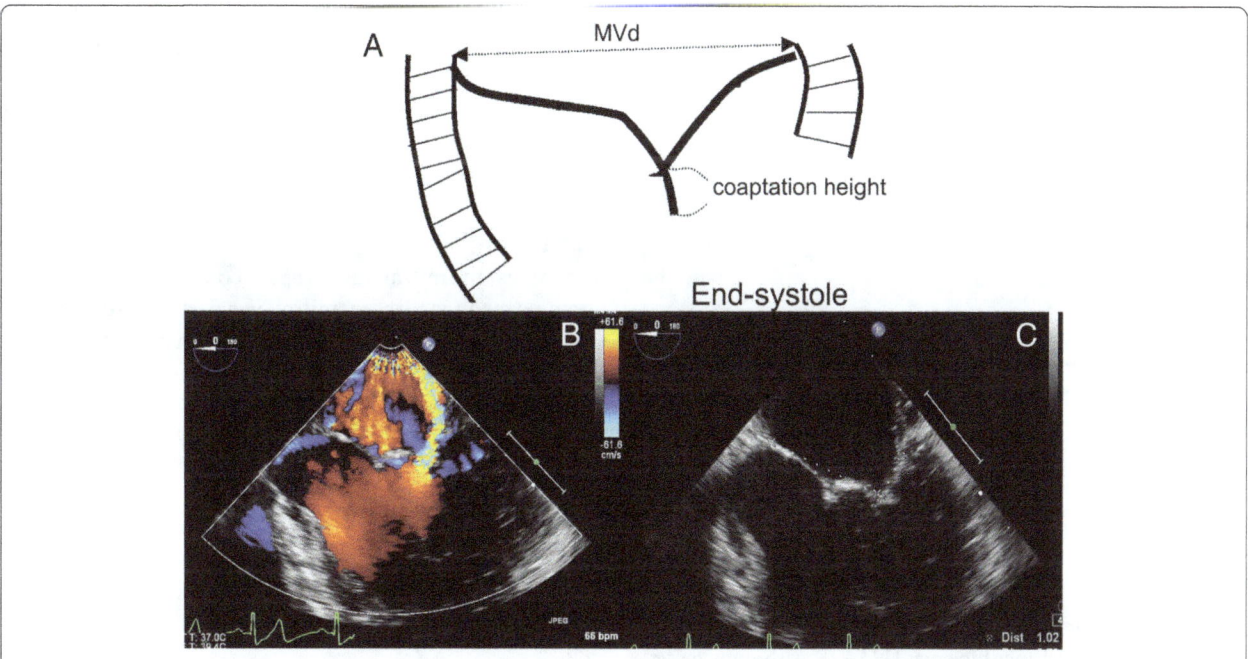

Fig. 1 The TEE view for measurement parameter. **a** Coaptation height measurement. **b** Measurement under TEE. **c** Coaptation height measurement by TEE

patients had a posterior middle scallop prolapse, the mean LVEF was 62.75 ± 7.94%. All patients underwent MVP with prosthetic ring. Pre-operative and operative data are shown in Table 1. In the 20 cases studied, mitral regurgitation was 0 in 14 patients, 1 in 3 cases, and 2 in 3 cases 12 months after the operation.

Leaflet morphologic change and Echocardiographic factor in regulating mitral regurgitation

Table 1 shows the preoperative and postoperative values of EF, MVd. The values of LVEF and MVd were not

significantly changed. However, MVd showed only increase trend after the surgery. In Fig. 2, CH of A1P1, A2P2, A3P3 was increased significantly. Among those stated index, the average values of CH (A1P1, A2P2, A3P3) after heart resuscitation showed a statistically significant negative correlation with degree of mitral regurgitation 12 months after the operation. ($p < 0.05$ $r = 0.81$) (Fig. 3).

Discussion

Surgical valve repair for mitral regurgitation (MR) has significant advantages over valve replacement and has acquired greater importance as a surgical treatment of MR.

Table 1 Measurement values

		MR ($n = 20$)
Age (years)		52.45 ± 14.26
Weight (kg)		67.8 ± 8.46
Height (cm)		164.7±8.20
Perfusion time (min)		40.4 ± 12.1
Cross-clamp time (min)		31.7 ± 14.2
LVEF (%)	Before the surgery	62.75 ± 7.94
	3 months after surgery	61.05 ± 9.00
	12 months after surgery	62.8 ± 10.52
MVd (mm)	Before the surgery	30.83 ± 3.48
	After heart resuscitation	31.95 ± 4.56
	3 months after surgery	33.33 ± 3.49
	12 months after surgery	33.78 ± 3.87

Left ventricular ejection fraction (LVEF), mitral valve short-axis dimension (MVd)
Values were shown as mean ± standard deviation

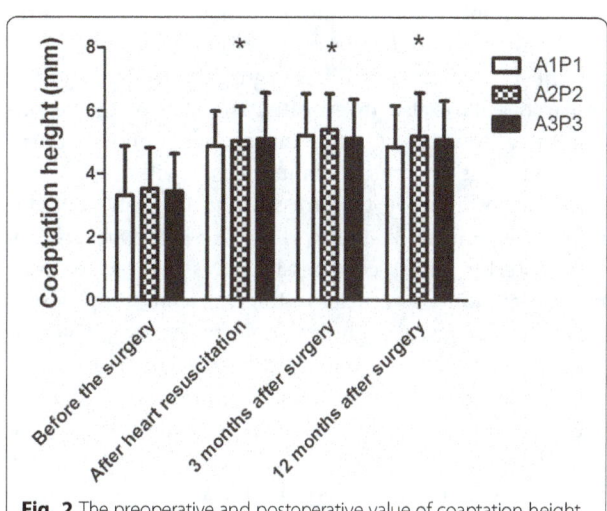

Fig. 2 The preoperative and postoperative value of coaptation height

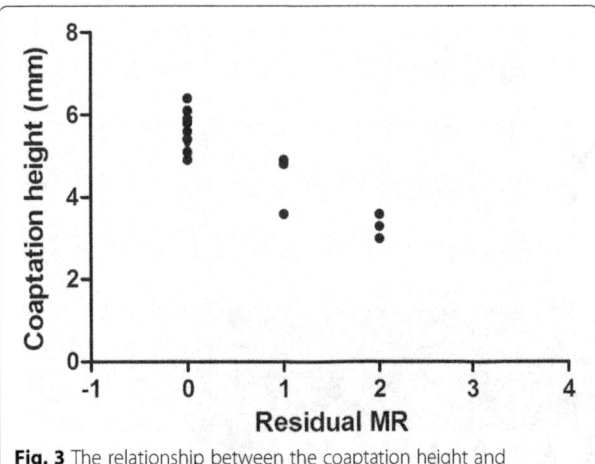

Fig. 3 The relationship between the coaptation height and residual regurgitaion

Some researches have already confirmed that the mitral valve repair could provided great long term results for the patients with mitral insufficiency [11, 12]. Although favorable clinical and functional results have been reported, the exact information of the valve leaflet morphology after those repairs is limited. The coaptation height was considered as an important morphologic index for mitral regurgitation. However, there are no uniform standards for the value of the coaptation height, which was mainly caused by the difficulty in measurement of the exact coaptation height in clinical practice, while even the exact point of the edge of free zone of leaflet at coaptation was difficult to obtained.

The main results of the our study showed that the LVEF and MVd were not significantly influenced after mitral valve repair. However, the coaptation height was significantly increased after the operation. Interestingly, CH after heart resuscitation showed a statistically significant negative correlation with degree of mitral regurgitation 12 months after operation, which meant CH after heart resuscitation may be an important predictive factor for the post-operative mitral regurgitation. Some other researches have also investigated the change of the mitral valve morphology after mitral annuloplasty. It was reported that the mitral annuloplasty with ring could significantly improve the stresses and the valve coaptation with annular dilatation [13]. The reconstruction of the posterior leaflet compressive stresses and nearnormal coaptation was crucial to the mitral annuloplasty. It was also reported that the anuloplasty ring could significantly improve the mitral valve coaptation by reducing the delayed action of the leaflet and preventing the mitral regurgitation in the case of acute left ventricular ischemia after ring implantation [14]. In a total, the normal coaptation is very important in the mitral annuloplasty.

There were also some limitations in our study. The number of the cases in our study is small. Further study with lager numbers is still needed. The differences of the surgery procedures and cardiac function were not excluded in this study, which may affect the measurement of mitral regurgitation.

Conclusion

In conclusion, mitral valve repair could induce the morphologic change of the mitral valve structure. The increase of CH after mitral valve repair may be one of the main factors in regulation of regurgitation after mitral valve repair.

Acknowledgements
We thanks all authors.

Funding
None.

Authors' contributions
XM was the guarantor of integrity of the entire study and designed the study concepts, prepared and edited the manuscript; DW and YL designed the study, done the literature research, gave the definition of intellectual content, CLX done the clinical studies and experimental studies, collected the data acquisition and analyzed statistical analysis; HBZ gave the definition of intellectual content JH also analyzed statistical analysis and reviewed the manuscript. All authors read and approved the final manuscript.

Competing interests
The authors declare that they have no competing interests.

References
1.   Carpentier A. Reconstructive valvuloplasty. A new technique of mitral valvuloplasty. Presse Med. 1969;77(7):251–3.
2.   Savage EB, Ferguson TB, DiSesa VJ. Use of mitral valve repair: analysis of contemporary United States experience reported to the Society of Thoracic Surgeons National Cardiac Database. Ann Thorac Surg. 2003;75:820–5.
3.   Gammie JS, Sheng S, Griffith BP, Peterson ED, Rankin JS, O'Brien SM, et al. Trends in mitral valve surgery in the United States: results from the Society of Thoracic Surgeons adult cardiac surgery database. Ann Thorac Surg. 2009;87:1431–7. discussion 1437-9
4.   Falk V, Seeburger J, Czesla M, Borger MA, Willige J, Kuntze T, et al. How does the use of polytetrafluoroethylene neochordae for posterior mitral valve prolapse (loop technique) compare with leaflet resection? A prospective randomized trial. J Thorac Cardiovasc Surg. 2008;136:1205.
5.   Gelsomino S, Lorusso R, Caciolli S, Capecchi I, Rostagno C, Chioccioli M, et al. 2008. Insights on left ventricular and valvular mechanisms of recurrent ischemic mitral regurgitation after restrictive annuloplasty and coronary artery bypass grafting. J Thorac Cardiovasc Surg. 2008;136:507–18.
6.   Hatle L, Angelsen B. Doppler ultrasound in cardiology: physical principles and clinical applications. Philadelphia, PA: Lea & Febiger; 1985. p. 97–176.
7.   Hatle L, Angelsen B, Thromsdal A. Non-invasive assessment of atrioventricular pressure half-time by Doppler ultrasound. Circulation. 1979;60:1096.
8.   Kronzon I, Tunick PA, Glassman E, Slater J, Schwinger M, Freedberg RS. Transesophageal echocardiography to detect atrial clot in candidates for percutaneous transseptal balloon valvuloplasty. JACC. 1990;16:1320–2.

9. Goldstein SA, Campbell AN. Mitral stenosis: evaluation and guidance of valvuloplasty by transesophageal echocardiography. Cardiol Clin. 1993;11:409–25.

10. Francis L, Finley A, Hessami W. Use of three-dimensional transesophageal echocardiography to evaluate mitral valve morphology for risk stratification prior to mitral valvuloplasty. Echocardiography. 2017;34(2):303–5.

11. Umesue M, Baba H, Kimura S. Immediate and mid-term result of restrictive mitral annuloplasty using a small semi-rigid ring. Gen Thorac Cardiovasc Surg. 2016;64(5):260–6.

12. Gillinov AM, Cosgrove DM III, Shiota T, Qin J, Tsujino H, Stewart WJ, et al. Cosgrove-Edwards Annuloplasty system: midterm results. Ann Thorac Surg. 2000;69:717–21.

13. Kunzelman KS, Reimink MS, Cochran RP. Variations in annuloplasty ring and sizer dimensions may alter outcome in mitral valve repair. J Card Surg. 1997;12:322–9.

14. Timek T, Glasson JR, Dagum P, Green GR, Nistal JF, Komeda M, et al. Ring annuloplasty prevents delayed leaflet coaptation and mitral regurgitation during acute left ventricular ischemia. J Thorac Cardiovasc Surg. 2000;119(4 Pt 1):774–83.

9

Control angiography for perioperative myocardial Ischemia after coronary surgery: meta-analysis

Fausto Biancari[1,2,3]*, Vesa Anttila[3], Angelo M. Dell'Aquila[4], Juhani K. E. Airaksinen[3] and Debora Brascia[1]

Abstract

Background: Perioperative myocardial ischemia (PMI) in patients undergoing coronary artery bypass grafting (CABG) is associated with poor outcome. The aim of this study was to pool the available data on the outcome after control angiography and repeat revascularization in patients with perioperative myocardial ischemia (PMI) after coronary artery bypass grafting (CABG).

Methods: A literature review was performed through PubMed, Scopus, ScienceDirect and Google Scholar to identify studies published since 1990 evaluating the outcome of PMI after CABG.

Results: Nine studies included 1104 patients with PMI after CABG and 1056 of them underwent control angiography early after CABG. Pooled early mortality after reoperation for PMI without control angiography was 43.6% (95%CI 29.7-57.6%) and 79.8% of them (95%CI 64.4-95.2%) had an acute graft failure detected at reoperation. Among patients who underwent control angiography for PMI, 31.7% had a negative finding at angiography (95%CI 25.6-37.8%) and 62.1% had an acute graft failure (95%CI 56.6-67.6%). Repeat revascularization was performed after early control angiography in 46.3% of patients (95%CI 39.9-52.6%; 54.2% underwent repeat surgical revascularization; 45.8% underwent percutaneous coronary intervention). Pooled early mortality after control angiography with or without repeat revascularization was 8.9% (95%CI 6.7-11.1%). Three studies reported on early mortality rates which did not differ between repeat surgical revascularization and PCI (11.7% vs. 9.2%, respectively; risk ratio 1.45, 95%CI 0.67-3.11). In these three series, early mortality after conservative treatment was 5.9% (95%CI 3.6-8.2%).

Conclusions: Control angiography seems to be a valid life-saving strategy to guide repeat revascularization in hemodynamically stable patients suffering PMI after CABG.

Keywords: Coronary artery bypass, Perioperative myocardial infarction, Angiography, Percutaneous coronary intervention

Background

Perioperative myocardial ischemia (PMI) in patients undergoing coronary artery bypass grafting (CABG) is associated with poor outcome [1–3]. Still, a reliable and clinically useful definition of this condition remains elusive and with it also the optimal treatment of patients suffering PMI [1]. Recently, the European Society of Cardiology endorsed a document suggesting new cutoff values for cardiac troponin levels for the diagnosis of PMI after CABG and proposed a treatment strategy for its treatment [1]. This document recognized the clinical importance of PMI in these patients, however it unclear whether postoperative control angiography and, when needed, prompt repeat revascularization is beneficial in these patients. We sought to investigate this issues by pooling the available data from the literature on the outcome of patients with PMI after CABG.

Methods

The present systematic review and meta-analysis is registered in the International prospective register of systematic reviews PROSPERO with the reference code CRD (ID=CRD42017076614).

---
* Correspondence: faustobiancari@yahoo.it
[1]Department of Surgery, University of Turku, Turku, Finland
[2]Department of Surgery, University of Oulu, Oulu, Finland
Full list of author information is available at the end of the article

Search Strategy

The guidelines for Preferred Reporting Items for Systematic reviews and Meta-Analyses (PRISMA) were applied [4]. A literature review was performed through PubMed, Scopus, ScienceDirect and Google Scholar on September 2017, to identify any study being published since 1990 evaluating the outcome of patients who underwent angiography and any treatment for PMI immediately after CABG. The retrieval terms were "perioperative myocardial ischemia", "perioperative myocardial infarction", "angiography" combined with "cardiac surgery" or "coronary artery bypass". The abstracts of retrieved studies were scrutinized and each study was independently evaluated by two investigators (D.B, F.B.) for inclusion or exclusion from this analysis. Reference lists of retrieved articles were examined as well to identify any article of fulfilling the pre-specified inclusion criteria.

Treatment Definition and Inclusion/Exclusion Criteria

Studies eligible for the present studies were those reporting on perioperative myocardial ischemia after CABG. Studies that met the Population, Interventions, Comparison and Outcomes (PICO) criteria (Tab. 1) were included in the present meta-analysis.

To enter this analysis, studies had to fulfil all these inclusion criteria: (1) provide data on patients who suffered PMI immediately after CABG according to the investigators' definition criteria; (2) include patients undergoing CABG as isolated procedure or associated with any other major cardiac procedure; (3) include patients aged 18 years or older; (4) be a prospective or retrospective observational study; (5) be published in English language as a full article; (6) include at least 10 patients with postoperative PMI; and (7) be published since 1990.

Articles were not eligible for study inclusion in case of (1) angiography and/or repeat revascularization performed after discharge from the hospital associated with the index procedure; (2) ambiguous or inaccurate data; (3) lack on information on in-hospital/30-day mortality; (4) data reported only in abstracts; (5) article published in non-English language.

Table 1 Participants, intervention, comparison and outcomes (PICO) of the present meta-analysis

PICO	Description
Population	Patients who developed perioperative myocardial ischemia immediately after coronary artery bypass grafting
Intervention	Coronary angiography and repeat myocardial revascularization
Comparison	None
Outcomes	In-hospital/30-day mortality

Data Extraction

Data was independently collected by two investigators (D.B, F.B.) and any disagreement on retrieved data was settled by consensus between these investigators. Specific or missing data were not asked to the authors of the original studies. The following data was collected in to a dedicated datasheet: first author, year of publication, study period, overall number of CABG procedures performed during the study period, type of primary procedure, number of patients with PMI, number of patients who underwent immediate control angiography, findings at angiography, type of repeat revascularization and in-hospital/30-day mortality. The quality of the included studies was assessed by two investigators (F.B., D.B.) using the National Heart, Lung, and Blood Institute (NHLBI) criteria for study quality assessment of case series (https://www.nhlbi.nih.gov/health-pro/guidelines/in-develop/cardiovascular-risk-reduction/tools/case_series; accessed on September 17, 2017).

Outcomes

The primary outcome of this study was in-hospital/30-day postoperative mortality. Acute graft failure (defined as stenotic or occluded grafts, or faulty site of anastomosis), incomplete revascularization and new lesions of the native coronary arteries were the secondary endpoints of this analysis.

Statistical Analysis

Statistical analysis was performed using the Open Meta-Analyst software (Brown University, Providence, RI, USA; *http://www.cebm.brown.edu/openmeta/*). Means and absolute values were pooled using random effects models because of anticipated heterogeneity of the retrieved studies. The results are expressed as untransformed proportions and means with their 95% confidence intervals (CI). Heterogeneity across studies was evaluated using the I^2 test. I^2 <40% was considered as acceptable heterogeneity. Leave-one-out sensitivity analysis was performed to confirm consistency of the overall analysis. The impact of risk factors on in-hospital/30-day mortality was evaluated by meta-regression analysis. A $p < 0.05$ was considered statistically significant.

Results

Overall data

Nine studies including 39 266 patients who underwent CABG (98.2% underwent isolated procedure) fulfilled the pre-specified selection criteria and were included in this analysis (Fig. 1). [2, 3, 5–11] Among these patients, a diagnosis of PMI was made in 1104 patients and 1056 underwent control angiography early after CABG. Angiography was performed within the same hospital stay in seven studies, within 48 hours from surgery in one study and

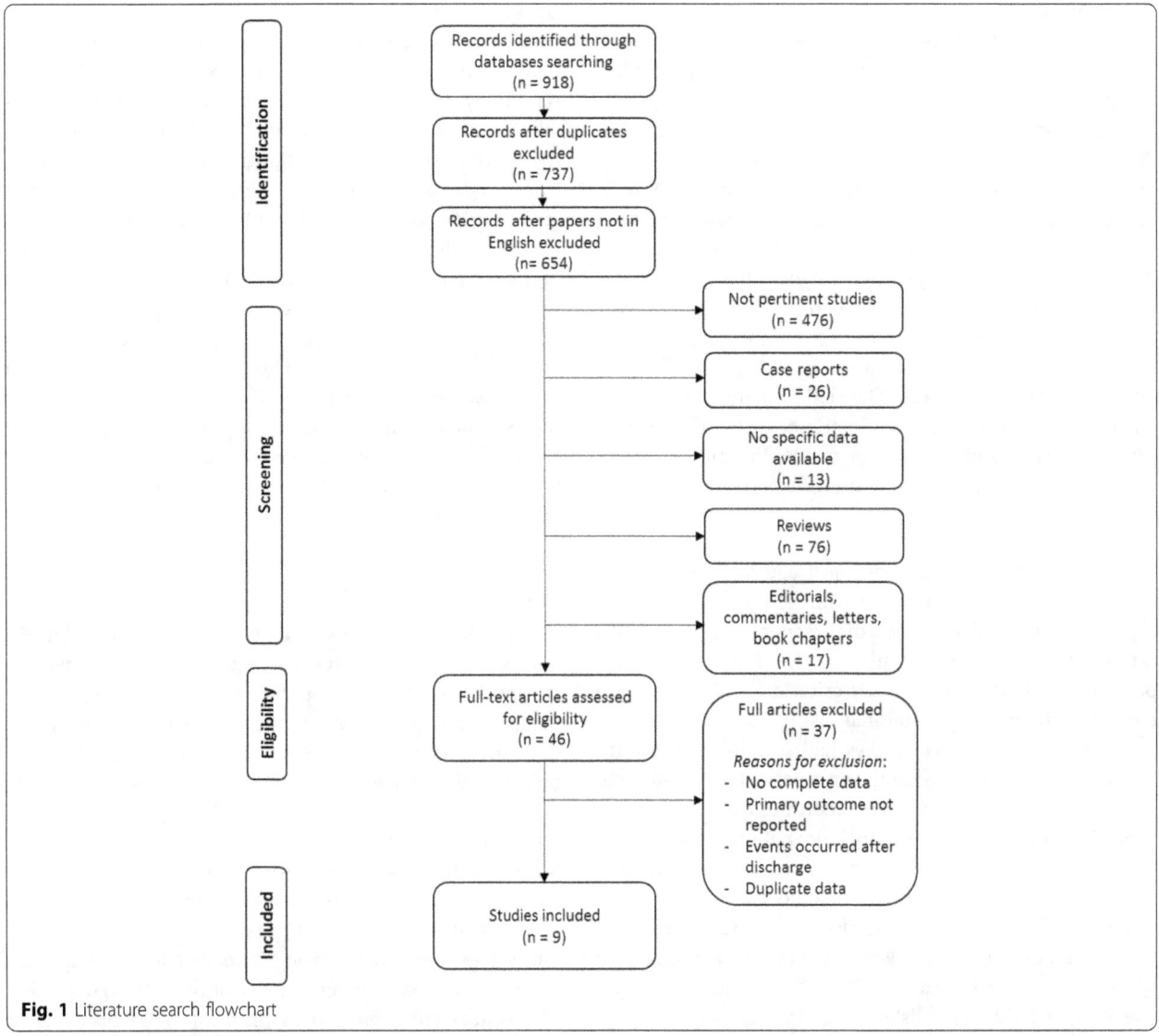

Fig. 1 Literature search flowchart

within 24 hours from surgery in another study (Tab. 2). Definition criteria for PMI used in these studies are summarized in Table 3. All these studies reported on in-hospital or 30-day mortality after angiography followed or not by repeat revascularization. Three studies [7, 9, 11] reported on 48 patients who underwent repeat CABG without early angiography because of unstable hemodynamic conditions. Characteristics and main data of these studies are summarized in Table 1. All studies were considered of fair quality according to the NHBLI criteria.

The pooled incidence of PMI requiring angiography or immediate reintervention without control angiography was 3.5% (95%CI 0.2-6.8%, I^2 91%, 3 studies, 9306 patients) and the related pooled in-hospital/30-day mortality of these patients was 12.6% (95%CI 8.8-16.4%, 3 studies, 286 patients).

Outcome of reoperation for PMI without control angiography

Pooled in-hospital/30-day mortality in patients who suffered perioperative myocardial ischemia and underwent reoperation without control angiography was 43.6% (95%CI 29.7-57.6%, I^2 81%, three studies, 48 patients). Among patients who underwent reoperation without control angiography, acute graft failure was detected in 79.8% of cases (95%CI 64.4-95.2%, I^2 49%, three studies, 48 patients).

Outcome of PMI with control angiography

Among patients who underwent control angiography for PMI after CABG, 31.7% of them had negative finding at angiography (95%CI 25.6-37.8%, I^2 75%, 9 studies, 1056 patients), 62.1% of patients had an acute graft failure (95%CI 56.6-67.6%, I^2 66%, 9 studies, 1056 patients), 6.1% had incomplete revascularization (95%CI 0.4-

Table 2 Characteristics and data of the included studies

Author	Year	Country	Type of study	Study period	NHLBI quality rating	No. of control angiography	Negative findings at angiography (%)	Graft failure at angiography (%)	Repeat revascularization (%)	Repeat CABG (%)	PCI (%)	Early mortality (%)
Rasmussen	1997	Denmark	P	1990-1995	Fair	59	27.1	72.9	45.8	45.8	0.0	5.1
Fabricius	2001	Germany	R	1999	Fair	108	41.7	58.3	39.8	31.5	8.3	9.3
Thielmann	2006	Germany	P	1999-2006	Fair	118	43.2	56.8	33.9	12.7	21.2	8.5
Karhunen	2010	Finland	R	2000-2007	Fair	23	47.8	52.2	43.5	21.7	21.7	8.7
Laflamme	2012	Canada	R	2003-2009	Fair	39	17.9	82.1	48.7	10.3	38.5	7.7
Szavits-Nossan	2012	Croatia	R	1999-2009	Fair	55	21.8	65.5	69.1	14.5	54.5	23.6
Davierwala	2013	Germany	P	2004-2010	Fair	399	36.1	61.2	41.1	32.6	8.5	7.3
Hultgren	2016	Sweden	R	2007-2012	Fair	87	31.0	59.8	44.8	28.7	16.1	11.5
Preußer	2017	Germany	R	2006-2013	Fair	168	23.2	52.4	53.6	17.9	35.7	10.7

R retrospective study, *P* prospective study, *NHLBI* National Heart, Lung, and Blood Institute, *CABG* coronary artery bypass grafting, *PCI* percutaneous coronary intervention

12.5%, I^2 91%, 5 studies, 624 patients) and 3.5% has a new lesion of the native coronary arteries (95%CI 1.4-5.7%, I^2 91%, 9 studies, 1056 patients).

Repeat revascularization was performed after control angiography in 46.3% of patients (95%CI 39.9-52.6%, I^2 74%, 9 studies, 1056 patients). Among these patients, 54.2% underwent repeat surgical revascularization (95%CI 33.7-74.8%, I^2 97%, 9 studies, 470 patients) and 45.8% underwent any percutaneous coronary intervention (PCI) (95%CI 25.2-66.3%, I^2 97%, 9 studies, 470 patients). Three studies (2,3,5) reported on the graft/native artery of repeat revacularization in 294 patients, which was on the left anterior descending artery territory in 56.0% of cases (95%CI 43.2-68.8%, I^2 78%), on the circumflex artery territory in 21.3% of cases (95%CI 9.3-33.3%, I^2 84), on the right coronary artery territory in 23.3% of cases (95%CI 16.6-30.0%, I^2 40%) and on the diagonal arteries territory in 4.8% of cases (95%CI 0.9-8.8%, I^2 58%).

Pooled in-hospital/30-day mortality in patients who underwent control angiography was 8.9% (95%CI 6.7-11.1%, I^2 28%, 9 studies, 1056 patients) (Fig. 2). Three studies reported on specific early mortality after repeat surgical revascularization and PCI after control angiography without any difference between the treatment methods (CABG 11.7% vs. PCI 9.2%; risk ratio 1.45, 95%CI 0.67-3.11, I^2 0%, 3 studies, 175 CABG patients vs. 119 PCI patients, respectively). These three series reported on early mortality after conservative treatment as well which was 5.9% (95%CI 3.6-8.2%, I^2 0%, 3 studies, 391 patients), without reporting separate rates of early mortality in patients with graft failure and in those with negative angiographic findings.

Discussion

The present pooled results suggest that severe PMI is rather uncommon, but its incidence may significantly vary between series (3.5%, 95%CI 0.2-6.8%). This estimate is also biased by the fact that most of series did not report on emergency reoperation performed without control angiography. Furthermore, the definition criteria of PMI as well as the policy of performing control angiography might vary between these series. Control angiography revealed problems of the graft or native vessels in two third of patients and it was valuable to guide a repeat revascularization in half of patients with PMI. This strategy of control angiography and, when indicated, repeat revascularization contributed to an early mortality rate of 8.9%. The lack of a control cohort with similar graft/native vessels problems treated conservatively prevents any estimation of the real benefits and possible harms of an active revascularization policy in patients with ongoing ischemia after CABG. The paucity of data on angiographic findings and on the outcome of patients treated conservatively because of negative angiographic findings or lack of suitable target vessels/grafts for repeat revascularization render the interpretation of these pooled results even more difficult. However, Karhunen et al. [9] showed that a policy of control angiography in PMI patients was associated with a dramatic decrease of postoperative mortality when compared with an historical control group who did not undergo any control

Table 3 Definition criteria for perioperative myocardial ischemia after coronary artery bypass grafting

Authors	Year of publication	Definition criteria
Rasmussen	1997	One or more of the following criteria:
		- new changes in the ST-segment in the ECG;
		- new Q-waves in the ECG;
		- CK-MB >80 U/L;
		- recurrent episodes of, or sustained ventricular tachyarrhythmia;
		- ventricular fibrillation;
		- hemodynamic deterioration and left ventricular failure.
Fabricius	2001	One or more of the following criteria:
		- increase in CK/CK-MB above 10%;
		- ischemic electrocardiographic episodes (new changes in ST-segment lasting at least 1 min and involving a shift from baseline of greater than or equal to 0.1 mV of ST-depression and a new postoperative Q;
		- recurrent episodes of, or sustained ventricular tachyarrhythmia or ventricular fibrillation;
		- hemodynamic deterioration despite adequate inotropic support.
Thielmann	2006	One or more of the following criteria:
		- cTnI serum level >20 ng/ml within 24 h after surgery;
		- ST-segment deviations at the J point in two or more contiguous leads with cut-off points ≥0.2 mV in leads V1, V2, or V3 and 0.1 mV in other leads or T-wave abnormalities in two or more contiguous leads as previously described;
		- hemodynamic instability despite intravenous inotropic support (>0.3 mg/kg/min).
Karhunen	2010	One or more of the following criteria:
		- ST-level changes in ECG and increased levels of cardiac biomarkers, creatine phosphokinase isoenzyme CK-MB or Tn;
		- ECG changes or findings of poor myocardial function or a new wall motion abnormality in echocardiography.
Laflamme	2012	One or more of the following criteria:
		- ECG modifications (new ST segment alterations or new Q wave);
		- refractory malignant arrhythmias;
		- elevation of cardiac biomarkers;
		- persistent low cardiac output syndrome;
		- new echocardiography wall motion abnormalities.
Szavits-Nossan	2012	One or more of the following criteria:
		- hemodynamical deterioration;
		- new ST segment depression or elevation greater than 1 mm;

Table 3 Definition criteria for perioperative myocardial ischemia after coronary artery bypass grafting (Continued)

Authors	Year of publication	Definition criteria
		- isoenzyme ratio of creatinine phosphokinase > 0.1;
		- cardiac troponin >0.1 mmol/L;
		- sustained ventricular tachycardia;
		- repeated nonsustained ventricular tachycardia and ventricular fibrillation.
Davierwala	2013	One or more of the following criteria:
		- electrocardiographic alterations;
		- CK-MB >2x normal;
		- new regional wall motion abnormalities on echocardiography;
		- repetitive ventricular arrhythmias;
		- hemodynamic instability.
Hultgren	2016	One or more of the following criteria:
		- ECG changes;
		- chest pain;
		- Aspartate aminotransferase (ASAT) on postoperative day 1 >2.5 µkat/l;
		- Troponin T measured 3-4 days after surgery > 2000 ng/L.
Preußer	2017	One or more of the following criteria:
		- progressive postoperative elevation of cardiac enzymes;
		- ECG changes suggestive of myocardial ischemia (such as ST segment alteration);
		- major ventricular arrhythmia of unclear cause.

ECG electrocardiogram, *CK-MB* creatine kinase-MB, *Tn* troponin

angiography for PMI (22.2% vs. 46.1%, p=0.015). Therefore, we may assume that in most of cases on-going severe myocardial ischemia secondary to any graft or new native vessels problem cannot be relieved by a conservative approach [6] and is associated with poor early and mid-term outcome.

The present findings indicate that control angiography may enable optimization of a reintervention strategy by identification of acute graft failure and/or new native vessels stenosis/occlusion amenable to surgical or catheter-based revascularization. Control angiography may identify also non-structural defects such as graft spam which are relievable by systemic or local administration of nitrates (9). Furthermore, angiographic findings may indicate PCI in conditions not amenable with repeat surgical revascularization. Finally, control angiography may guide toward prompt optimization of inotropic and mechanical circulatory support in patients with normal angiographic findings or poor run-off contraindicating any repeat revascularization.

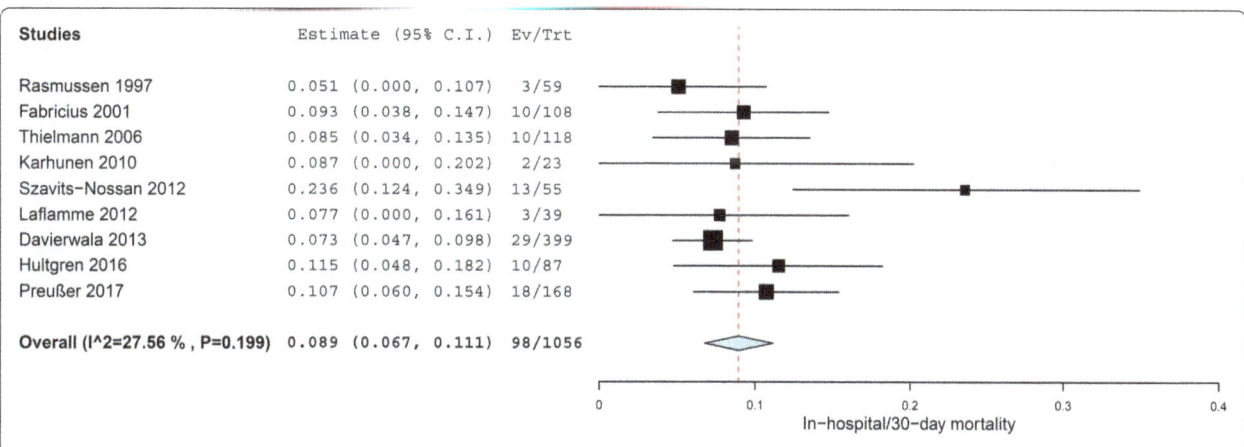

Fig. 2 Forest plot of pooled in-hospital/30-day mortality in patients with or without perioperative myocardial ischemia after coronary artery bypass grafting

This study showed that a valid and easy-to-use definition of type V myocardial infarction is needed for a prompt identification and treatment of patients with severe PMI. The present results showed that one third of patients do not have structural defects of the grafts or new stenosis/occlusions of native vessels at angiography. These patients most likely suffered of PMI because of suboptimal myocardial protection, distal coronary embolization, or subclinical myocardial injury secondary to intraoperative manipulation of the heart. The angiographic evaluation of the patients represents a unique opportunity for a practical definition of type V myocardial infarction because it may identify clinical, biochemical, electrocardiographic and echocardiographic parameters underlying PMI secondary to structural defects of the grafts and native vessels.

Control angiography for PMI has some drawbacks, which may induce clinicians to avoid prompt invasive imaging of the coronary arteries and grafts. Although coronary angiography in a patient with recent CABG may not be technically difficult, moving a patients in hemodynamically unstable conditions from the intensive care unit to the catheterization angiography laboratory can be difficult and requires major efforts from personnel. Furthermore, the use of contrast agent during control angiography may expose the patents to a significant risk of severe acute kidney injury. These important drawbacks should be weighed against the possible benefits of prompt treatment of ongoing PMI.

This meta-analysis has a number of limitations. First, the included studies are of fair quality, but do not provide all details on the characteristics and outcome of patients with PMI with negative angiographic findings and of those with graft or native vessels problems who did not undergo any repeat revascularization. Second, only three studies reported on the outcome of patients who underwent straightly a reoperation, whilst this

information was not provide in the other studies. Third, we may expect that prompt recognition and treatment of PMI has a prognostic impact on the outcome of these patients, but only two study assessed the timing of angiography in this setting [2, 3]. Fourth, the included studies failed to report data on any method employed to verify intraoperatively the patency of vascular grafts [12] and whether these findings might correlate with the development of PMI. Finally, there is paucity of data comparing the impact of PCI and surgical revascularization in patients with PMI after CABG.

Conclusions

In conclusion, control angiography seems to be a valid life-saving strategy to guide repeat revascularization in hemodynamically stable patients suffering PMI after CABG. However, a throughout assessment of the harms and benefits associated with this strategy is prevented by the lack of any possible control cohort. Further studies are needed to assess the prognostic impact of the timing of control angiography and repeat revascularization as well as to identify clinical, biochemical, electrocardiographic and echocardiographic parameters associated with PMI secondary to acute graft failure or new native vessels lesions after CABG.

Abbreviations
PMI: perioperative myocardial infarction; CABG: coronary artery bypass grafting; PRISMA: Preferred Reporting Items for Systematic reviews and Meta-Analyses; PICO: Population, Interventions, Comparison and Outcomes; NHLBI: National Heart, Lung, and Blood Institute; CI: confidence interval; PCI: percutaneous coronary intervention

Acknowledgements
Not applicable.

Funding
This study was not financially supported.

Authors' contributions

FB participated in the design of the study, data collection, statistical analysis, writing and revision of the manuscript. VA participated in the design of the study, writing and revision of the manuscript. AMD participated in the design of the study, writing and revision of the manuscript. JKEA participated in the design of the study, writing and revision of the manuscript. DB participated in the design of the study, data collection, writing and revision of the manuscript. All authors read and approved the final manuscript.

Competing interests

The authors declare that they have no competing interests.

Author details

[1]Department of Surgery, University of Turku, Turku, Finland. [2]Department of Surgery, University of Oulu, Oulu, Finland. [3]Heart Center, Turku University Hospital and University of Turku, Hämeentie 11, 20521 Turku, PL 52, Finland. [4]Department of Cardiac Surgery, University Hospital, Münster, Germany.

References

1. Thielmann M, Sharma V, Al-Attar N, Bulluck H, Bisleri G, Bunge J, et al. Perioperative myocardial injury and infarction in patients undergoing coronary artery bypass graft surgery. Eur Heart J. 2017;38:2392–407.
2. Davierwala PM, Verevkin A, Leontyev S, Misfeld M, Borger MA, Mohr FW. Impact of expeditious management of perioperative myocardial ischemia in patients undergoing isolated coronary artery bypass surgery. Circulation. 2013;128(11 Suppl 1):S226–34.
3. Preußer MJ, Landwehrt J, Mastrobuoni S, Biancari F, Dakkak AR, Alshakaki M, et al. Survival results of postoperative coronary angiogram for treatment of perioperative myocardial ischemia following coronary artery bypass grafting: a single centre experience. Interact Cardiovasc Thorac Surg. 2018;26:237–42.
4. Moher D, Liberati A, Tetzlaff J, Altman DG. PRISMA group. Preferred reporting items for systematic reviews and meta-analyses: the PRISMA statement. Ann Intern Med. 2009;151:264–9.
5. Thielmann M, Massoudy P, Jaeger BR, Neuhauser M, Marggraf G, Sack S, et al. Emergency re-revascularization with percutaneous coronary intervention, reoperation, or conservative treatment in patients with acute perioperative graft failure following coronary artery bypass surgery. Eur J Cardiothorac Surg. 2006;30:117–25.
6. Szavits-Nossan J, Stipić H, Sesto I, Kapov-Svilicić K, Sipić T, Bernat R. Angiographic control and percutaneous treatment of myocardial ischemia immediately after CABG. Coll Antropol. 2012;36:1391–4.
7. Rasmussen C, Thiis JJ, Clemmensen P, Efsen F, Arendrup HC, Saunamaki K, et al. Significance and management or early graft failure after coronary artery bypass grafting. Feasibility and results of acute angiography and re-revascularization. Eur J Cardiothorac Surg. 1997;12:847–52.
8. Laflamme M, DeMey N, Bouchard D, Carrier M, Demers P, Pellerin M, et al. Management of early postoperative coronary artery bypass graft failure. Interact Cardiovasc Thorac Surg. 2012;14:452–6.
9. Karhunen J, Raivio P, Maasilta P, Sihvo E, Suojaranta-Ylinen R, Vento A, et al. Impact of early angiographic evaluation on the frequency of emergency reoperations after coronary bypass surgery. Scand J Surg. 2010;99:173–9.
10. Hultgren K, Andreasson A, Axelsson TA, Albertsson P, Lepore V, Jeppsson A. Acute coronary angiography after coronary artery bypass grafting. Scand Cardiovasc J. 2016;50:123–7.
11. Fabricius AM, Gerber W, Hanke M, Garbade J, Autschbach R, Mohr FW. Early angiographic control of perioperative ischemia after coronary artery bypass grafting. Eur J Cardiothorac Surg. 2001;19:853–8.
12. Leacché M, Balaguer JM, Byrne JG. Intraoperative grafts assessment. Semin Thorac Cardiovasc Surg. 2009;21:207–12.

10

Correlation of structural defects in the ascending aortic wall to ultrasound parameters: benefits for decision-making process in aortic valve surgery

Saša D. Borović[1*], Milica M. Labudović Borović[2], Ivan V. Zaletel[2], Vera N. Todorović[3], Petar A. Dabić[1], Jelena T. Rakočević[2], Jelena M. Marinković-Erić[4] and Predrag S. Milojević[1]

Abstract

Background: Histopathological changes in the ascending aorta wall in patients with severe tricuspid aortic valve (TAV) stenosis were graded and correlated to echocardiographic parameters. Objective was to associate threshold echocardiographic values with structural defects in the ascending aorta providing a tool to improve decision-making process in cases when simultaneous aortic valve replacement (AVR) and ascending aorta replacement is considered.

Methods: Biopsies from 108 TAV stenosis patients subjected to AVR were graded into three grades according to severity of aortic wall changes. Echocardiographic parameters obtained preoperatively and correlated to grade, age, gender and risk factors, were diameters of ventriculo-aortic junction (AA), sinus Valsalva (SV), sinotubular junction (STJ), the largest diameter of the visualized ascending aorta (AscA) as well as indexes: sinus Valsalva (SVI), sinotubular junction (STJI), AscA/AA and STJ/AA.

Results: Two echocardiographic parameters portrayed grades with statistical significance: STJ ($F = 5.417$; $p = 0.006$ ($p < 0.05$)) and AscA ($F = 3.924$; $p = 0.023$ ($p < 0.05$)). By using multiple predictors in the setting of Regression analysis, statistically significant differences among grades were reached for AA, SV, STJ, AscA and SVI. With further ROC curves analysis, threshold values for different grades were recognized. Grade 2 is identified in patients with AscA > 3.3 cm, while Grade 3 is identified in patients with values of AscA > 3.5 cm, STJ > 2.9 cm and STJI > 1.

Conclusions: Hemodynamic stress induced by TAV stenosis leads to elastic lamellae disruption in the aortic wall. Those changes could be graded and correlated with echocardiographic parameters of the aortic root and ascending aorta, providing a tool for decision to replace ascending aorta concomitantly with AVR.

Keywords: Aortic stenosis, Ascending aorta replacement, Aortic valve replacement, Aging, Remodeling

Background

In the present study, we investigated the spectrum of structural changes in the ascending aortic wall in patients with severe degenerative, calcific aortic stenosis of the tricuspid aortic valve (TAV), and correlated them to echocardiographic parameters. It is important to understand the evolution of aortic wall changes due to aortic stenosis, for tailoring guidelines for surgical treatment of aortic stenosis. Current guidelines recommend that simultaneous surgery of the aortic root and ascending aorta should be considered in patients with degenerative TAV stenosis, when maximal ascending aortic diameter is ≥55 mm. The main goal of our study is to determine when is the replacement of the ascending aorta warranted simultaneously with the aortic valve replacement (AVR), from the histological perspective.

We addressed several issues in this paper. The influence of severe TAV stenosis on structural changes in the wall of ascending thoracic aorta. Design and application of the grading system that identifies gradual progression

* Correspondence: sborovic@lecenjerana.com
[1]Dedinje Cardiovascular Institute, Belgrade, Serbia, 1 Heroja Milana Tepića Street, Belgrade 11000, Serbia
Full list of author information is available at the end of the article

of aortic wall changes caused by hemodynamic disturbances in the setting of the aortic stenosis. Definition of irreversible changes in the ascending aorta wall in patients with severe aortic stenosis, Correlation of histological grades with echocardiographic parameters in order to obtain reliable insight into the aortic wall structure by means of non-invasive diagnostics.

The answers to issues are particularly complex because aortic stenosis and hemodynamic derangement that it causes, is not the only factor influencing the structure of the ascending aorta. Other factors including aging, arterial hypertension, atherosclerosis and diabetes mellitus may act synergistically resulting in definitive changes [1–3]. Finally, we analyzed are there any gender-related differences in the remodeling process.

We focused exclusively on the severe TAV stenosis and its influence on the ascending aorta wall. The chosen method was to compare grades of elastic skeleton defects, assessed by light microscopy, with the echocardiographic parameters. Grading of the structural changes was done according to accepted grading systems.

Methods
Overall patients data
We performed analysis of wall segments of the ascending aorta of 108 patients who were undergoing AVR because of severe, symptomatic TAV stenosis. All patients were operated at Dedinje Cardiovascular Institute. There were 56 (51.9%) males and 52 (48.1%) female patients. The mean age of patients was 67.56 ± 8.23 years. The mean age of male patients was 67.23 ± 8.49 years (median 68.5 (60–74)), while for the female patients it was 67.92 ± 8.01 years (median 70 (59.75–74)). There was no statistical significance in the mean age of male and female patients in the aortic stenosis group (Mann-Whitney U test: 1403.500; $p = 0.747$ (> 0.05)).

Diameter of the ascending aorta was <5 cm in all patients, with the mean value of 3.33 ± 0.54 cm. The minimal diameter was 2.2 cm and the maximal diameter 4.7 cm.

Excluded from this study group were (1) patients with moderate or severe aortic regurgitation, (2) patients with aortic stenosis and acute or chronic aortic dissection, (3) patients who had had a previous cardiac operation and (4) patients who had had aortic stenosis combined with a connective tissue disorder, bicuspid or congenitally malformed aortic valve.

Intraoperative Aortic Wall sampling
The diagnosis of a severe TAV stenosis was established by preoperative echocardiography. Transverse aortotomy was made approximately 1 cm above the take-off of the right coronary artery, slightly above the level of the sinotubular junction. The aortic wall specimens were taken from the distal lip of the incision at the convexity of the

ascending aorta, 2 to 4 cm above the level of the aortic valve annulus [4]. Samples of the aortic wall with the minimal dimensions 1 mm × 9 mm and maximal dimensions 5 mm × 20 mm were excised, immediately fixed in 4% neutral buffered formaldehyde by the immersion procedure, and subsequently processed for the morphological and morphometric analysis.

Echocardiographic parameters
Echocardiographic parameters of the aortic root and the ascending aorta were determined preoperatively from parasternal longitudinal section with standard 2D procedure. Diameters at the level of ventriculo-aortic junction (AA), sinus Valsalva (SV), sinotubular junction (STJ) and the largest diameter of visualized ascending aorta (AscA) were measured.

Index of sinus Valsalva (SVI) was calculated as the ratio between measured and predicted diameter (pSV) at the level of the sinus of Valsalva. Predicted diameter at the level of the sinus Valsalva (pSV) was calculated according to regression formula $pSV(cm) = 1{,}92 + 0{,}74 \times BSA(m^2)$, where BSA stands for body surface area [5]. Sinotubular junction index (STJI) was calculated as the ratio between measured and predicted diameter at the level of sinotubular junction. Predicted diameter at the level of sinotubular junction was calculated according to regression formula $pSTJ(cm) = 1{,}69 + 0{,}62 \times BSA(m^2)$ [5].

Indexes AscA/AA and STJ/AA were calculated as the ratio between AscAA or STJ diameters and AA diameter, respectively.

Preparation of arterial samples for analysis
Preparation of tissue for light microscopy and Histomorphometry
The tissue was prepared for morphological and morphometric analysis according to the procedure described in the previously published studies of our group [6–8]. Out of 30 serial sections per patient, three sections were chosen for the analysis with respect to following rules: oblique sections were excluded from the analysis, as well as sections with major technical flaws. In addition, minimal distance between chosen sections must be at least 100 μm.

Sections were stained with the application of selective techniques for elastic fibers: Weigert van Gieson technique with resorcin fuchsine, Verhoeff van Gieson method or Pincus' staining with acid orcein.

Grading of morphological changes
Grading of morphological changes in the ascending aorta was established to test the hypothesis that aortic stenosis induces progressive histopathological changes and that subsequent grades follow the natural history of

these alterations. All sections were graded according to the principle described by Schlatmann and Becker [9] for gradation of aortic wall changes during aging and Niwa et al. [10] for the gradation of congenital aortic stenosis.

Using both methods for morphometric analyses of elastic skeleton parameters, we found statistically significant differences among the grades (data not shown). However, we decided to proceed with Schlatmann and Becker gradation system since criteria for grading were more precise, hence, the reproducibility of the results was also higher with this system.

The grades were established according to the most severe changes at the magnification ×200 of the Olympus BX41 microscope.

Grade 1 slides had fewer than five foci of elastic lamellae fragmentation in one microscopic field. Focus

of elastic lamellae fragmentation comprises 2 to 4 neighboring elastic lamellae (Fig. 1a-b).

Grade 2 sections had 5 to 10 foci of elastic lamellae fragmentation in one microscopic field and foci were confluent or scattered throughout the media of the aorta (Fig. 1c-d).

Grade 3 sections were distinguished by the presence of foci with elastic fragmentation in 10 or more neighboring elastic lamellae, irrespective of the number of foci per microscopic field, with disorganization of smooth muscle cells layers (Fig. 1e-f).

Pathologist, who performed the analysis, was blinded for patients' data. The slides were reexamined twice to obtain the final data as advised in previous similar studies [11].

Atherosclerosis was graded according to established classification systems [12].

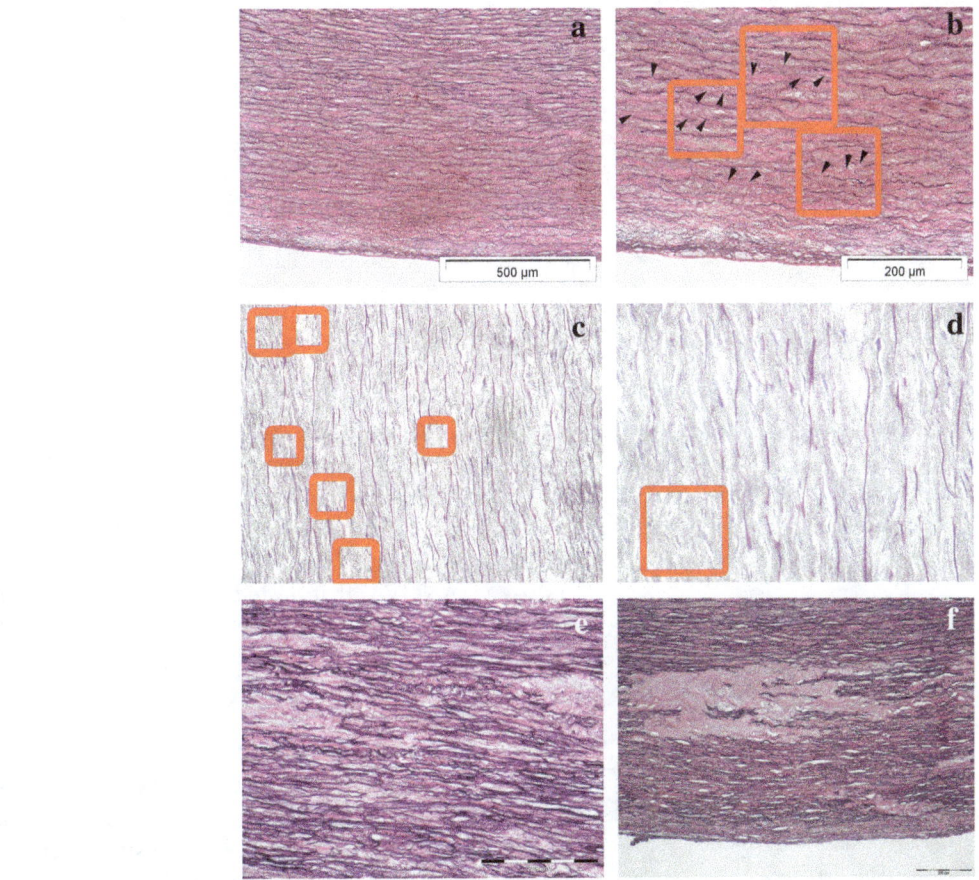

Fig. 1 The ascending aorta in patients with severe aortic stenosis – **a)** and **e)** (Weigert van Gieson staining, original magnification ×100, bar = 500 µm); **b)** and **f)** (Weigert van Gieson staining, original magnification ×200, bar = 200 µm); **c)** (PTAH staining, original magnification ×200, bar = 200 µm); **d)** (PTAH staining, original magnification, ×400): **a) – b)** grade 1; three foci of elastic lamellae fragmentation in 1 microscopic field of the Olympus BX41 microscope, magnification ×200; focus of elastic lamellae fragmentation comprises 2 to 4 neighboring elastic lamellae; **c)** grade 2; eight foci of elastic lamellae fragmentation in 1 microscopic field of the Olympus BX41 microscope, magnification ×200; confluent or scattered foci throughout the media of the aorta; **d) - f)** the presence of foci with elastic fragmentation in 10 or more neighboring elastic lamellae. As opposite to control aortas, aortas of aortic stenosis patients have thin subendothelial connective tissue with numerous elastic fibers. These samples are atherosclerosis free or with low grade atherosclerosis (types I – III atherosclerotic lesions)

Statistical analysis

Descriptive statistics included the mean values or the median with 25th – 75th percentile values, the standard deviation (SD), the standard error (SE) and a 95% confidence interval (95% C.I.).

The tests were performed with the SPSS version 10.0 for Windows. Following tests were used where appropriate: One-Sample Kolmogorov-Smirnov Test, ANOVA, Mann-Whitney test, Bonferroni Post Hoc Multiple Comparison test, Tukey Post Hoc, Pearson Correlation and Spearman's Rho, ROC Curves and Regression Analysis. The value of $p < 0.05$ was considered statistically significant.

Data are presented as the means ± SD or the median with 25th – 75th percentile value.

Data distribution pattern – Echocardiographic parameters

Values of echocardiographic parameters conform normal distribution as confirmed with the One-Sample Kolmogorov-Smirnov Test, hence they were analyzed with parametric tests.

Results

Overall patients' data

Overall patients' data are systematized in Table 1.

The distribution of grades are presented in Table 2.

Echocardiographic parameters and grades

Values of echocardiographic parameters are given in Table 3. With the increase in grade and severity of histopathological defect, values of echocardiographic parameters increase (Fig. 2). Statistical significance was confirmed with ANOVA among echocardiographic parameters of different grades for STJ (F = 5.417; $p = 0.006$ ($p < 0.05$)) and AscA (F = 3.924; $p = 0.023$ ($p < 0.05$)) (Table 2 and Fig. 2). By using Bonferroni Post Hoc Analysis statistical significance among grades was confirmed

Table 1 Baseline clinical characteristics

Number of patients (n)	108	
Age (years) (mean ± SD)	67.56 ± 8.23	
Males (years) (median (25th – 75th percentile))	68.5 (60–74)	
Females (years) (median (25th – 75th percentile))	70 (59.75–74)	
Parameter	Number of patients (n)	Percentage (%)
Arterial hypertension (HTA)	80	74.1
Diabetes mellitus (DM)	26	24.1
Coronary artery disease (CAD)	35	32.4
Chronic renal disease (ChRD)	18	16.7
Chronic pulmonary disease (ChPD)	11	10.2
Peripheral vascular disease (PVD)	22	20.4

Table 2 Grades distribution

Grades	Number of patients (n)	Percentage (%)
Grade 1	63	58.3
Grade 2	27	25
Grade 3	18	16.7
Gender		
Males (total)	56	51.9
Grade 1	29	51.79
Grade 2	13	23.21
Grade 3	14	25
Females (total)	52	48.1
Grade 1	34	65.38
Grade 2	14	26.92
Grade 3	4	7.69
Number of patients (n)	108	

for STJ, but not for AscA (GR1 vs GR2 $p = 0.079$; GR 1vs GR3 $p = 0.093$; GR2vs GR3 $p = 1.000$).

Additional testing with Spearman Correlation Coefficient test confirmed the ANOVA results. Statistically significant and positive correlations were established between grades and parameters STJ and AscA. Testing also revealed significant positive association of echocardiographic parameter STJI and the defined grades (Table 4).

Influence of aging

Patients age did not differ significantly among different grades as confirmed with ANOVA and post hoc Tukey HSD analysis (F = 0.398; $p = 0.673$ ($p > 0.05$)). Also, when distribution of grades was counted in a group <65 years and ≥65 years, Pearson Chi-square test revealed no statistically significant difference (Pearson Chi-square = 0.405; $p = 0.817$ (p > 0.05)).

Two-way ANOVA that tested influence of age and grade to different echocardiographic parameters revealed no statistically significant difference (Fig. 3).

Influence of gender

Distribution of grades did not differ among genders as confirmed with Pearson Chi-Square test (5.849; $p = 0.054$ (p > 0.05)). All echocardiographic parameters except indexes STJ/AA and AscA/AA were statistically significantly higher in males than in females, but simultaneous effects of grade and gender to echocardiographic parameters was not statistically significant as confirmed with Two-Way ANOVA (Fig. 4).

Multifactorial analysis

Echocardiographic parameters had no differences when tested for the presence or absence of arterial

Table 3 Echocardiographic parameters of different morphological grades

Parameter	Grades	N	Mean	SD	SE	95% C.I.	Min.		Max.	p
AA	1.00	63	2.7122	0.35304	0.04448	2.6233	2.8011	2.00	3.50	0.062
	2.00	27	2.8344	0.42827	0.08242	2.6650	3.0039	2.20	4.20	
	3.00	18	2.9578	0.52635	0.12406	2.6960	3.2195	1.97	4.10	
	Total	108	2.7837	0.41178	0.03962	2.7052	2.8623	1.97	4.20	
SV	1.00	63	2.9519	0.42024	0.05294	2.8461	3.0577	2.00	3.90	0.190
	2.00	27	3.1219	0.49951	0.09613	2.9243	3.3195	2.10	4.40	
	3.00	18	3.1067	0.51923	0.12238	2.8485	3.3649	2.40	4.50	
	Total	108	3.0202	0.46087	0.04435	2.9323	3.1081	2.00	4.50	
STJ	1.00	63	2.6830	0.38806	0.04889	2.5853	2.7807	2.00	3.60	0.006*
	2.00	27	2.8570	0.53146	0.10228	2.6468	3.0673	2.00	3.80	
	3.00	18	3.0594	0.49402	0.11644	2.8138	3.3051	2.40	4.20	
	Total	108	2.7893	0.46341	0.04459	2.7009	2.8777	2.00	4.20	
AscA	1.00	63	3.2124	0.49394	0.06223	3.0880	3.3368	2.20	4.60	0.023*
	2.00	27	3.4767	0.56276	0.10830	3.2540	3.6993	2.60	4.70	
	3.00	18	3.5289	0.57376	0.13524	3.2436	3.8142	2.67	4.70	
	Total	108	3.3312	0.53931	0.05190	3.2283	3.4341	2.20	4.70	
SVI	1.00	63	0.8935	0.12078	0.01522	0.8631	0.9239	0.63	1.22	0.199
	2.00	27	0.9493	0.15402	0.02964	0.8883	1.0102	0.64	1.28	
	3.00	18	0.9194	0.15345	0.03617	0.8431	0.9958	0.71	1.34	
	Total	108	0.9118	0.13609	0.01309	0.8858	0.9377	0.63	1.34	
STJI	1.00	63	0.9489	0.14145	0.01782	0.9133	0.9845	0.68	1.44	0.073
	2.00	27	1.0100	0.19365	0.03727	0.9334	1.0866	0.71	1.37	
	3.00	18	1.0317	0.15143	0.03569	0.9564	1.1070	0.84	1.44	
	Total	108	0.9780	0.15997	0.01539	0.9474	1.0085	0.68	1.44	
STJ/AA	1.00	63	0.9954	0.11409	0.01437	0.9667	1.0241	0.79	1.40	0.585
	2.00	27	1.0096	0.14103	0.02714	0.9538	1.0654	0.75	1.32	
	3.00	18	1.0294	0.14210	0.03349	0.9588	1.1001	0.76	1.39	
	Total	108	1.0046	0.12547	0.01207	0.9807	1.0286	0.75	1.40	
AscA/AA	1.00	63	1.1933	0.17621	0.02220	1.1490	1.2377	0.79	1.65	0.486
	2.00	27	1.2448	0.24061	0.04631	1.1496	1.3400	0.87	2.00	
	3.00	18	1.2017	0.12045	0.02839	1.1418	1.2616	0.94	1.45	
	Total	108	1.2076	0.18665	0.01796	1.1720	1.2432	0.79	2.00	

AA ventriculo-aortic junction, *AscA* ascending aorta, *SV* sinus Valsalva, *SVI* sinus Valsalva index, *STJ* sinotubular junction, *STJI* sinotubular junction index

hypertension, diabetes mellitus and atherosclerosis (data not shown).

Application of Regression Analysis by using multiple predictors: age, gender, presence of arterial hypertension, diabetes mellitus, atherosclerosis with changes of grade identified statistically significant differences among echocardiographic parameters (Table 5).

Based on the regression analysis ROC Curves were constructed to test the sensitivity and specificity of different echocardiographic parameters for different grades (Fig. 5).

According to ROC Curves analysis following threshold values were detected to identified specific grades (Table 6).

Discussion

The debate about concomitant replacement of ascending aorta with aortic valve replacement spins around aortic diameter, etiology of valve disease, structural changes in the aortic wall and the influence of mechanical stress on the aortic wall. Our study focuses on TAV stenosis and structural derangements in the aortic wall that it causes.

According to the current guidelines, surgery should be considered in patients who have aortic root disease (whatever the severity of aortic regurgitation or stenosis) with maximal ascending aortic diameter ≥ 45 mm for patients with Marfan syndrome with risk factors, ≥50 mm

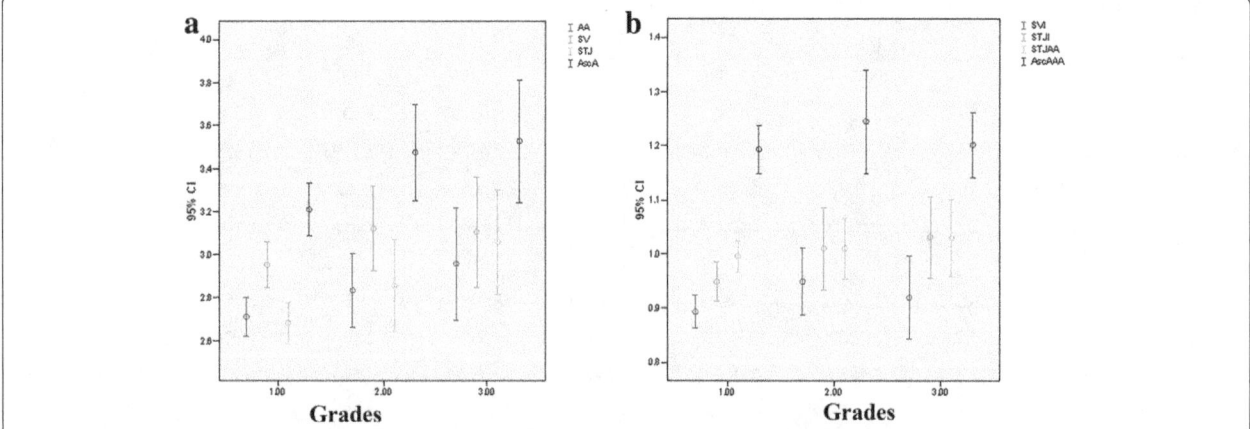

Fig. 2 Values of echocardiographic parameters in different grades: **a**) values of diameters at the level of ventriculo-aortic junction (AA), sinus Valsalva (SV), sinotubular junction (STJ) and the largest diameter of visualized ascending aorta (AscA); **b**) values of sinus Valsalva index (SVI), sinotubular junction index (STJI), STJ/AA and AscA/AA

for patients with bicuspid valve with risk factors, and ≥55 mm for other patients [13].

Aortic valve disease is associated with the ascending aortic dilatation because of the "hemodynamic burdens caused by forceful jets" [14, 15]. Due to mechanical stress, the size of the dilatation is related to the degree of turbulence induced by the stenotic valve and the severity of stenosis [16]. However, it seems that there is no independent association between the severity of aortic stenosis and the aortic diameter, indicating that factors other than the aortic stenosis itself (geometry of aortic orifice, flow distribution pattern and histopathological changes in the aortic wall) could affect the echocardiographic parameters of the aorta [17].

Gaudino et al. [16] published the results of follow-up study of patients submitted to AVR only and showed moderate dilatation of the ascending aorta with the expansion rate of 0.3 ± 0.2 mm/year after 10 years postoperatively [16]. Similarly, Yasuda et al. [18] reported a mean ascending aorta expansion rate of 0.08 mm/m^2/year in a series of 14 patients followed for 9.7 years after surgery [18]. They speculated that correction of the aortic stenosis in these patients stabilized the hemodynamics and prevented further development of the aortic wall changes. Andrus et al. [19] reported results of a vast study that comprised 107 patients with an aortic diameter ≥ 3.5 cm. He found no evidence of further dilation in the first 3 years after isolated AVR, and concluded that in patients with aortic valve stenosis and with

accompanying mild or moderate ascending aortic dilatation (3.5 cm to 4.9 cm) AVR alone may be reasonable [19].

Botzenhardt et al. [20] have even described a reduction of the aortic diameter in 10 patients with pre-operative aortic diameter ≥ 4 cm, 4.8 years after the isolated valve surgery [20].

As opposite to these studies, Matsuyama et al. [21] concluded that the clinical course of patients with a dilated ascending aorta is unpredictable and that aortic events may occur in patients with an aortic diameter of <5 cm. The author also found that patients with TAV stenosis and a slightly dilated aorta are at risk of late aortic events. Therefore, suggested preventive aortic surgery and AVR, even in patients with slightly dilated ascending aorta with a diameter of 4 cm to 5 cm, except in cases of high operative risk [21].

Ergin et al. [22] advocate more liberal ascending aorta replacement in conjunction with AVR since it significantly improves postoperative outcome in comparison to patients with AVR and already dilated aorta [22].

Only few studies investigated histopathological defects of aortic wall elastic skeleton in patients with the aortic valve dysfunction, utilizing limited number of elastic skeleton parameters. Roberts et al. [11] using a semi-quantitative method, found that there is no significant loss of elastic fibers in patients with stenosis of the TAV as compared to the control group [11]. Bauer et al. [4] showed that the thickness of elastic lamellae is decreased and the distance between elastic lamellae is increased significantly in patients with dilatation of the ascending aorta and with TAV stenosis [4]. Bechtel et al. [23] found that patients with TAV stenosis and the ascending aorta dilatation have more severe defects of the ascending aorta than patients with bicuspid valve and the same degree of dilatation [23].

Von Kodolitsch et al. [24] concluded that any patient at aortic valve replacement with an aortic diameter ≥ 43 mm and the presence of aortic wall fragility, aortic

Table 4 Spearman Correlation Coefficient for correlation of grades and echocardiographic parameters

	AA	SV	STJ	AscA	SVI	STJI	STJAA	AscAA
Grade	0.189	0.132	0.268**	0.250**	0.095	0.203*	0.085	0.076

*$p < 0.05$; **$p < 0.01$

AA ventriculo-aortic junction, *AscA* ascending aorta, *SV* sinus Valsalva, *SVI* sinus Valsalva index, *STJ* sinotubular junction, *STJI* sinotubular junction index

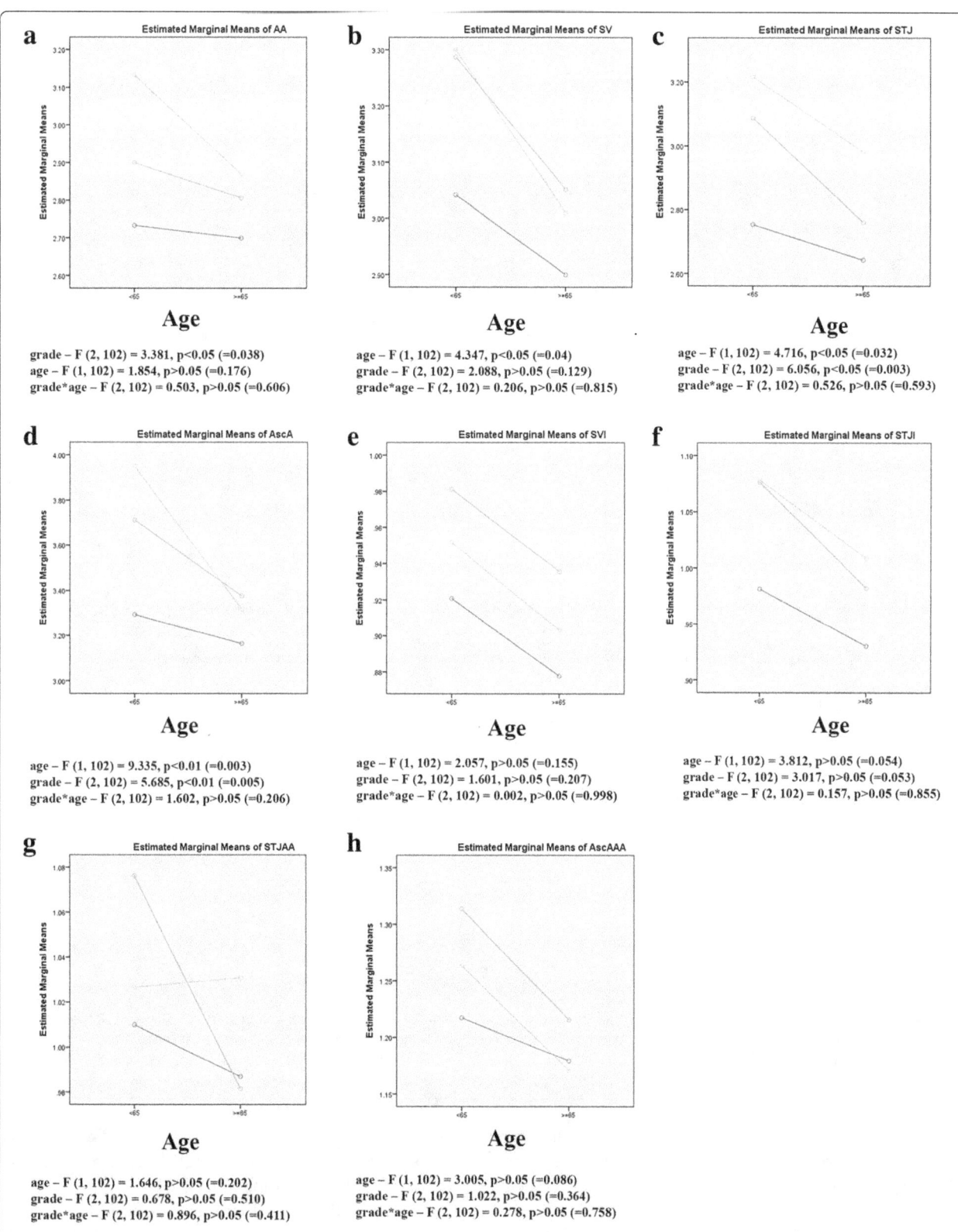

Fig. 3 Influence of age and grade to echocardiographic parameters – there is an increase in values of echocardiographic parameters with grade and a decrease with age. However differences are not statistically significant (blue - grade 1; green – grade 2; beige – grade 3): simultaneous effects of age and grade to **a)** diameters at the level of ventriculo-aortic junction (AA), **b)** diameters at the level of sinus Valsalva (SV), **c)** diameters at the level of sinotubular junction (STJ), **d)** the largest diameter of visualized ascending aorta (AscA), **e)** values of sinus Valsalva index (SVI), **f)** values of sinotubular junction index (STJI), **g)** STJ/AA and **h)** AscA/AA

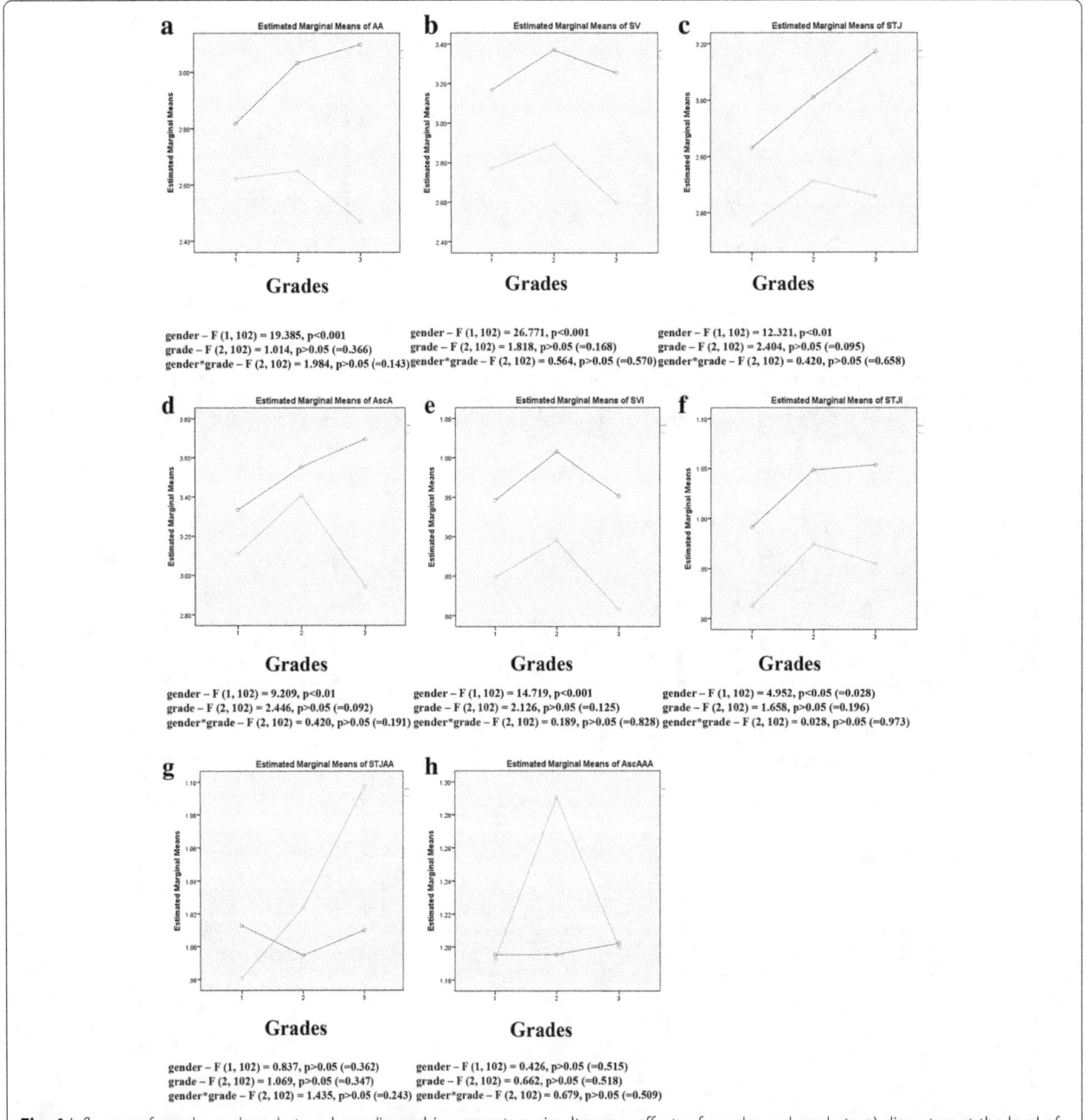

Fig. 4 Influence of gender and grade to echocardiographic parameters: simultaneous effects of gender and grade to **a**) diameters at the level of ventriculo-aortic junction (AA), **b**) diameters at the level of sinus Valsalva (SV), **c**) diameters at the level of sinotubular junction (STJ), **d**) the largest diameter of visualized ascending aorta (AscA), **e**) values of sinus Valsalva index (SVI), **f**) values of sinotubular junction index (STJI), **g**) STJ/AA and **h**) AscA/AA

thinning or aortic regurgitation, will likely benefit from prophylactic aortic surgery. The combined presence of these parameters identifies a disease process of the entire aortic root rather than isolated valve disease [24].

Tsutsumi et al. [25] portrayed clinical entity of the patients prone to postsurgical aortic complications. They suggested that patients with aortic regurgitation combined with systemic hypertension, male sex, and thinned or fragile aortic walls in patients with ascending aortic

dilatation (≥45 mm diameter) at the time of aortic valve replacement, should be considered for concomitant replacement of the ascending aorta [25].

Beller et al. [26] found that, in cases of aortic stenosis, restored aortic valve competence (by replacing the diseased valve) is associated with increased aortic root motion, theoretically heightening the threat of dissection posed to the aortic wall by mechanical stress. Mechanical principles command to include the higher magnitude of

Table 5 Regression Analysis predicting significance of multiple variables and grades to values of echocardiographic parameters

Predictors	Dependant variable										
	AA			SV			STJ			AscA		
	B	95% C.I.		B	95% C.I.		B	95% C.I.		B	95% C.I.	
HTA (arterial hypertension)	0.089	−0.078	0.256	0.030	−0.151	0.211	0.079	−0.105	0.263	0.162	−0.058	0.382
DM (diabetes mellitus)	−0.051	−0.226	0.124	−0.009	−0.198	0.181	0.017	−0.176	0.210	−0.186	−0.416	0.045
Atherosclerosis	0.092	−0.042	0.226	0.028	−0.117	0.173	0.030	−0.117	0.178	0.070	−0.106	0.246
Grade	0.080	−0.018	0.178	0.036	−0.070	0.142	0.148	0.039	0.256	0.134	0.005	0.263
Gender	−0.289	−0.440	−0.139	−0.428	−0.591	−0.265	−0.298	−0.464	−0.132	−0.265	−0.463	−0.067
Age	−0.003	−0.012	0.006	−0.006	−0.016	0.003	−0.009	−0.019	0.001	−0.013	−0.025	−0.002
F	4.249			5.705			5.107			3.995		
p	0.001			<0.001			<0.001			0.001		

Predictors	Dependant variable										
	SVI			STJI			STJ/AA			AscA/AA		
	B	95% C.I.		B	95% C.I.		B	95% C.I.		B	95% C.I.	
HTA (arterial hypertension)	0.024	−0.032	0.024	0.035	−0.033	0.102	−0.016	−0.071	0.040	0.162	−0.058	0.382
DM (diabetes mellitus)	−0.002	−0.061	−0.002	0.005	−0.066	0.076	0.028	−0.030	0.086	−0.186	−0.416	0.045
Atherosclerosis	0.013	0.032	0.013	0.008	−0.046	0.061	−0.030	−0.074	0.015	0.070	−0.106	0.246
Grade	0.007	−0.026	0.007	0.036	−0.004	0.075	0.019	−0.014	0.051	0.134	0.005	0.263
Gender	−0.100	−0.151	−0.100	−0.075	−0.135	−0.014	0.000	−0.050	0.050	−0.265	−0.463	−0.067
Age	−0.001	−0.004	−0.001	−0.003	−0.007	0.000	0.002	−0.005	0.001	−0.013	−0.025	−0.002
F	3.268			2.701			1.055			0.800		
p	0.006			0.018			0.395			0.572		

aortic root motion during follow-up of patients after AVR as an additional risk factor for dissection [26].

We have previously found significant thinning of the ascending aorta wall and all its tunics in patients with aortic stenosis [27]. Similar changes have already been described in a different model of exaggerated hemodynamic forces and its influence to the arterial wall [28]. Rabkin, Jue and Tsang [29] proved echocardiographically that after the adjustment for body surface area, wall thickness of the sinus Valsalva is a good indicator of the aortic wall stress associated with the aortic valve sclerosis even in those cases when luminal diameters of the aorta are not dilated [29].

We applied Schlatmann and Becker grading system to demonstrate three different histopathological grades. Furthermore, our supposition is that these three grades follow the natural progression and evolution of aortic stenosis and its hemodynamic impact to the aortic wall. In our previous study, we confirmed significant progress of elastic lamellae disruption through different grades as well as spatial distribution of these changes in the aortic wall as they affect the internal media first [27]. These

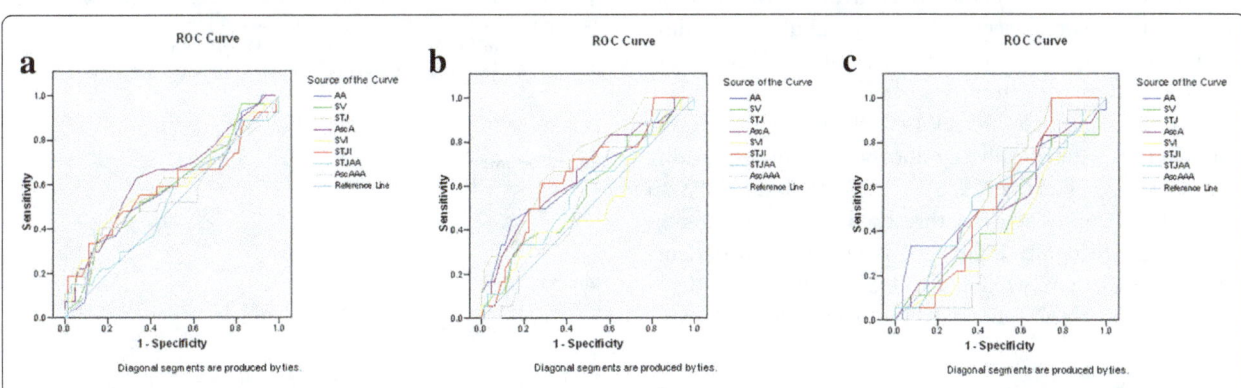

Fig. 5 ROC Curves test the sensitivity and specificity of different echocardiographic parameters for different grades for parameters AscA (**a**), STJ (**b**) and STJI (**c**)

Table 6 Threshold values of echocardiographic parameters that identify different grades

Variable Classification variable	Criterion	Sensitivity	95% CI	Specificity	95% CI	+LR	95% CI	-LR	95% CI
AscA Grade 2 vs. 1	>3.3 *	62.96	42.4–80.6	66.67	53.7–78.0	1.89	1.3–2.6	0.56	0.3–1.0
AscA Grade 3 vs 1	>3.5 *	50.00	26.0–74.0	77.78	65.5–87.3	2.25	1.4–3.6	0.64	0.3–1.2
STJ Grade 3 vs. 1	>2.9 *	61.11	35.7–82.7	73.02	60.3–83.4	2.26	1.5–3.4	0.53	0.3–1.1
STJI Grade 3 vs 1	>1 *	61.11	35.7–82.7	71.43	58.7–82.1	2.14	1.4–3.2	0.54	0.3–1.1

*statistically significant
AscA ascending aorta, *STJ* sinotubular junction, *STJI* sinotubular junction index

observations are in keeping with previous similar studies [6–8, 30, 31].

Grade 3 with destructive changes in numerous elastic lamellae and disorganization of smooth muscles resembled irreversible changes in the aortic wall.

Morphological and morphometric characteristics of elastic skeleton are changing during aging. Even the "perfect" internal thoracic artery is prone to elastic skeleton changes induced by aging [6, 7]. Nakashima et al. [30] proved that the number of elastic lamellae fenestrations increase with aging, as does the number of interlamellar elastic fibers, their ramifications and the number of their fenestrations [30]. It was very important to prove that the observed grades are not merely effects of aging. Our study showed there is no difference between patient age distribution in different histological grades. Dividing patients in two age groups ('65 and ≥65), there is no difference in the distribution of grades. Described changes persisted in both groups of patients, younger and older than 65 years, they are potentiated with aging, but they are not the effect of aging entirely.

Combined effect of gender and grade had no effect to echocardiographic parameters and the distribution of grades among genders did not differ significantly.

Girdauskas et al. [32], using cardiac magnetic resonance imaging, showed that systolic transvalvular flow jet is hitting the right-lateral segment of the tubular ascending aorta, in patients with aortic valve stenosis. This finding confermed that we sampled aorta from the right place [32]. By using multiple predictors in the setting of Regression analysis, statistically significant differences among grades were reached for AA, SV, STJ, AscA and SVI. With further ROC curves analysis, threshold values for different grades were recognized. Grade 2 is identified in patients with AscA > 3.3 cm, while grade 3 is identified in patients with values of AscA > 3.5 cm, STJ > 2.9 cm and STJI > 1.

Limitations of the study

Our study obviously lacks *post festum* echo analisys – to determine what happens with aortas in patients with different grades, following AVR. Nevertheless, we focused on proving the existence of different, progressive, histological changes in the aortic wall, and to correlate them with various echo parameters, in patients exclusively with severe stenosis of tricuspid aortic valve.

Conclusion

Our findings strongly support the view that aortas of patients with TAV stenosis are submitted to hemodynamic stress that subsequently leads to gradual elastic lamellae disruption that could be histologically identified and graded. The changes in the aortic wall correlated statistically significant with echocardiographic parameters. Grade 2 is identified in patients with AscA > 3.3 cm, while grade 3 is identified in patients with values of AscA > 3.5 cm, STJ > 2.9 cm and STJI > 1. Although current guidelines suggest simultaneous replacement of ascending aorta with AVR when aortic diameter is ≥55 mm, we propose more radical approach, with diameter > 3.5 cm as a cutoff, in patients with severe TAV stenosis, especially in patients with long life expectancy.

Abbreviations

AA: Ventriculo-aortic junction; AscA: Ascending aorta; AVR: Aortic valve replacement; BSA: Body surface area; GR: Grade; pSTJ: Predicted diameter at the level of sinotubular junction; pSV: Predicted diameter at the level of the sinus of Valsalva; STJ: Sinotubular junction; STJI: Sinotubular junction index; SV: Sinus Valsalva; SVI: Sinus Valsalva index; TAV: Tricuspid aortic valve

Acknowledgments

Not applicable.

Funding

The research activities were supported by grants No. 175005, 175,061, III45005, III41002 and III41022 from the Ministry of Education, Science and Technological Development of Republic of Serbia. The Ministry of Education, Science and Technological Development was not involved in study design, the collection, analysis and interpretation of data, the writing of the report and the decision to submit the article for publication.

Authors' contributions

SB and MLB made study concept and design, SB and MLB collected the data, SB, MLB, IZ and JME performed analysis and interpretation, SB, MLB and VT drafted the manuscript, SB, MLB, PM, VT, JR, IZ and PD performed critical revision of the manuscript. All authors read and approved the final manuscript.

Competing interests

The authors declare that they have no competing interests.

Author details

[1]Dedinje Cardiovascular Institute, Belgrade, Serbia, 1 Heroja Milana Tepića Street, Belgrade 11000, Serbia. [2]Institute of Histology and Embryology "Aleksandar Đ. Kostić", Faculty of Medicine, University of Belgrade, 26 Višegradska Street, Belgrade 11000, Serbia. [3]Faculty of Stomatology, University Business Academy in Pančevo, Novi Sad, Serbia. [4]Institute of Medical Statistics, Faculty of Medicine, University of Belgrade, Belgrade, Serbia.

References

1. Taghizadeh H, Tafazzoli-Shadpour M, Shadmehr MB. Analysis of arterial wall remodeling in hypertension based on lamellar modeling. J Am Soc Hypertens. 2015;9(9):735–44.
2. Yapei Y, Xiaoyan R, Sha Z, Li P, Xiao M, Shuangfeng C, Lexin W, Lianqun C. Clinical significance of arterial stiffness and thickness biomarkers in type 2 diabetes mellitus: an up-to-date meta-analysis. Med Sci Monit. 2015;21: 2467–75.
3. Kohn JC, Chen A, Cheng S, Kowal DR, King MR, Reinhart-King CA. Mechanical heterogeneities in the subendothelial matrix develop with age and decrease with exercise. J Biomech. 2016;49(9):1447–53.
4. Bauer M, Pasic M, Meyer R, Goetze N, Bauer U, Siniawski H, Hetzer R. Morphometric analysis of aortic media in patients with bicuspid and tricuspid aortic valve. Ann Thorac Surg. 2002;74:58–62.
5. Lang RM, Bierig M, Devereux RB, Flachskampf FA, Foster E, Pellikka PA, Picard MH, Members of the Chamber Quantification Writing Group. Recommendations for chamber quantification: a report from the American Society of Echocardiography's guidelines and standards committee and the chamber quantification writing group, developed in conjunction with the European Association of Echocardiography, a branch of the European Society of Cardiology. J Am Soc Echocardiogr. 2005, 18:1440–63.
6. Labudović BM, Borović S, Marinković-Erić J, Todorović V, Puškaš N, Kočica M, Radak Đ, Lačković V. A comprehensive morphometric analysis of the internal thoracic artery with emphasis on age, gender and left-to-right specific differences. Histol Histopathol. 2013a;28:1299–314.
7. Labudović BM, Borović S, Perić M, Vuković P, Marinković-Eric J, Todorović V, Radak Đ, Lačković V. The internal thoracic artery as a transitional type of artery: a morphological and morphometric study. Histol Histopathol. 2010; 25:561–76.
8. Labudović Borović M., Borović S., Radak Đ., Marinković-Erić J., Maravić-Stojković V., Vučević D., Stojšić Z., Milićević Ž., Čolić M., 2013b. Morphometric model of abdominal aortic aneurysms and the significance of the structural changes in the Aortic Wall for rupture risk assessment, In: Fischhof D. and Hatig F., editors. Aortic aneurysms: risk factors, diagnosis, surgery and repair. Hauppauge, New York: Nova Science Publishers, Inc.; pp. 81-117.
9. Schlatmann TJM, Becker AE. Histological changes in the normal aging aorta: implications for dissecting aortic aneurysm. Am. J Cardiol. 1977;39:13–20.
10. Niwa K, Perloff JK, Bhuta SM, Laks H, Drinkwater DC, Child JS, Miner PD. Structural abnormalities of great arterial walls in congenital heart disease: light and electron microscopic analyses. Circulation. 2001;103:393–400.
11. Roberts WC, Vowels TJ, Ko JM, Filardo G, Hebeler RF Jr, Henry AC, Matter GJ, Hamman BL. Comparison of the structure of the aortic valve and ascending aorta in regurgitation and resection of the ascending aorta for aneurysm. Circulation. 2011;123:896–903.

12. American Heart Association Committee on Vascular Lesions of the Council of Atherosclerosis, Stary H.C. (chair). A definition of advanced types of atherosclerosis lesions and a histological classification of atherosclerosis. Circulation. 1995;92:1355–74.
13. Vahanian A, et al. Guidelines on the management of valvular heart disease (version 2012). Eur J Cardiothorac Surg. 2012;42:S1–S44.
14. Robiscek F. Editorial: bicuspid versus tricuspid aortic valves. J. Heart Valve Dis. 2003;12:52–3.
15. Glower DD. Indications for ascending aortic replacement. Size alone is not enough. J Am Coll Cardiol. 2011;58:585–6.
16. Gaudino M, Anselmi A, Morelli M, Pragliola C, Tsiopoulos V, Glieca F, Possati G. Aortic expansion rate in patients with dilated post-stenotic ascending aorta submitted only to aortic valve replacement. J Am Coll Cardiol. 2011;58:581–4.
17. Linhartová K, Beránek V, Šefrna F, Hanisová I, Sterbáková G, Pesková M. Aortic stenosis severity is not a risk factor for poststenotic dilatation of the ascending aorta. Circ J. 2007;71:84–8.
18. Yasuda H, Nakatani S, Stugaard M, Tsujita-Kuroda Y, Bando K, Kobayashi J, Yamagishi M, Kitakaze M, Kitamura S, Miyatake K. Failure to prevent progressive dilatation of ascending aorta by aortic valve replacement in patients with bicuspid aortic valve: comparisons with tricuspid valve. Circulation. 2003;108:II291–4.
19. Andrus BW, O'Rourke DJ, Dacey LJ, Palac RT. Stability of ascending aortic dilatation following aortic valve replacement. Circulation. 2003;108:II295–9.
20. Botzenhardt F, Hoffmann E, Kemkes BM, Gansera B. Determinants of ascending aortic dimensions after aortic valve replacement with a stented bioprosthesis. J. Heart Valve Dis. 2007;16:19–26.
21. Matsuyama K, Usui A, Akita T, Yoshikawa M, Murayama M, Yano T, Takenaka H, Katou W, Toyama M, Okada M, Sawaki M, Ueda Y. Natural history of a dilated ascending aorta after aortic valve replacement. Circ J. 2005;69:392–6.
22. Ergin MA, Spielvogel D, Apaydin A, Lansman SL, McCullough JN, Galla JD, Griepp RB. Surgical treatment of the dilated ascending aorta: when and how? Ann Thorac Surg. 1999;67:1834–9.
23. Bechtel JFM, Noack F, Sayk F, Erasmi AW, Bartels C, Sievers HH. Histopathological grading of ascending aortic aneurysm: comparison of patients with bicuspid versus tricuspid aortic valve. J Heart Valve Dis. 2003;12:54–61.
24. Von Kodolitsch Y, et al. Predictors of proximal aortic dissection at the time of aortic valve replacement. Circulation. 1999;100(suppl II):II-287–94.
25. Tsutsumi K, et al. Risk factor analysis for acute type a aortic dissection after aortic valve replacement. Gen Thorac Cardiovasc Surg. 2010;58:601–5.
26. Beller C, et al. Aortic root motion remodeling after aortic valve replacement – implications for late aortic dissection. Interact Cardiovasc Thorac Surg. 2008;7:407–11.
27. Borović S. Korelacija između ehokardiografskih parametara i histoloških promena u zidu ascendentne aorte kod bolesnika sa degenerativnom stenozom aortne valvule [correlation between echocardiographic parameters and histological changes in the ascending aorta wall in patients with degenerative aortic valve stenosis], Master of Sciences Thesis, University of Belgrade, Belgrade, 2009; pp. 47-55.
28. Masuda H, Zhuang YJ, Singh TM, Kawamura K, Murakami M, Zarins CK, Glagov S. Adaptive remodeling of internal elastic lamina and endothelial lining during flow-induced arterial enlargement. Arterioscler Thromb Vasc Biol. 1999;19:2298–307.
29. Rabkin SW, Jue J, Tsang MY. Aortic valve sclerosis is associated with an echocardiographically determined thinner aortic wall. J Heart Valve Dis. 2006;15:158–64.
30. Nakashima Y, Shiokawa Y, Sueishi K. Alterations of elastic architecture in human aortic dissecting aneurysm. Lab Investig. 1990;62:751–9.
31. Agozzino L, Ferraraccio F, Esposito S, Trocciola A, Parente A, Della Corte A, De Feo M, Cotrufo M. Medial degeneration does not involve uniformly the whole ascending aorta: morphological, biochemical and clinical correlations. Eur J Cardiothorac Surg. 2002;21:675–82.
32. Girdauskas et al. Functional aortic root parameters and expression of aortopathy in bicuspid versus tricuspid aortic valve stenosis, 2016. J Am Coll Cardiol. 19;67(15):1786-1796.

11

Positive impact of retrograde autologous priming in adult patients undergoing cardiac surgery: a randomized clinical trial

Britt Hofmann[1*] (ID), Claudia Kaufmann[1], Markus Stiller[1], Thomas Neitzel[1], Andreas Wienke[2], Rolf-Edgar Silber[1] and Hendrik Treede[1]

Abstract

Background: Adult cardiac surgery with extracorporeal circulation is known to be associated with increased risk of blood transfusion leading to adverse outcomes. Procedures like retrograde autologous priming (RAP) may reduce these negative side effects. This randomized prospective study was initiated to assess whether RAP using specifically designed RAP bag (Terumo) has immediate effects on patient outcome.

Methods: One hundred eighteen adults undergoing elective CABG or elective aortic valve replacement were randomly assigned by a computer program into two groups: the RAP group ($n = 54$) in which the retrograde autologous priming was applied and the non-RAP ($n = 64$) group in which the same setting was used without the possibility to save priming volume. Patient demographics, preoperative characteristics and postoperative outcomes were analyzed for both groups.

Results: The primary endpoint defined as rate of intraoperative blood transfusion was significantly reduced in the RAP-group ($p = 0.04$). The absolute risk reduction for RAP managed patients was 13.5 percent points. There were no significant differences in operation time and blood loss. No deaths and no myocardial infarctions were observed. The number of patients needed to treat to prevent at least one red blood cell transfusion was around 8 (NNT = 7.42).

Conclusions: Retrograde autologous priming is a safe and less invasive procedure which achieves clear benefits for adult cardiac surgery patients. In the light of increasing red blood cell transfusion risks and costs and the wish of patients to avoid a transfusion implementation of retrograde autologous priming is an interesting option.

Keywords: Retrograde autologous priming (RAP), Cardiac surgery, Perioperative management, Blood transfusion

Background

Despite notable advances in extracorporeal circulation during the last decade, cardiac surgery with cardiopulmonary bypass (CPB) is still associated with an increased risk of blood transfusions [1]. Today, using the gold-standard technique of CPB, elective coronary artery revascularization and aortic valve replacement can be performed with a mortality rate of less than 3% (https://iqtig.org/berichte/strukturierter-qualitaetsbericht/2015/). The primary setup of the CPB circuit demands a priming volume of approximately 1500 mL of crystalloid solution [2], which leads to a relevant hemodilution. Hemodilution resulting in low hematocrit levels during CPB is known to be responsible for impaired hemostasis, detrimental effects on end-organ function and on cognitive outcome [3–5]. In consequence, nearly 50% of all cardiac surgery patients [6] receive a transfusion of red blood cells and cardiac surgery accounts for a significant amount of blood product consumption worldwide [7]. Blood transfusions have been associated with several serious complications, like transfusion related acute lung injury, modulation of the immune system and increased post-operative infection risk [6]. Furthermore, blood transfusions are an independent risk factor for morbidity

* Correspondence: britt.hofmann@uk-halle.de
[1]Department of Cardiac Surgery, University Hospital Halle, Ernst-Grube-Strasse 40, 06120 Halle, Germany
Full list of author information is available at the end of the article

and mortality after cardiac surgery [8] and responsible for considerable healthcare costs [9–11]. Therefore, the Society of Thoracic Surgeons and the Society of Cardiovascular Anesthesiologists guidelines recommend efforts to reduce blood transfusion in cardiac surgery [12]. The measures employed in our institution to reduce hemodilution intraoperatively include cell salvage procedures, reduction of CPB priming volume and retrograde autologous priming (RAP). RAP was first introduced in 1959 by Panico and Neptune [13], in 1998 Rosengart et al. [14] refined and reintroduced the technique in clinical practice. The modern RAP procedure minimizes hemodilution by displacing the crystalloid priming volume of arterial and venous lines via passive exsanguination of native blood prior to CPB initiation. Procedures like retrograde autologous priming may further reduce the negative side effects of ECC and transfusion related healthcare costs. Several studies focusing on RAP have documented varying effectiveness in reducing transfusion rates and equivalent or improved outcomes associated with this technique [7, 14–19]. This randomized prospective study was initiated to assess whether RAP using specifically designed RAP bag (TERUMO, Europe NV, Leuven, Belgium) has immediate effects on hemodilution, blood transfusions and patient outcome. Our study is the first

randomized trial were the effect measure number needed to treat for clinical decision making was calculated. Furthermore, we focused on cost-effectiveness of the RAP procedure, as well as on other factors predicting postoperative blood transfusions.

Methods
Study patients
In the present study, 118 adults undergoing first-time elective CABG or elective aortic valve replacement between August 2012 and July 2015 were randomly assigned by a computer program into two groups: the RAP group ($n = 54$) in which the retrograde autologous priming was applied and the non-RAP ($n = 64$) group in which the same setting was used without the possibility to save priming volume (Fig. 1). All patients were admitted to our unit the day before the planned operation. All patients received aspirin 100 mg/d until the day before the operation. Exclusion criteria were age < 18 years, LVEF $\leq$ 20%, emergency operations, reoperations, combined procedures, myocardial infarction 24 h before surgery, preoperative cortisone, coumarin, dual platelet inhibitor, or IV heparin therapy, thrombocytopenia (< 100 Gpt/l), liver disease, preoperative dialysis, hematological or oncological systemic disease or systemic infection. As an

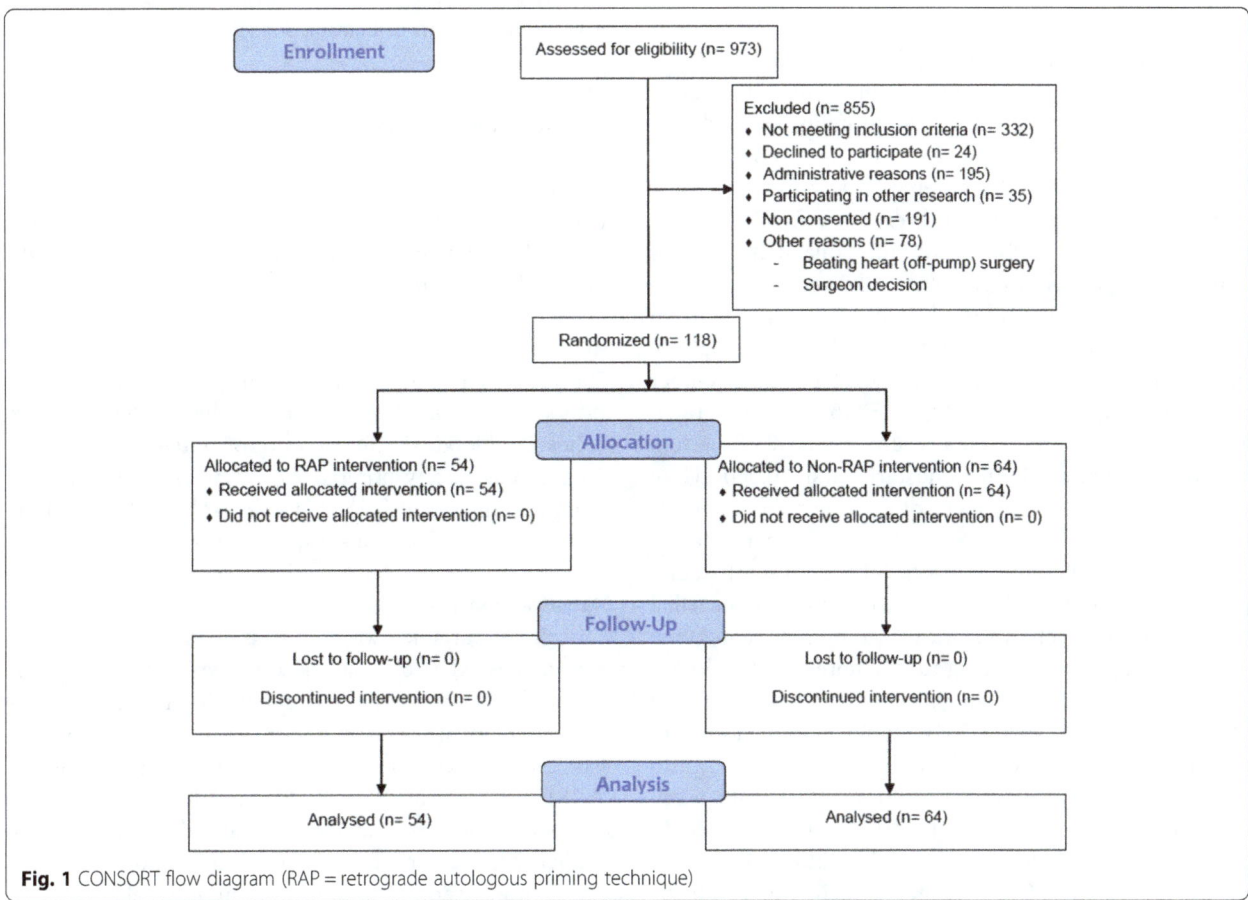

Fig. 1 CONSORT flow diagram (RAP = retrograde autologous priming technique)

investigator initiated project, the trial was registered as RAP 18080 at the local research portal of the federal state of Saxony-Anhalt (https://forschung-sachsen-anhalt.de/) on August 18th, 2012.

Randomization

Consenting patients meeting inclusion criteria were randomly assigned at the day of surgery. The randomization was computerized by software. This software generated a binary result by chance. Each was strictly associated with one study group and was linked to the subject's ID. The ID, the time of randomization, and the assigned study group were stored in a MySQL database.

Anticoagulation management

The Heparin concentration management system has been used in our institution since the year 2010 and we developed a protocol for the rational use of the device. Both study groups were managed according to this protocol [20]. In all patients, tranexamic acid (Cyklokapron®) was used as a standard perioperative bleeding prophylaxis to prevent hyperfibrinolysis. According to our institutional standards all patients received a cumulative dosage of 4 g tranexamic acid.

Anesthesia and cardiopulmonary bypass circuit

Anesthesia was initiated using an intravenous technique with propofol, fentanyl and pancuronium bromide on demand. After initiation anaesthesia was performed as balanced anesthesia, administered as low fresh gas flow with inhalational sevoflurane over the ventilator or the oxygenator of the CPB system; additional fentanyl was administered intravenously. Normothermic extracorporeal circulation was accomplished in all patients with an open non-heparin-coated system including a poly-2-methoxyethyl-acrylate (PMEA) coated hollow-fiber membrane oxygenator (CAPIOX® FX15) with integrated arterial filter, and reservoir (Terumo). The CPB system was primed with 850 ml Jonosteril® and 10.000 IU of porcine heparin. Management of CPB included systemic temperature of 36 °C, α-stat pH management, target mean perfusion pressure between 50 and 70 mmHg, and pump flow rates of $\geq$ 2.4 l/min/m^2. Myocardial protection was achieved with intermittent antegrade warm cardioplegia according to Calafiore's protocol [21]. All patients received an intraoperative infusion of tranexamic acid (bolus of 2 g after the administration of the initial heparin bolus and another 2 g were given into the CPB circuit during reperfusion). In all patients, a cell saver (Medtronic autoLog™ or Sorin Xtra®) was used to collect wound blood prior to CPB, blood from the pleural space and CPB volume, which could not be

reinfused before protamine administration. This blood was processed if the collected volume exceeded 600 ml.

Retrograde autologous priming

The only structural difference to the standard CPB circuit is a RAP bag (CE, Terumo, Belgium). Before RAP started, mean arterial pressure was elevated to approximately 80 mmHg using small doses of i.v. noradrenaline. Then priming fluid in the arterial line of the heart-lungmachine was displaced with patient's blood using arterial pressure, the venous line was drained by slowly rotating the arterial pump. The priming fluid of the CPB circuit was slowly drained into the RAP bag. The RAP bag stayed connected with the venous reservoir for crystalloid fluid replacement during CPB. The retrograde priming procedure took approximately 3 to 5 min.

Transfusion guidelines

Packed red blood cells (PRB) were transfused when hemoglobin concentration (Hb) was < 7.0 g/dl or hematocrit (Hk) < 21% during CPB, and after cardiac surgery if Hb < 8.0 g/dl or Hk < 24% [22–24]. The transfusion of fresh frozen plasma (FFP) and platelet concentrates was based on the clinical decision of the anesthetist. According to the departmental protocol a hemorrhage of over 1000 ml within the first 6 postoperative hours was an indication for surgical re-exploration.

Data collection

Patient demographics, preoperative characteristics and postoperative outcomes were analyzed for both groups. For all patients, more than 200 variables were entered in a database. All clinical laboratory parameters were assessed by the central department of Laboratory Medicine of the University Hospital.

Study endpoints

The primary endpoint for this study was determined as intraoperative blood transfusion. Other endpoints were in-hospital blood transfusion (intraoperative or postoperative), defined safety criteria like intra- and postoperative complications (renal failure, stroke, prolonged ventilation, reintubation, ICU stay, in-hospital stay, death).

Statistical analyses

Categorical variables were expressed as frequencies and percentages. Metric variables were expressed as mean ± standard deviation (SD). The benefit of the RAP use over the control was tested with the chi-square test and was further expressed as the absolute risk reduction (ARR). For clinical decision making the effect measure number needed to treat (NNT) was calculated [25]. To predict risk factors for intraoperative and in-hospital blood transfusion, simple and multivariable logistic regression analyses were done to estimate the odds ratios (OR) with their 95% confidence intervals (CI). Discrimination was assessed using the area under the receiver operating characteristic curve (AUROC). AUROC analysis was also utilized to calculate cut off values. Sample size calculation was based on a two-sided chi-square-test with significance level alpha = 5%, a power of 90% and expected intraoperative transfusion rates of 5% in the RAP group and 25% in the non-RAP group, respectively, and resulted in $n = 65$ patients per group. However, the study had to be terminated due to relevant changes in value measurement procedures of the central department of Laboratory Medicine. Especially, the change from troponin I to troponin T measurement as well as the change of the measurement methods for kidney, liver, hematological and hemolysis parameters was critical. Because it was not possible to establish a trouble-free conversion, we felt that the clear analysis of the study was too heavily biased, so we decided to terminate the enrolment. The authors did not look into the data before terminating the enrolment.

Results

Patients

In the present prospective randomized study, we assessed 118 patients (mean age: 69.74 ± 8.74 years, range 42–87 years). Eighteen (15.25%) of the 118 patients were females and they were slightly older (70.3 ± 7.1 years) than males (69.6 ± 9 years). The pre-operative left ventricular ejection fraction was normal with 58.9 ± 10.3% in the overall patient population. Further demographic and clinical data of the study individuals are shown in Table 1. There was no clinically relevant difference between the two groups with exception for BMI and hematocrit. Most patients had comorbidities and risk factors for coronary artery disease. All patients had first time cardiac surgery. Surgical details are shown in Table 2. Ninety-five patients underwent isolated coronary artery bypass grafting (80%), 21 patients underwent isolated aortic valve surgery (18%) and 2 patients underwent combined single CABG and aortic valve surgery (2%). The two patients with combined procedures were initially planned for aortic valve replacement. However, in both cases the surgeon decided intraoperatively, that the patients would profit from a venous bypass graft (one case CABG-D1, other case CABG-RCA). Both patients were in the RAP group. There were no other differences between the groups regarding the type of operation or other surgical details, including the number of bypass grafts performed and the cardiopulmonary bypass, aortic cross-clamp and total surgical times (Table 2). RAP could reduce the priming volume of the ECC by 357 ± 57 mL.

Table 1 Baseline characteristics of study patients

Variables	RAP patients ($n = 54$)	Non-RAP ($n = 64$)
Age (years)	69.94 ± 8.65	69.56 ± 8.90
Male gender	81.48 (44/54)	87.50 (56/64)
Height (cm)	172.04 ± 8.12	172.44 ± 7.32
Weight (kg)	87.52 ± 16.07	83.16 ± 12.42
BMI (kg/m^2)	29.57 ± 5.36	27.88 ± 3.52
Hypertension	92.59 (50/54)	95.31 (61/64)
Diabetes mellitus	38.89 (21/54)	40.63 (26/64)
Diabetes Type		
IDDM	33.33 (7/21)	23.08 (6/26)
NIDDM	66.67 (14/21)	76.92 (20/26)
Hypercholesterolemia	79.63 (43/54)	79.69 (51/64)
Renal disease	16.67 (9/54)	15.63 (10/64)
Smoking Status		
Currently	12.96 (7/54)	20.31 (13/64)
Never	64.81 (35/54)	65.63 (42/64)
Previously	22.22 (12/54)	14.06 (9/64)
Chronic Lung Disease	7.41 (4/54)	17.19 (11/64)
PAD	16.67 (9/54)	4.69 (3/64)
Atrial Fibrillation	11.11 (6/54)	7.81 (5/64)
NYHA class		
I	11.32 (6/53)	11.48 (7/61)
II	43.40 (23/53)	52.46 (32/61)
III	43.40 (23/53)	31.15 (19/61)
IV	1.89 (1/53)	4.92 (3/61)
CCS class		
I	16.67 (6/36)	14.89 (7/47)
II	44.44 (16/36)	46.81 (22/47)
III	38.89 (14/36)	38.30 (18/47)
LVEF (%)	59.93 ± 10.37	57.95 ± 10.16
CAD		
1 vessel CAD	20.37 (11/54)	17.19 (11/64)
2 vessel CAD	22.22 (12/54)	14.06 (9/64)
3 vessel CAD	57.41 (31/54)	68.75 (44/64)
Aortic valve stenosis	24.07 (13/54)	15.63 (10/64)
Baseline Hct (%)	37.7 ± 3.9	38.2 ± 4.1
Baseline creatinine (μmol/L)	79.00 ± 19.07	76.84 ± 19.10
Logistic EuroSCORE	3.81 ± 2.21	3.41 ± 2.51
EuroSCORE II	1.44 ± 0.70	1.27 ± 0.88

Values are mean ± SD or n (%). *Baseline Hct* preoperative hematocrit, *BMI* body mass index, *CAD* Coronary artery disease, *CABG* coronary artery bypass grafting, *CCS class* Canadian Cardiovascular Society classification, *IDDM* insulin dependent diabetes mellitus, *NIDDM* non-insulin dependent diabetes mellitus, *NYHA class* New York Heart Association classification, *LVEF* left ventricular ejection fraction, *PAD* peripheral artery disease

Table 2 Relevant intraoperative details of study patients

Variables	RAP patients (n = 54)	Non-RAP (n = 64)
CABG distal Anastomoses	2.41 ± 1.38	2.63 ± 1.33
AVR	24.07 (13/54)	15.63 (10/64)
Total surgical procedure (min)	172.41 ± 27.48	175.09 ± 35.00
Cardiopulmonary bypass (min)	84.98 ± 14.08	87.13 ± 22.60
Aortic cross-clamp time (min)	52.67 ± 12.06	52.16 ± 14.78
Reperfusion (min)	25.15 ± 7.76	26.19 ± 9.81
Total crystalloid volume (mL)	2065.74 ± 978.97	1942.19 ± 1142.27
Plasma expanders administered	61.11 (33/54)	53.13 (34/64)
Cellsaver volume harvest (mL)	710.22 ± 538.21	659.77 ± 541.88
Cellsaver volume wash (mL)	163.87 ± 245.51	146.97 ± 235.04
MAP (mmHg)	75.8 ± 5.1	77.6 ± 4.7
Adrenalin dose (µg/kg/min)	0.005 ± 0.02	0.009 ± 0.03
Noradrenalin dose (µg/kg/min)	0.06 ± 0.06	0.06 ± 0.05

Values are mean ± SD or n (%). AVR aortic valve replacement, MAP mean arterial pressure

Primary endpoint

The intraoperative transfusion rate was 3.7% (2 of 54 patients) in the RAP group and 17.2% (11 of 64 patients) in the non-RAP group. The primary endpoint defined as rate of intraoperative blood transfusion was significantly reduced in the RAP group ($p = 0.04$). The absolute risk reduction for RAP managed patients was 13.5 percent points. Non-RAP managed patients had an increased relative risk for an intraoperative red blood cell transfusion of 4.6 (95% CI, 1.07 to 20.03; $p = 0.039$) compared to RAP managed patients. The number of patients needed to treat to prevent at least one red blood cell transfusion was around 8 (NNT = 7.42). With regard to the fact, that in most of the cases two red blood cell concentrates (costs per RCC: 272 € [11]) are administered, the RAP procedure (costs per RAP bag: 60 €) with 480 € costs for the treatment of eight patients versus 544 € costs for two RCC is cost-effective.

Additional analyses

As we noticed an imbalance between the two patient groups regarding body mass index and preoperative hematocrit value, we adjusted for these potential confounders in a multivariable logistic regression analysis for the primary endpoint intraoperative blood transfusion (Table 3).

Secondary endpoints and additional analyses

Also, we did a multivariable logistic regression analysis for in-hospital blood transfusion and adjusted for the potential confounders body mass index, preoperative hematocrit value and blood loss 12 h post-operative (Table 4). As independent predictors of the outcome

Table 3 Multivariable logistic regression analysis for intraoperative blood transfusion

Variables	Multivariable Logistic Regression		
	OR	95%-CI	p
BMI (kg/m²)	0.99	0.84–1.16	0.88
Baseline Hct (%)	0.75	0.62–0.91	0.003
Non-RAP	6.93	1.34–35.74	0.02

OR Odds Ratio, 95%-CI 95%- confidence interval for OR, BMI body mass index, Hct hematocrit, RAP retrograde autologous priming

blood transfusion throughout the hospital stay we identified a body mass index > 29 kg/m^2 (AUROC ± SE, 0.68 ± 0.05; 95%-CI, 0.58–0.76; $p = 0.0007$), a preoperative hematocrit value ≤ 36% (AUROC ± SE, 0.8 ± 0.04; 95%-CI, 0.72–0.87; $p < 0.0001$), blood loss 12 h post-operative > 450 mL (AUROC ± SE, 0.63 ± 0.05; 95%-CI, 0.54–0.72; $p = 0.01$) and RAP ≤ 350 mL (AUROC ± SE, 0.7 ± 0.08; 95%-CI, 0.54–0.81; $p = 0.01$).

The postoperative MAP was 79.8 ± 9.7 mmHg in the RAP group and 81.2 ± 9.2 mmHg in the Non-RAP group. The noradrenalin dose up to 16 h postoperative was 2505 ± 3087 µg in RAP patients and 2465 ± 2929 µg in Non-RAP patients. Postoperative adrenalin was used in 7.41% (4/54; 195.3 ± 745.3 µg) of RAP and 12.5% (8/64; 604.4 ± 1989.8 µg) of Non-RAP managed patients.

Data on postoperative complications are shown in Table 5. There were no perioperative deaths, defined as a death within 30 days of surgery or prior to discharge following surgery.

Discussion

In the present study, we could show that retrograde autologous priming is a safe, simple to use and effective procedure to reduce blood transfusions in elective adult cardiac surgery. RAP managed patients had a significantly reduced rate of intraoperative red blood cell transfusions, the number of patients needed to treat with RAP to prevent one red blood cell transfusion was around 8. With regard to the fact, that in most of the cases two red blood cell concentrates are administered, the RAP procedure with a cost of 480 € for the treatment of eight patients versus 544 € costs for two red

Table 4 Multivariable logistic regression analysis for in-hospital blood transfusion

Variables	Multivariable Logistic Regression		
	OR	95%-CI	p
BMI (kg/m²)	1.26	1.11–1.42	0.0004
Baseline Hct (%)	0.62	0.52–0.75	< 0.0001
Blood loss 12 h post-op. (mL)	1.01	1.002–1.01	0.008
Non-RAP	3.38	1.13–10.12	0.03

OR Odds Ratio, 95%-CI 95%- confidence interval for OR, BMI body mass index, Hct hematocrit, RAP retrograde autologous priming

Table 5 Postoperative complications of the study patients

Postoperative complication	RAP patients (n = 54)	Non-RAP (n = 64)	p value
Prolonged ventilation > 48 h	0	4.69 (3/64)	0.31
Re-intubation	1.85 (1/54)	4.69 (3/64)	0.74
Bleeding	7.41 (4/54)	4.69 (3/64)	0.81
Myocardial infarction	0	0	
Reoperation	0	0	
Renal failure	0	0	
Stroke	0	0	
Mediastinitis	0	0	
Perioperative death	0	0	
Length of stay in ICU (d)	2.02 ± 2.8	2.3 ± 2.6	0.57
Length of in-hospital stay (d)	15.4 ± 4.75	15.02 ± 6.4	0.72

Values are mean ± SD or n (%)

blood cell concentrates [11] is also cost-effective. A major concern with RAP is the possible need for vasopressor support during volume reduction. However, we noticed that this is only transient with no long-term impact for patients. In this randomized study, the RAP technique was performed safely in patients undergoing ECC without adding evident additional time to the procedure.

Further analyses revealed a body mass index over 29 kg/m^2, a preoperative hematocrit value of ≤ 36% and a 12 h postoperative blood loss of over 450 mL as independent predictors for in-hospital blood transfusion after elective adult cardiac surgery. To be effective in avoiding in-hospital blood transfusion the RAP volume had to be at least 350 mL. We did not find a difference in postoperative complications or operative mortality between groups.

A low baseline hematocrit was identified as risk factor for intraoperative transfusion and was an independent predictor for in-hospital blood transfusion in general. According to the new 2017 EACTS/EACTA Guidelines on patient blood management for adult cardiac surgery [26, 27], 48% of our RAP managed patients and 45% of the control group had a mild anemia (women, Hb 100–120 g/L; men, Hb 100–130 g/L). For future optimal preoperative management of red blood cells in line with the guidelines and available data [28, 29] we need to elucidate reasons for preoperative anemia (e.g. iron deficiency, vitamin D or folate deficiency) and implement erythropoietin (EPO) treatment with or without iron supplementation (class IIa, level B recommendation) in our subsequent work.

The results of our randomized trial are in line with data reported by Rosengart et al. [14] and current data from Teman et al. [7], Trapp et al. [19] and a meta-analysis by Sun et al. [30]. This growing body of data supports the findings of our study that RAP decreases intraoperative and postoperative blood transfusion rates without increasing peri- or postoperative complications, leading to comparable or even favorable outcomes. Our study is the first randomized trial were the effect measure number needed to treat for clinical decision making was calculated, showing that eight patients need to be treated with RAP to avoid at least one intraoperative blood transfusion. We also showed for the first time that a minimum RAP volume of 350 mL is needed for the procedure to be effective. Furthermore, known factors influencing the transfusion rate, such as the preoperative hematocrit, were confirmed. Despite these results the use of RAP technique in adult cardiac surgery has only been given a level II B recommendation from the practice guidelines of the Society of Thoracic Surgeons and the Society of Cardiovascular Anesthesiologists [12]. Considering all the reported data and the findings of the current study confirming safety and efficacy of the technique, RAP should potentially be used in all patients undergoing cardiopulmonary bypass. With regard to Likosky et al. [1], we also feel that blood conservation in cardiac surgery needs more efforts and a team approach. Our goal should be to avoid considerable hemodilution due to ECC, especially in the growing body of patients with high body mass index and low preoperative hematocrit. We are convinced that particularly in these patients saving blood products by avoiding hemodilution will have huge consequences regarding postoperative infection rates and morbidity. This will be implemented within our subsequent work.

Study limitations

Our study is subject to the limitations inherent in studies from a single center. Furthermore, the treatment group variable (non-RAP vs. RAP) is associated with large confidence intervals (Tables 3 and 4). This is mainly a consequence of the binary nature of this variable compared to the more informative continuous variables BMI, baseline hematocrit, and blood loss. Additionally, because of the small sample population and numbers of complications, the uses of body mass index, preoperative hematocrit value, blood loss 12 h postoperative and RAP as predictors for in-hospital blood transfusions in cardiac surgery require further evaluation.

Conclusions

In conclusion, this randomized study observed in non-RAP managed patients an increased relative risk for intraoperative red blood cell transfusion. The number of patients needed to treat with RAP to prevent one red blood cell transfusion was around 8. To our knowledge, this is the first study to confirm that RAP is cost-effective relating to intraoperative blood transfusions. In addition, our data revealed RAP, BMI, preoperative hematocrit and 12 h postoperative blood loss as independent predictors for in-hospital blood transfusions after elective adult cardiac surgery. Adopting the RAP technique into the daily perfusion routine does not require sophisticated or expensive pharmacologic or technical modifications and is not related to increased peri- or postoperative patient risks. Therefore, we recommend considering this method in adult patients scheduled for elective cardiac surgery.

Abbreviations

AUROC: Area under the receiver operating characteristic curve; BMI: Body mass index; CI: Confidence interval; CPB: Cardiopulmonary bypass; ECC: Extracorporeal circulation; NNT: Number of patients needed to treat; RAP: Retrograde autologous priming; RCC: Red blood cell concentrates; SD: Standard deviation; SE: Standard error

Acknowledgements

We thank our anesthesiologists and intensivists for their contribution to the study.
We acknowledge the financial support of the Open Access Publication Fund of the Martin-Luther-University Halle-Wittenberg.

Funding

TERUMO Europe NV, Leuven, Belgium was the sponsor of this study and participated with the investigators in the design of the study. The authors had full control of the data collection, analysis, and interpretation of data and in writing the manuscript.

Authors' contributions

BH drafted and reviewed the manuscript, participated in the design of the study and performed data collection and analysis; CK reviewed the manuscript, reviewed the analysis and performed data collection for the study; MS reviewed the manuscript, reviewed the data analysis and performed data collection for the study; TN reviewed the manuscript and performed data collection for the study; AW reviewed the manuscript and performed data analysis for the study; RES reviewed the manuscript and participated in the design and coordination of the study; HT reviewed the manuscript, reviewed the data analysis and performed data collection for the study. All authors read and approved the final manuscript.

Competing interests

The authors declare that they have no competing interests.

Author details

[1]Department of Cardiac Surgery, University Hospital Halle, Ernst-Grube-Strasse 40, 06120 Halle, Germany. [2]Institute of Medical Epidemiology, Biostatistics and Informatics, Martin-Luther-University Halle-Wittenberg, 06097 Halle, Germany.

References

1. Likosky DS, Dickinson TA, Paugh TA. Blood conservation-a team sport. J Extra Corpor Technol. 2016;48(3):99–104.
2. Neitzel T, Stiller M, Bushnaq H. Statistische Analyse der in Deutschland durchgeführten Perfusionen - Ergebnisse einer Umfrage 2013. Kardiotechnik. 2014;10:12–22.
3. Habib RH, Zacharias A, Schwann TA, Riordan CJ, Durham SJ, Shah A. Adverse effects of low hematocrit during cardiopulmonary bypass in the adult: should current practice be changed? J Thorac Cardiovasc Surg. 2003; 125(6):1438–50.
4. Karkouti K, Beattie WS, Wijeysundera DN, Rao V, Chan C, Dattilo KM, Djaiani G, Ivanov J, Karski J, David TE. Hemodilution during cardiopulmonary bypass is an independent risk factor for acute renal failure in adult cardiac surgery. J Thorac Cardiovasc Surg. 2005;129(2):391–400.
5. Loor G, Li L, Sabik JF 3rd, Rajeswaran J, Blackstone EH, Koch CG. Nadir hematocrit during cardiopulmonary bypass: end-organ dysfunction and mortality. J Thorac Cardiovasc Surg. 2012;144(3):654–62. e654
6. Horvath KA, Acker MA, Chang H, Bagiella E, Smith PK, Iribarne A, Kron IL, Lackner P, Argenziano M, Ascheim DD, et al. Blood transfusion and infection after cardiac surgery. Ann Thorac Surg. 2013;95(6):2194–201.
7. Teman N, Delavari N, Romano M, Prager R, Yang B, Haft J. Effects of autologous priming on blood conservation after cardiac surgery. Perfusion. 2014;29(4):333–9.
8. Ranucci M, Baryshnikova E, Castelvecchio S, Pelissero G. Major bleeding, transfusions, and anemia: the deadly triad of cardiac surgery. Ann Thorac Surg. 2013;96(2):478–85.
9. Stokes EA, Wordsworth S, Bargo D, Pike K, Rogers CA, Brierley RC, Angelini GD, Murphy GJ, Reeves BC. Are lower levels of red blood cell transfusion more cost-effective than liberal levels after cardiac surgery? Findings from the TITRe2 randomised controlled trial. BMJ Open. 2016; 6(8):e011311.
10. Murphy GJ, Pike K, Rogers CA, Wordsworth S, Stokes EA, Angelini GD, Reeves BC. Liberal or restrictive transfusion after cardiac surgery. N Engl J Med. 2015;372(11):997–1008.
11. Honemann C, Bierbaum M, Heidler J, Doll D, Schoffski O. Costs of delivering allogenic blood in hospitals. Chirurg. 2013;84(5):426–32.
12. Ferraris VA, Brown JR, Despotis GJ, Hammon JW, Reece TB, Saha SP, Song HK, Clough ER, Shore-Lesserson LJ, Goodnough LT, et al. 2011 update to the Society of Thoracic Surgeons and the Society of Cardiovascular Anesthesiologists blood conservation clinical practice guidelines. Ann Thorac Surg. 2011;91(3):944–82.
13. Panico FG, Neptune WB. A mechanism to eliminate the donor blood prime from the pump-oxygenator. Surg Forum. 1960;10:605–9.
14. Rosengart TK, DeBois W, O'Hara M, Helm R, Gomez M, Lang SJ, Altorki N, Ko W, Hartman GS, Isom OW, et al. Retrograde autologous priming for cardiopulmonary bypass: a safe and effective means of decreasing hemodilution and transfusion requirements. J Thorac Cardiovasc Surg. 1998; 115(2):426–38. discussion 438-429
15. Eising GP, Pfauder M, Niemeyer M, Tassani P, Schad H, Bauernschmitt R, Lange R. Retrograde autologous priming: is it useful in elective on-pump coronary artery bypass surgery. Ann Thorac Surg. 2003;75(1):23–7.
16. Sobieski MA 2nd, Slaughter MS, Hart DE, Pappas PS, Tatooles AJ. Prospective study on cardiopulmonary bypass prime reduction and its effect on intraoperative blood product and hemoconcentrator use. Perfusion. 2005; 20(1):31–7.
17. Reges RV, Vicente WV, Rodrigues AJ, Basseto S, Alves Junior L, Scorzoni Filho A, Ferreira CA, Evora PR. Retrograde autologous priming in cardiopulmonary bypass in adult patients: effects on blood transfusion and hemodilution. Rev Bras Cir Cardiovasc. 2011;26(4):609–16.
18. Severdija EE, Heijmans JH, Theunissen M, Maessen JG, Roekaerts PH, Weerwind PW. Retrograde autologous priming reduces transfusion requirements in coronary artery bypass surgery. Perfusion. 2011;26(4):315–21.
19. Trapp C, Schiller W, Mellert F, Halbe M, Lorenzen H, Welz A, Probst C. Retrograde autologous priming as a safe and easy method to reduce Hemodilution and transfusion requirements during cardiac surgery. Thorac Cardiovasc Surg. 2015;63(7):628–34.
20. Hofmann B, Bushnaq H, Kraus FB, Raspe C, Simm A, Silber RE, Ludwig-Kraus B. Immediate effects of individualized heparin and protamine management on hemostatic activation and platelet function in adult patients undergoing

cardiac surgery with tranexamic acid antifibrinolytic therapy. Perfusion. 2013; 28(5):412–8.

21. Calafiore AM, Teodori G, Mezzetti A, Bosco G, Verna AM, Di Giammarco G, Lapenna D. Intermittent antegrade warm blood cardioplegia. Ann Thorac Surg. 1995;59(2):398–402.

22. Cross-Sectional Guidelines for Therapy with Blood Components and Plasma Derivates - 4th revised edition. Transfus Med Hemother. 2009;36(6):345–492.

23. Hoppe JD, Scriba PC, Kluter H. Cross-sectional guidelines for therapy with blood components and plasma derivatives (4th revised edition, 2008) - suspension of chapter 5 'Human albumin. Transfus Med Hemother. 2011;38(1):71.

24. Muller MM, Geisen C, Zacharowski K, Tonn T, Seifried E. Transfusion of packed red cells: indications, triggers and adverse events. Dtsch Arztebl Int. 2015;112(29–30):507–17. quiz 518

25. Schechtman E. Odds ratio, relative risk, absolute risk reduction, and the number needed to treat–which of these should we use? Value Health. 2002; 5(5):431–6.

26. Boer C, Meesters MI, Milojevic M, Benedetto U, Bolliger D, von Heymann C, Jeppsson A, Koster A, Osnabrugge RL, Ranucci M, et al. 2017 EACTS/EACTA guidelines on patient blood management for adult cardiac surgery. J Cardiothorac Vasc Anesth. 2017;

27. Pagano D, Milojevic M, Meesters MI, Benedetto U, Bolliger D, von Heymann C, Jeppsson A, Koster A, Osnabrugge RL, Ranucci M, et al. 2017 EACTS/EACTA guidelines on patient blood management for adult cardiac surgery. J Cardiothorac Vasc Anesth. 2018;32(1):88–120. https://doi.org/10.1053/j.jvca.2017.06.026.

28. Weltert L, Rondinelli B, Bello R, Falco M, Bellisario A, Maselli D, Turani F, De Paulis R, Pierelli L. A single dose of erythropoietin reduces perioperative transfusions in cardiac surgery: results of a prospective single-blind randomized controlled trial. Transfusion. 2015;55(7):1644–54.

29. Hogan M, Klein AA, Richards T. The impact of anaemia and intravenous iron replacement therapy on outcomes in cardiac surgery. Eur J Cardiothorac Surg. 2015;47(2):218–26.

30. Sun P, Ji B, Sun Y, Zhu X, Liu J, Long C, Zheng Z. Effects of retrograde autologous priming on blood transfusion and clinical outcomes in adults: a meta-analysis. Perfusion. 2013;28(3):238–43.

12

A standardized approach to treat complex aortic valve endocarditis

Anna Gomes[1]* (iD), Jayant S. Jainandunsing[2], Sander van Assen[3], Peter Paul van Geel[4], Bhanu Sinha[1], Sandro Gelsomino[5], Daniel M. Johnson[5] and Ehsan Natour[5,6]

Abstract

Background: Surgical treatment of complicated aortic valve endocarditis often is challenging, even for experienced surgeons. We aim at demonstrating a standardized surgical approach by stentless bioprostheses for the treatment of aortic valve endocarditis complicated by paravalvular abscess formation.

Methods: Sixteen patients presenting with aortic valve endocarditis (4 native and 12 prosthetic valves) and paravalvular abscess formation at various localizations and to different extents were treated by a standardized approach using stentless bioprostheses. The procedure consisted of thorough debridement, root replacement with reimplantation of the coronary arteries and correction of accompanying pathologies (aortoventricular and aortomitral dehiscence, septum derangements, Gerbode defect, total atrioventricular conduction block, mitral and tricuspid valve involvement).

Results: All highly complex patients included (14 males and 2 females; median age 63 years [range 31–77]) could be successfully treated with stentless bioprostheses as aortic root replacement. Radical surgical debridement of infected tissue with anatomical recontruction was feasible. Although predicted operative mortality was high (median logarithmic EuroSCORE I of 40.7 [range 12.8–68.3]), in-hospital and 30-day mortality rates were favorable (18.8 and 12.5% respectively).

Conclusions: Repair of active aortic valve endocarditis complicated by paravalvular abscess formation and destruction of the left ventricular outflow tract with stentless bioprosthesis is a valuable option for both native and prosthetic valves. It presents a standardized approach with a high success rate for complete debridement, is readily available, and yields comparable clinical outcomes to the historical gold standard, repair by homografts. Additionally, use of one type of prosthesis reduces logistical issues and purchasing costs.

Keywords: Infective endocarditis, Stentless bioprostheses, Abscess, High-risk, Surgery

Background

Infective endocarditis causes in-hospital mortality of 20% and 40% after 1-year, rising further to 79% for aortic valve endocarditis [1, 2]. This high rate is largely due to extended local destruction of heart tissue, e.g. paravalvular abscess formation, with secondary heart failure. Risk factors for endocarditis include rheumatic, congenital, and degenerative valve lesions, intracardiac prosthetic material, intravenous drug use, and healthcare contact [3]. Diagnosis of endocarditis is based on the modified Duke criteria, bearing a sensitivity and specificity of 80% for the total patient population [4]. As this is not optimal, the expert opinion of a multidisciplinairy team is essential for diagnosis. Therapy of endocarditis relies on antimicrobial therapy and surgery for cardiac anatomical damage (vegetation, abscess, fistula, shrunken valve, valve tears or holes, prosthetic valve detachment), as well as uncontrolled infection. In this way, 25–50% of patients are operated upon in the acute phase of infection and an additional 20–40% later in the course due to haemodynamic complications [5].

Paravalvular abscess formation complicates aortic valve endocarditis. Early surgical treatment of complicated endocarditis improves outcome when compared to

* Correspondence: a.gomes@umcg.nl
[1]Department of Medical Microbiology, University of Groningen, University Medical Center Groningen, Groningen, Netherlands
Full list of author information is available at the end of the article

medical therapy alone, reducing 6-month mortality from 33 to 16% [6] and the composite endpoint of death/ embolic events/ recurrence of endocarditis from 28 to 3% [7]. Aortic valve paravalvular abscess formation and root destruction requires radical resection of infected tissue with subsequent reconstruction of the left ventricular outflow tract (LVOT) (modified Bentall procedure) [8]. Therefore, surgical treatment of complicated aortic valve endocarditis is considered challenging, bearing high operative (11–40% in-hospital) and late (60% in 5 years) mortality rates [9].

Various surgical techniques are used to treat complicated aortic valve endocarditis, depending on the surgical preference and with differing results: patch, prosthesis, homograft. Historically, cryopreserved homografts were considered as the gold standard for these patients [10–12]. Homografts offer low recurrence rates, acceptable valve-related morbidity and mortality, and their low transvalvular gradient is associated with improved left ventricular mass regression [13, 14]. Homografts also have disadvantages, including demanding surgical techniques, the need for reoperation due to calcification, limited availability and shelf life [8, 9, 15]. Nowadays, biological stentless valves are more often used in complicated aortic valve endocarditis [8, 9]. Using these prostheses, the surgical versatility of homografts is reached due to their comparable durability, shape and pliability [8]. In addition, stentless bioprostheses have advantages, such as a rather long shelf life and being readily available in various sizes, uniform in quality, technically easier to implant and furnished with anticalcification properties [8, 13, 14, 16–18].

Guidelines support the use of both homografts and stentless bioprostheses in aortic valve endocarditis with paravalvular abscess formation [2, 10, 19]. The choice of prosthesis depends on patient characteristics, technical considerations, and surgeon preferences [8, 14]. In this illustrated series of sixteen patients with aortic valve endocarditis and complicating paravalvular abscess formation, we show that the use of stentless bioprostheses provides a more standardized surgical procedure that consists of thorough debridement, root replacement with reimplantation of the coronary arteries, and treatment of accompanying pathologies.

Methods
Patients
In this case series we aimed at providing evidence for the standardized use of a stentless bioprostheses in complex aortic valve endocarditis. "Standardized use" refers to the use of one type of stentless bioprosthesis for a variety of anatomical problems complicating aortic valve endocarditis. Clinical data and high quality macroscopic pictures from sixteen patients with active aortic valve endocarditis

and paravalvular abscess formation were collected between 2006 and 2015. In this time period, a total of 85 patients underwent aortic valve surgery for endocarditis in our center. Here, we report on those patients treated with stentless bioprostheses. Their endocarditis was not limited to the cusps but also involved the annulus with formation of large paravalvular abscesses at various anatomical locations. Consequently, complications arose, such as root disarrangement with loss of aortaventricular or aortomitral continuity, atrioventricular conduction disturbance, or infection of the septum or the right ventricle. Despite their poor clinical condition, these patients were deemed eligible for surgical valve repair and LVOT reconstruction using stentless bioprostheses.

Definitions
Infective endocarditis was diagnosed based on the modified Duke criteria [4] and expert opinion of a multidisciplinairy team. Prosthetic valve endocarditis was considered early if it occurred during the first year after valve replacement, otherwise it was considered late [2]. Causative microorganisms were identified by culture and molecular testing on peripheral blood and tissue or prosthetic material collected during surgery [2]. Functional cardiac derangements as described by the guidelines were important indications for surgery [2, 19]. Macroscopically visible pathological findings considered an indication for the use of stentless bioprostheses were presence of destructive lesions, including annular abscess, paravalvular leak and cusp perforation. Re-thoracotomy was defined as reopening of the sternum after implantation of the bioprosthesis. Reoperation was defined as any surgical procedure involving the implanted bioprosthesis. Recurrence was used as a combined term for both relapse (repeat episodes of endocarditis caused by the same microorganism) and reinfection (infection caused by a different microorganism) [2].

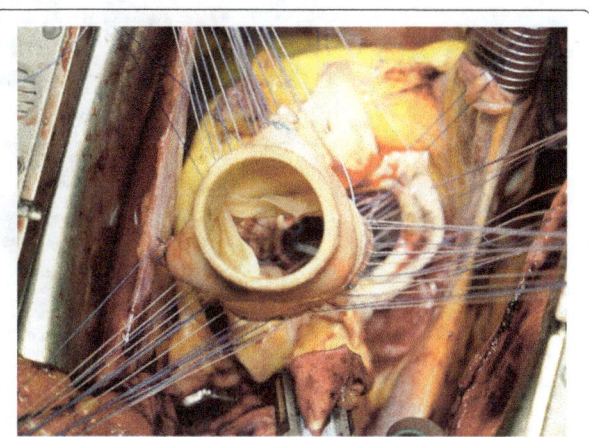

Fig. 1 Stentless bioprosthesis

Prosthesis

The Freestyle® bioprosthesis (Medtronic Inc., Minneapolis, MN, USA) is a stentless porcine aortic root prosthesis with ligated coronary arteries and a thin skirt over the porcine septal myocardium. The bioprosthesis is fixed with low pressure applied to the aortic wall, and zero-net pressure across the leaflets (Fig. 1). Pre-implantation, the bioprosthesis underwent an anticalcification treatment using alpha-amino-oleic acid. The device can be implanted by various techniques: subcoronary valve replacement, root inclusion, or complete aortic root replacement.

Surgical technique

The standard surgical approach was a median (re)sternotomy with mild/moderate hypothermic (32–34 °C) cardiopulmonary bypass and cardioplegic cardiac arrest (retrograde blood cardioplegia). Cardiopulmonary bypass was performed using aortic cannulation and right atrial or bicaval cannulation for venous drainage.

The aorta was transected above the sinotubular junction. After the aortotomy exposure, the abscess regions were inspected (Fig. 2) and infected native cusps or prosthesis as well as any aortic aneurysms were removed with extensive tissue debridement. The aortic sinuses were resected with

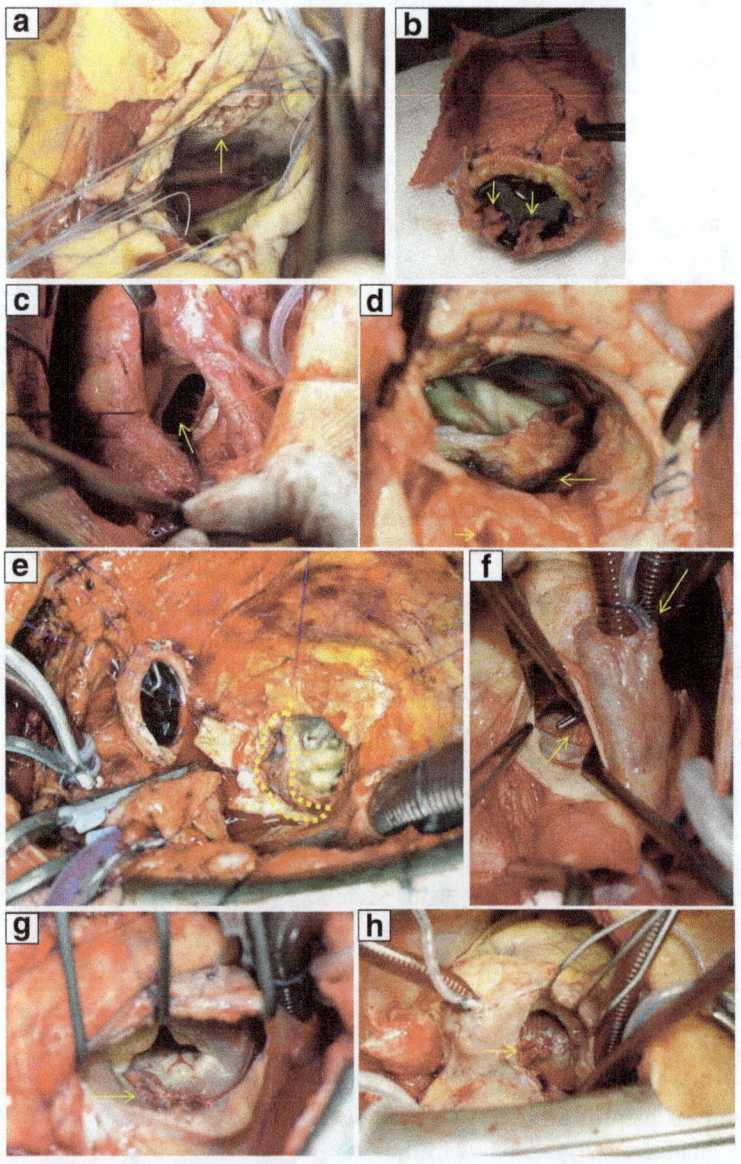

Fig. 2 Aortic valve endocarditis with paravalvular abscess formation, surgical view: **a** view from aortic root, ventricular septal defect, **b** valved conduit with vegetations, **c** total aorto-ventricular dehiscence, with left ventricular outflow tract discontinuity, **d** abscess cavity (large arrow) with left main coronary visible (small arrow), **e** retro-aortal abscess cavity with aorto-mitral involvement and mitral annulus dehiscence, **f** aorto-atrial fistula, Gerbode-like defect, **g** atrial view, tricuspid valve annular abscess with torn septal leaflet and paravalvular leak, **h** tricuspid valve deformity with vegetational mass

trumpet-shaped recesses of the coronary ostia. More specifically, a ventricular septum defect just under the membranous septum was identified in Fig. 2a. In this case a pericardial patch was used, which was distally sutured on the septum covering both the defect and the membranous septum, proximally attached at the level of the aortic annulus. Figure 2b and c depict chronic dehiscence of a mechanical prosthesis (implanted after a Bentall procedure) as a result of abcess formation at the annular level. Interestingly, the prosthesis was found floating above the annulus, only attached by the coronary arteries. Hence, the adhesions surrounding the annulus kept the prosthesis in place. Following resection of the infected prosthesis and clearance of the abcess, the stentless bioprosthesis was sutured on the annulus using a single-stitch technique. Given the chronic nature of disease in this case, the bioprosthesis was parachutted downwards towars the subannular plane to minimize traction of the chronically anchored anterior mitral leaflet (AML). In contrast, Fig. 2d and e illustrate acute subannular abcess formation. In this case, the AML was detached from the annulus while the prosthesis attachment site remained intact. In this case, due to the recent onset of infection, traction of the AML to the annulus plane and a neo-annulus were created after clearance of the abcess and other inflammatory tissue. Afterwards the stentless bioprosthesis was sutured to the annulus. Figure 2f to h depict Gerbode lesions with tricuspid valve involvement. Gerbode(–like) lesions encompass fistulas formed between the left ventricle(aorta) and the right side of the heart, appearing above or below the septal leaflet of the tricuspid valve. Repair of the subvalvular fistula from the right side included temporary resection of the spetal leaflet of the tricupid valve, which was thereafter re-attached.

After debridement, restoration and sizing of the aortic annulus the proximal anastomosis was performed using 20–25 interrupted sutures of Ticron 3–0 in a single plane. If required, the coronary ostia were mobilised using diathermy. After completion of the proximal suture line, the patient's coronary ostia were reimplanted end-to-side to the corresponding sinus of Valsalva of the prosthesis using a continuous 5–0 polyproylene suture. Finally, the bioprosthesis was anastomosed with the aorta using continuous 4–0 polyproylene. If further resection of the ascending aorta was required, a vascular tube graft was interposed.

Ethical considerations

The institutional medical ethical review board of the University Medical Center Groningen approved the use of retrospective patient data for our study and waived informed consent (METc2015/033; February 2015).

Results

Patient characteristics

This series consecutively included 14 males and 2 females with a median age of 63 years (Tables 1 and 2). All patients had an urgent indication for cardiothoracic surgery with implantation of a stentless bioprosthesis as root replacement due to uncontrolled infection and abscess formation (evidence class I and level B [2]). Median New York Heart Association score was III, and median logarithmic EuroSCORE I score was 40.7. Median follow-up for survivors was 4.6 years. All survivors were followed for at least 2 years, 36% were followed for 5 years, and 9% for 10 or more years. In 4 patients (25%) the endocarditis involved native aortic valves, with 2 identified bicuspid valves. In 12 patients (58%) the endocarditis involved prosthetic aortic valves: in 7 patients the aortic valve was replaced once and in 1 patient twice before, in 5 patients a Bentall procedure had been

Table 1 Patient characteristics (*n* = 16

Characteristic	Value
Age: median [range] (years)	63 [31–77]
Gender: male; female, n (%)	14 (87.5); 2 (12.5)
Reoperation / PVE (%)	75
Follow-up survivors: median [range] (years)	4.6 [2.3–11.7]
NYHA score: median [range]	III [II-IV]
Logarithmic EuroSCORE I: median [range]	40.7 [12.8–68.3]
Microbiology	
PVE	
• *Staphylococcus* spp.: 5 CoNS, 1 *S. aureus*	*n* = 6 (50%)
• *Streptococcus* spp.: 1 viridans group, 1 *S. bovis*, 1 *S. agalactiae*	*n* = 3 (25%)
• *Enterococcus* spp.: 2 *E. faecalis*	*n* = 2 (17%)
• no micro-organism identified	*n* = 1 (8%)
NVE	
• *Staphylococcus* spp.: *S. aureus*	*n* = 1 (25%)
• *Streptococcus* spp.: 2 viridans group	*n* = 2 (50%)
• *Enterococcus* spp.: *E. faecalis*	*n* = 1 (25%)

Outcome	Value
Cardiopulmonary bypass perfusion time: median [range] (minutes)	358 [186–731]
Aortic cross-clamping time: median [range] (minutes)	266 [107–389]
Intensive care unit stay: median [range] (days)	1.5 [1–21]
Hospital stay: median [range] (days)	55 [29–90]
In-hospital mortality: n (%)	3 (18.8)
30 day mortality: n (%)	2 (12.5)

CoNS coagulase negative staphylococci, *COPD* chronic obstructive pulmonary disease, *e.c.i.* e cause ignota, *NVE* native valve endocarditis, *NYHA* New York Heart Association, *PVE* prosthetic valve endocarditis, *SD* standard deviation

Table 2 Characteristics of included patients

#	Age (yr)	sex	Previous surgery	Micro-organism	Indication for surgery	Euro SCORE	Remarks during stentless bioprosthesis implantation	Outcome			
								rethoracotomy	re-IE	permanent dialysis	PPM
1	66	M	2 yr. bio	*Streptococcus sanguinis*	aortic root abscess	38.92	pericard patch to support MV, 1 RBC	Recovery initially, but death 7.5 months post surgery			
								−	+	−	+
2	70	M	1 yr. bio	*Staphylococcus epidermidis*	aortic root abscess, mycotic aneurysm, loose prosthesis, septic emboli, AV block	65.87	aorta annulus support with pledges and transseptal stiches, CABG, 5 RBC	In-hospital death 40 days post surgery			
								−			+
3	71	M	1 yr. bio	*Streptococcus agalactiae*	aortic root abscess with Gerbode defect, AV block	47.06	pericard patch reconstruction aorta annulus, atriotomy, TVP and Devega plasty, 14 RBC	Recovery > 6 years post surgery			
								−	−	−	+
4	31	M	−	*Streptococcus mitis*	totally destructed LVOT with Gerbode defect, AV block	42.52	pericard patch reconstruction aorta annulus, TVP, Devega plasty, 0 RBC	Recovery > 4 years post surgery			
								−	−	−	+
5	71	M	29 yr. mech	*Enterococcus faecalis*	aortic root abscess, septic emboli	47.06	3 RBC	Recovery > 3 years post surgery			
								−			
6	36	M	2 yr. mech	not identified	aortic root abscess, septic emboli	28.55	0 RBC	Recovery > 4 years post surgery			
								−			−
7	64	M	−	*Staphylococcus aureus*	aortic root abscess, multiple septic emboli, cardiac decompensation	23.42	aorta annulus support with pledges, 2 RBC	Recovery > 2 year (20 months) post surgery			
								−	−	−	+
8	72	M	3mo bio	*Staphylococcus epidermidis*	loose prosthesis, cardiac decompensation	64.48	closure of destructed coronary ostia, CABG, 0 RBC	In-hospital death 14 days post surgery			
								−			
9	45	M	12 yr. mech	*Staphylococcus aureus*	aortic root abscess, mycotic aneurysm	28.55	multiple vegetations AV, pericard patch reconstruction aorta annulus, 0 RBC	Recovery initially, but death 13 months post surgery			
								−	+	−	+
10	60	F	4mo bio	*Staphylcoccus epidermidis*	progressive aortic root abscess with Gerbode defect, septic emboli, blood cultures persistantly positive, AV-block	37.28	removal of vegetation from right atrium with affected AML and PPM implantation, 4 RBC	Recovery > 2 years post surgery			
								−	−	−	+
11	55	M	−	*Enterococcus faecalis*	aortic root abscess, mycotic aneurysm, conduction disturbance	26.62	pericard patch reconstruction aorta annulus and AML, 1 RBC	Recovery > 4 years post surgery			
								−	−	−	−
12	42	M	−	*Streptococcus mutans*	mycotic aneurysm, large vegetation	12.79	MVP, 0 RBC	Recovery > 5 years post surgery			
								−	−	−	−
13	75	F	1 yr. bio	*Staphylococcus epidermidis*	aortic wall thickening, septic emboli, AV block	61.76	mobilization of tightly adhered coronary ostia, 2 RBC	Recovery > 8 years post surgery			
								−	−	−	+
14	77	M	2 yr. bio	*Enterococcus faecalis*	septal mycotic aneurysm with fistula and threatened anatomy	52.33	urgent surgery with two times reanimation setting and persistant instability for which	In-hospital death directly post surgery			
								−	−		

Table 2 Characteristics of included patients *(Continued)*

#	Age (yr)	sex	Previous surgery	Micro-organism	Indication for surgery	Euro SCORE	Remarks during stentless bioprosthesis implantation	Outcome			
								rethoracotomy	re-IE	permanent dialysis	PPM
							sternum left open, 0 RBC				
15	62	M	1 yr. mech	coagulase negative Staphylococci	aortic root abscess, progressive mycotic aneurysm, aortoventricular dehiscence	68.31	4 RBC	Recovery > 11 years post surgery			
								–	–	–	–
16	60	M	7 yr. mech	*Streptococcus bovis*	aortic root abscess, mycotic aneurysm, aortoventricular dehiscence, cardiac decompensation	60.7	drainage of 1 L pleural effusion at both sides, 0 RBC	Recovery > 5 years post surgery			
								–	–	–	–

 # patient number, AML anterior mitral leaflet, AV aortic valve, AV block atrio-ventricular block, bio biological prosthetic valve inplanted, CABG coronary artery bypass grafting, EuroSCORE logarithimic I, F female, LVOT left ventricular outflow tract, M male, mech mechanical prosthetic valve inplanted, mo months, MV mitral valve, PPM placement of permanent pacemaker, RBC number of bags with red blood cells given during surgery, re-IE recurrence of endocarditis, rethoracotomy for bleeding or tamponade, TVP tricuspid valve plasty, yr. years

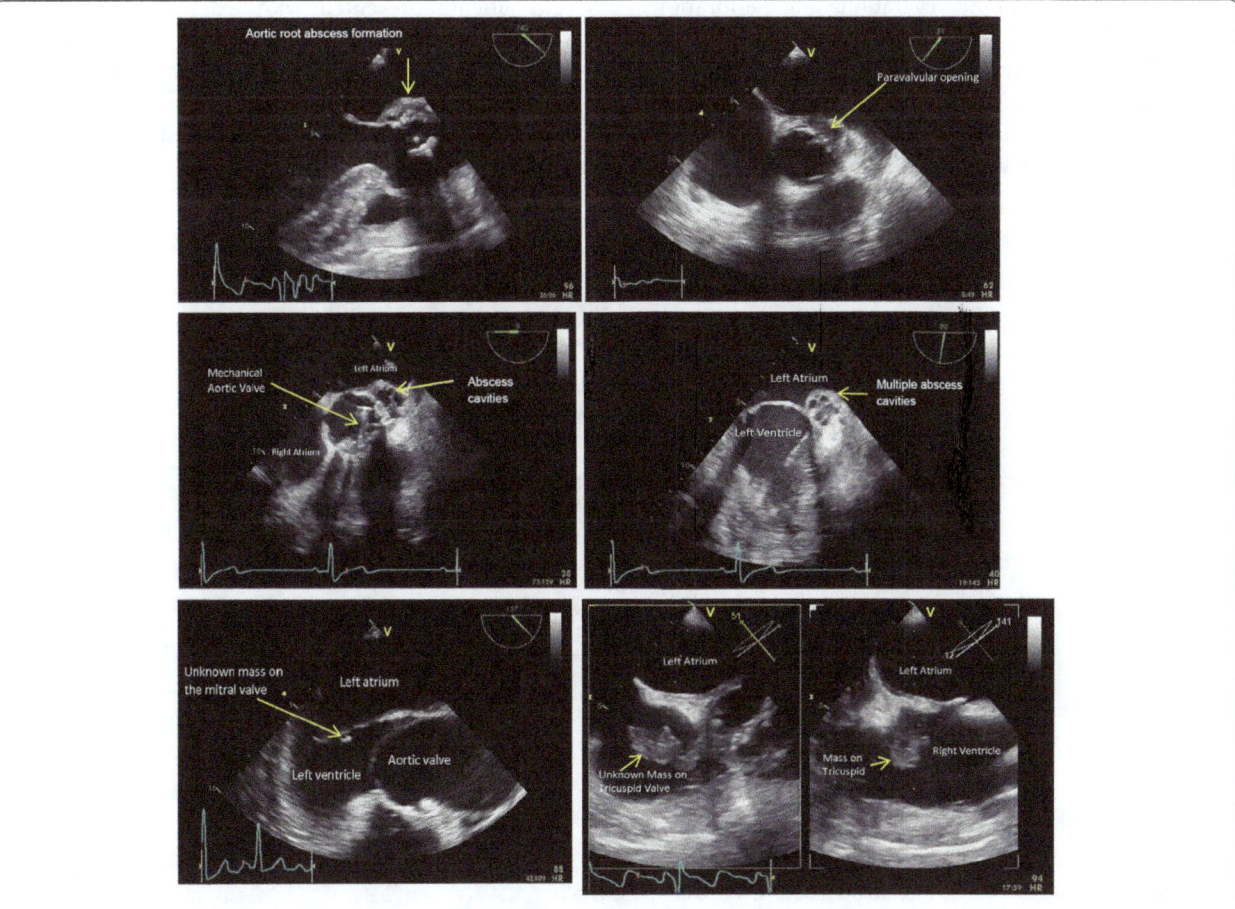

Fig. 3 Aortic valve endocarditis with paravalvular abscess formation, transesophageal echocardiographic view

performed. Of the patients with prosthetic valves, 2 patients had early (3–4 months after surgery) and 10 patients late endocarditis (1–29 years after surgery). In-hospital and 30 day mortality were 18.8% and 12.5%, respectively; 2-year recurrence rate was 14%.

Infectious cardiac anatomical compliations eligible for stentless bioprostheses repair

Several situations of active aortic valve endocarditis with paravalvular abscess formation and accompanying pathologies were deemed eligible for valve repair and LVOT reconstruction with a stentless bioprosthesis (Figs. 2, 3, 4 and 5).

Aortoventricular dehiscence

Seven patients with a prosthetic valve presented with aortoventricular dehiscence. Pathogens included coagulase-negative staphylococci, *Staphylococcus aureus*, *Streptococcus* bovis, *Enterococcus faecalis*. 29% (2/7) of these patients also had extention of infection towards their mitral valve.

Septum derangements

Seven patients presented with infectious derangements of their septum, including vegetations and perforations. Four of these patients had a prosthetic valve. Pathogens included *Staphylococcus epidermidis*, *Staphylococcus aureus*, *Streptococcus agalactiae*, *Streptococcus mitis*, and *Enterococcus faecalis*. 71% (5/7) of these patients had a permanent pacemaker (PPM) implanted and 43%

(3/7) had extention of infection towards the right side of the heart through a Gerbode(–like) defect.

Total atrioventricular conduction block

Six patients presented with a total or third degree atrioventricular conduction block. Five of these patients had a prosthetic valve. Pathogens included *Staphylococcus epidermidis*, *Streptococcus sanguinis*, *Streptococcus agalactiae*, and *Streptococcus mitis*. All these patients had a PPM implanted, 50% had extention of infection towards their right ventricle through a Gerbode(–like) defect, and 50% had extention of infection towards their mitral valve.

Gerbode defect (with tricuspid valve involvement)

Three patients presented with a Gerbode(–like) defect, a left ventricular (aorta) to right atrial shunt [20], causing an infection of their tricuspid valve due to local spread. Two of these patients had a prosthetic valve. Pathogens included *Staphylococcus epidermidis*, *Streptococcus agalactiae* and *Streptococcus mitis*. All patients had a PPM implanted, and needed a tricuspid valve plasty.

Mitral valve involvement (with aortomitral dehiscence)

Seven patients presented with extension of infection towards their mitral valve. Five of these patients had a prosthetic valve. Pathogens included *Staphylococcus epidermidis*, *Streptococcus sanguinis*, *Streptococcus mutans*, and *Enterococcus faecalis*. 57% (4/7) of these patients had septic emboli.

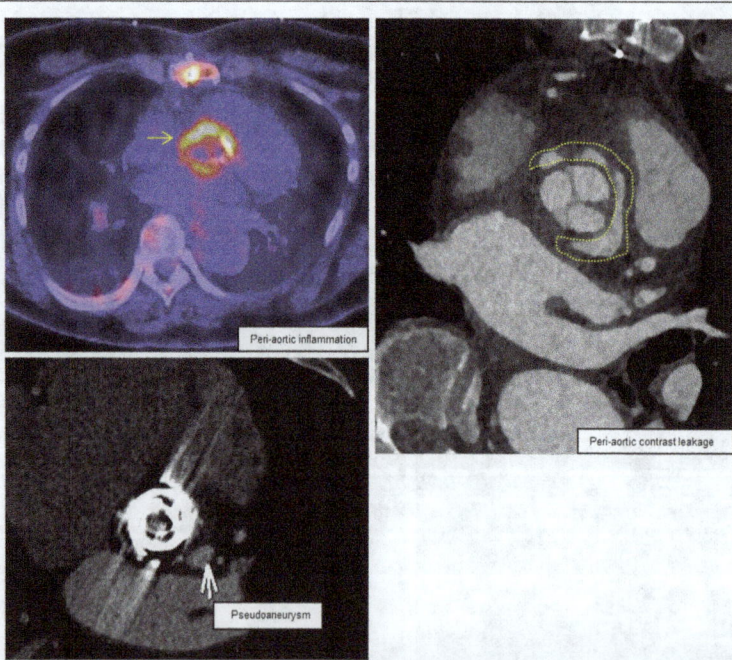

Fig. 4 Aortic valve endocarditis with paravalvular abscess formation, nuclear/radiological view with ^{18}F-fluorodeoxyglucose positron emission tomography/computed tomography

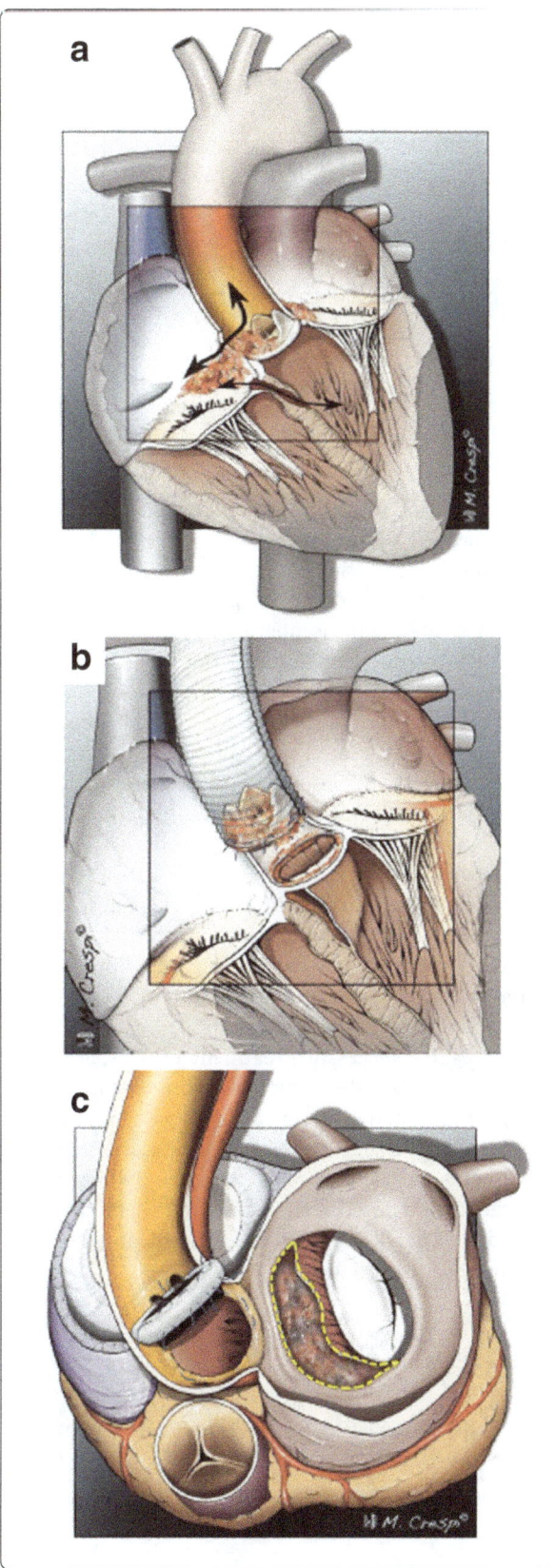

Fig. 5 Aortic valve endocarditis with paravalvular abscess formation, illustrations: **a** coronal view on the heart showing a ventricular septum defect, Gerbode defect (communication between the left ventricle and the right atrium), Gerbode-like defect (communication between the aorta and the right atrium) and tricuspid valve deformity; **b** coronal view on the proximal heart showing total aorto-ventricular dehiscence; **c** horizontal view on the proximal heart showing a retro-aortal abscess cavity with aorto-mitral involvement and mitral annulus dehiscence

Extracardiac complications due to endocarditis

Infective endocarditis is a cardiac disease with extracardiac complications due to hematogenous and embolic spread. In our series, the three most common complications were: mycotic aneurysm ($n = 3$), cerebral emboli ($n = 2$), and vertebral osteomyelitis ($n = 2$).

Patient survival

Figure 6 shows the survival of included patients for 11 years. Five patients died during this period (Table 2), due to: end-stage heart failure 227 days post-surgery; recurrent respiratory insufficiency resulting from sputum retention, encephalopathy and extended postoperative wound infection 40 days post-surgery; active intracerebral bleeding without therapeutic options 14 days post-surgery; re-infection of the prosthesis with cerebral embolization, mediastinitis and kidney failure 388 days post-surgery; severe hemodynamic instability immediately post-surgery.

Discussion

We have described and illustrated a series of patients with aortic valve endocarditis, paravalvular abscess formation and accompanying pathologies. All patients underwent cardiothoracic surgery with thorough debridement and restoration of cardiac anatomy using stentless bioprostheses. Patients with native and several types of prosthetic valves were included. Pathogens varied, including staphylococci ($n = 7$), streptococci ($n = 5$) and enterococci ($n = 3$). Predicted mortality was high (median logarithmic EuroSCORE I of 40.7 [range 12.8–68.3]) but actual mortality was relatively low (in-hospital 18.8% [3/16] and 30-day 12.5% [2/16]), showing that the stentless bioprostheses can be successfully used in a variety of surgically challenging situations and allows for a standardized approach. Figures 2, 3 and 4 show the cases of aortic valve endocarditis with various paravalvular abscesses from a surgical (Fig. 2), echocardiographic (Fig. 3) and nuclear/radiological (Fig. 4) view.

Due to its design, it is possible to use the stentless bioprostheses for subcoronary valve replacement, for inclusion of the root, or full root replacement [13, 16]. Using the prostheses for a full root replacement, enables exclusion of abscess cavities and the rebuilding of the LVOT. Furthermore, it maintains root geometry and the integrity of the "leaflet, sinus and root" as a functional entity, both

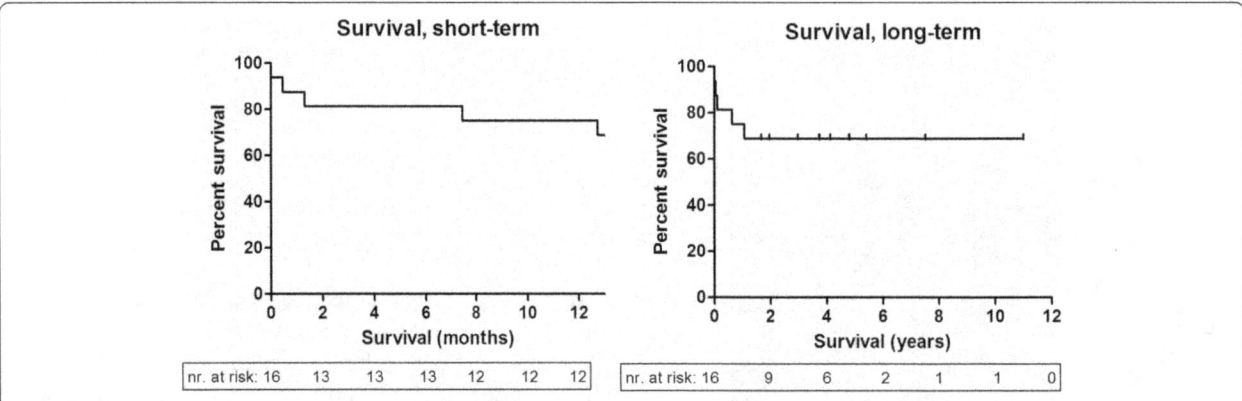

Fig. 6 Kaplan-Meier curves. The short-term curve depicts the survival of included patients over 12 months post surgery and the long-term curve depicts the survival of included patients during the total follow-up time (maximum 11 years)

increasing durability of the bioprostheses [8, 21]. Implantation with the single suture technique is believed to allow placement of the stentless bioprosthesis as full root replacement without narrowing of the LVOT nor obstruction by any rigid structures such as pledgets [21]. Using the stentless bioprothesis as a full root replacement in complex endocarditis was previously reported in 5 patients [22] and now supported with our data of 16 patients with various well described paravalvular abscesses.

Survival rates for the use of stentless bioprostheses when active native or prosthetic aortic valve endocarditis is complicated by extensive destruction of the LVOT have been reported as 81–89%, 76–83%, 62–70%, and 54% at 30 days, 1 year, 5 years, and 10 years, respectively [8, 13, 14, 16, 17]. Although early mortality remains considerably high in the group presented, studies show that stentless bioprostheses yield clinical outcomes, postoperative echocardiographic data, long-term recurrence and survival rates comparable to those of cryopreserved homografts [8, 9, 13, 14, 16, 17]. Indeed, the recurrence rates of homografts (3.8–6.8%) and stentless valves (3.7–8.6%) are similar and lower than that of standard prostheses (33%) [13]. However, as compared with standard aortic valve replacement, the need for reimplantation of coronary arteries conveys an increased risk of atrioventricular conduction block. Also, the use of bioprosthesis conveys an increased risk of reoperation in juvenile patients. Even though stentless and stented valves show equal performance with regard to clinical parameters and valve-related mortality, stentless valves have more favorable hemodynamic and biomechanical characteristics and significantly higher long-term survival rates (78% versus 66% in 8-years) [8, 14, 16]. Compared to homografts, progression of valve dysfunction (37% versus 86%, $p < 0.01$) [23] and need for reoperations are lower for stentless bioprostheses [14, 18, 23]. Furthermore, implantation is less challenging and demanding for stentless bioprostheses and reoperation of a calcified prosthesis may be easier as compared to homografts [9].

A limitation of this study is its retrospective nature. Furthermore, we did not directly compare the Freestyle® bioprosthesis with other stentless bioprostheses, nor with homografts. The described patient group had been previously treated with homografts, but we did not consider it useful to compare results from 10 years ago with recent results. Prospective studies should examine durability and long-term valve-related complication free survival of patients treated with various models of stentless bioprostheses. Experience with reoperation for replacing a bioroot also needs further examination [21].

Conclusion

Aortic valve endocarditis with paravalvular abscess formation remains a therapeutic challenge for which stentless bioprosthesis is a credible surgical option. This prosthesis allows a radical and uniform approach with a good surgical overview and use of limited prosthetic material. It enables successful treatment of complex aortic valve endocarditis with complete debridement, elimination of shunts and anatomical deviations, reconstruction of the LVOT and aortomitral continuity. Stentless bioprostheses yield comparable clinical outcomes as the historical gold standard – the homograft – and are readily available. Of note, use of one type of prosthesis reduces logistical issues and purchasing costs.

Abbreviations
AML: Anterior mitral leaflet; LVOT: Left ventricular outflow tract; PPM: Permanent pacemaker

Acknowledgements
We thank Jakob Wilkens for the high-quality macroscopic pictures. We thank Andor Glaudemans and Niek Prakken for the FDG-PET and CTA images. We thank Massimiliano Crespi for the illustrations of intracardiac pathology. We thank Igor van der Weide for the total number of aortic valve endocarditis surgeries in our center. We thank Sebastian-Patrick Sommer for valuable discussions.

Funding
This work was supported by INTERREG project EurHealth-1Health [grant number 202085]; http://www.eurhealth-1health.eu/nl/home/. INTERREG had not intellectual role.

Authors' contributions

AG composed the report. JJ, SVA, PPVG, BS, SG, DMJ, EN supervised the report. All authors wrote, edited, and reviewed the manuscript. All authors read and approved the final manuscript.

Competing interests

The authors declare that they have no competing interests.

Author details

[1]Department of Medical Microbiology, University of Groningen, University Medical Center Groningen, Groningen, Netherlands. [2]Department of Anesthesiology, University of Groningen, University Medical Center Groningen, Groningen, Netherlands. [3]Department of Internal Medicine, Infectious Diseases, Treant Care Group, Hoogeveen, Netherlands. [4]Department of Cardiology, University of Groningen, University Medical Center Groningen, Groningen, Netherlands. [5]Department of Thoracic Surgery, Maastricht University Medical Center, Maastricht, Netherlands. [6]Department of Cardio-Thoracic Surgery, University of Groningen, University Medical Center Groningen, Groningen, Netherlands.

References

1. Murdoch DR, Corey GR, Hoen B, Miro JM, Fowler VG, Jr BAS, et al. Clinical presentation, etiology, and outcome of infective endocarditis in the 21st century: the international collaboration on endocarditis-prospective cohort study. Arch Intern Med. 2009;169(5):463–73.

2. Habib G, Lancellotti P, Antunes MJ, Bongiorni MG, Casalta JP, Del Zotti F, et al. 2015 ESC guidelines for the management of infective endocarditis: the task force for the management of infective endocarditis of the European Society of Cardiology (ESC). Endorsed by: European Association for Cardio-Thoracic Surgery (EACTS), the European Association of Nuclear Medicine (EANM). Eur Heart J. 2015;36(44):3075–128.

3. Moreillon P, Que YA. Infective endocarditis. Lancet. 2004;363(9403):139–49.

4. Li JS, Sexton DJ, Mick N, Nettles R, Fowler VG, Jr RT, et al. Proposed modifications to the Duke criteria for the diagnosis of infective endocarditis. Clin Infect Dis. 2000;30(4):633–8.

5. Prendergast BD, Tornos P. Surgery for infective endocarditis: who and when? Circulation. 2010;121(9):1141–52.

6. Vikram HR, Buenconsejo J, Hasbun R, Quagliarello VJ. Impact of valve surgery on 6-month mortality in adults with complicated, left-sided native valve endocarditis: a propensity analysis. JAMA. 2003;290(24):3207–14.

7. Kang DH, Kim YJ, Kim SH, Sun BJ, Kim DH, Yun SC, et al. Early surgery versus conventional treatment for infective endocarditis. N Engl J Med. 2012; 366(26):2466–73.

8. Schneider AW, Hazekamp MG, Versteegh MI, Bruggemans EF, Holman ER, Klautz RJ, et al. Stentless bioprostheses: a versatile and durable solution in extensive aortic valve endocarditis. Eur J Cardiothorac Surg. 2016;49(6): 1699–704.

9. Sponga S, Daffarra C, Pavoni D, Vendramin I, Mazzaro E, Piani D, et al. Surgical management of destructive aortic endocarditis: left ventricular outflow reconstruction with the Sorin Pericarbon freedom stentless bioprosthesis dagger. Eur J Cardiothorac Surg. 2016;49(1):242–8.

10. Byrne JG, Rezai K, Sanchez JA, Bernstein RA, Okum E, Leacche M, et al. Surgical management of endocarditis: the society of thoracic surgeons clinical practice guideline. Ann Thorac Surg. 2011;91(6):2012–9.

11. Bonow RO, Carabello BA, Chatterjee K, de Leon AC Jr, Faxon DP, Freed MD, et al. 2008 focused update incorporated into the ACC/AHA 2006 guidelines for the management of patients with valvular heart disease: a report of the American College of Cardiology/American Heart Association task force on practice guidelines (writing committee to revise the 1998 guidelines for the management of patients with valvular heart disease). Endorsed by the Society of Cardiovascular Anesthesiologists, Society for Cardiovascular Angiography and Interventions, and Society of Thoracic Surgeons. J Am Coll Cardiol. 2008;52(13):e1–142.

12. Sabik JF, Lytle BW, Blackstone EH, Marullo AG, Pettersson GB, Cosgrove DM. Aortic root replacement with cryopreserved allograft for prosthetic valve endocarditis. Ann Thorac Surg. 2002;74(3):650–9.

13. Perrotta S, Lentini S. In patients with severe active aortic valve endocarditis, is a stentless valve as good as the homograft? Interact Cardiovasc Thorac Surg. 2010;11(3):309–13.

14. Heinz A, Dumfarth J, Ruttmann-Ulmer E, Grimm M, Muller LC. Freestyle root replacement for complex destructive aortic valve endocarditis. J Thorac Cardiovasc Surg. 2014;147(4):1265–70.

15. Savage EB, Saha-Chaudhuri P, Asher CR, Brennan JM, Gammie JS. Outcomes and prosthesis choice for active aortic valve infective endocarditis: analysis of the Society of Thoracic Surgeons adult cardiac surgery database. Ann Thorac Surg. 2014;98(3):806–14.

16. Miceli A, Croccia M, Simeoni S, Varone E, Murzi M, Farneti PA, et al. Root replacement with stentless freestyle bioprostheses for active endocarditis: a single Centre experience. Interact Cardiovasc Thorac Surg. 2013;16(1):27–30.

17. Edlin P, Sartipy U. Freestyle xenograft for aortic valve endocarditis. J Thorac Cardiovasc Surg. 2014;147(1):542–3.

18. El-Hamamsy I, Clark L, Stevens LM, Sarang Z, Melina G, Takkenberg JJ, et al. Late outcomes following freestyle versus homograft aortic root replacement: results from a prospective randomized trial. J Am Coll Cardiol. 2010;55(4):368–76.

19. Nishimura RA, Otto CM, Bonow RO, Carabello BA, Erwin JP 3rd, Guyton RA, et al. 2014 AHA/ACC guideline for the management of patients with valvular heart disease: a report of the American College of Cardiology/ American Heart Association task force on practice guidelines. J Am Coll Cardiol. 2014;63(22):e57–185.

20. Davies A, Lai K, Bastian B. Acquired Gerbode defects associated with infective endocarditis. Heart Lung Circ. 2016;25(3):e59–61.

21. Dapunt OE, Easo J, Holzl PP, Murin P, Sudkamp M, Horst M, et al. Stentless full root bioprosthesis in surgery for complex aortic valve-ascending aortic disease: a single center experience of over 300 patients. Eur J Cardiothorac Surg. 2008;33(4):554–9.

22. Bozbuga N, Erentug V, Erdogan HB, Kirali K, Ardal H, Tas S, et al. Surgical treatment of aortic abscess and fistula. Tex Heart Inst J. 2004;31(4):382–6.

23. Borger MA, Prasongsukarn K, Armstrong S, Feindel CM, David TE. Stentless aortic valve reoperations: a surgical challenge. Ann Thorac Surg. 2007;84(3): 737–44.

13

Mid-term results of mitral valve repair using flexible bands versus complete rings in patients with degenerative mitral valve disease: a prospective, randomized study

Alexandr V. Bogachev-Prokophiev, Alexandr V. Afanasyev[*], Sergei I. Zheleznev, Vladimir M. Nazarov, Ravil M. Sharifulin and Alexandr M. Karaskov

Abstract

Background: We aimed to compare the outcomes of mitral valve repair with flexible band (FB) versus complete semirigid ring (SR) in degenerative mitral valve disease patients.

Methods: From September 2011 to 2014, 171 patients were randomized and underwent successful mitral valve repair using a SR ($n = 85$) or FB ($n = 86$). There were no significant between-group differences at baseline.

Results: There were no early mortalities. The mean follow up was 24.7 months. The 2-year survival was $96.0 \pm 2.3\%$ (95% confidence interval [CI], 88.6–98.7%) and $94.3 \pm 2.8\%$ (95% CI, 85.5–97.9%) in the SR and FB groups, respectively ($p = 0.899$). The left ventricle remodeling was similar between the groups. Higher transmitral peak (8.5 [3.9–17] vs. 6 [2.1–18] mmHg, $p < 0.001$), mean pressure gradients (3.7 [1.3–8] vs. 2.8 [0.6–6.8] mmHg, $p = 0.001$), and systolic pulmonary artery pressure (34.5 [20–68] vs. 29.5 [8–48] mmHg, $p < 0.001$) was observed in the SR group. The 2-year freedom from recurrence of significant mitral regurgitation was significantly higher in the FB group than the SR group ($p = 0.002$). Residual mitral regurgitation was an independent prognostic factor of recurrence of mitral regurgitation. The 3-year freedom from reoperation was significantly higher in the FB group than the SR group ($p = 0.044$).

Conclusion: Patients with degenerative mitral valve disease may benefit from valve repair with FBs. Residual mitral regurgitation before discharge is an independent risk factor of late insufficiency recurrence.

Keywords: Degenerative mitral valve disease, Mitral regurgitation, Mitral valve repair

Background

In 1957, Lillehei et al. [1] proposed the mitral annuloplasty technique, a new concept in valve surgery. Remodeling annuloplasty, developed by Carpentier in 1983, increases leaflet coaptation, prevents future annular dilatation, and preserves leaflet mobility in patients with degenerative mitral valve (MV) disease [2, 3]. Currently, there are many commercially available mitral annuloplasty devices in the market, including complete or partial, rigid or flexible, and flat or saddle-shaped rings. However, no single annuloplasty device has been proven to have a clinical benefit above the others [4]. Theoretically, the flexible band does remodel mitral annulus providing reduction annuloplasty only. However, the rigid ring does not have enough flexibility for physiological annular motion during the cardiac cycle. A systematic review of clinical trials [5] showed comparable clinical outcomes between rigid and flexible rings. Currently, mitral ring selection is based on a surgeon's preference rather than evidence [6]. Semirigid rings combine flexibility and stability; however, their clinical benefit has not been completely clarified. The present study aimed to compare the outcomes of MV repair with a flexible posterior annuloplasty band versus complete semirigid ring in patients with degenerative MV disease.

* Correspondence: av.afanasyev@icloud.com
Heart Valves Surgery Department, Meshalkin National Medical Research Center Ministry of Health Russian Federation, 15 Rechkunovskaya street, Novosibirsk, Russian Federation630055

Methods

Study design

In this prospective, randomized study, 171 patients with degenerative MV disease who were scheduled for isolated MV repair in our Institute from September 2011 through September 2014 were enrolled (CONSORT flow diagram, Figure 1). Participants were randomly assigned following a simple randomization procedure to complete semirigid ring (SR group) or flexible posterior annuloplasty band (FB group), according to computerized random numbers on the day before surgery. Eligible participants were adults aged 18 years or more with degenerative MV disease [7] who met the indications for MV operation according to the American College of Cardiology/American Heart Association guidelines [8]. Exclusion criteria were previous open cardiac surgery, indication for concomitant aortic valve replacement, or left ventricle (LV) impairment (ejection fraction <40%). The Local Ethics Committee approved the study design, and all the patients provided informed consent. The present study was conducted in compliance with the Declaration of Helsinki.

Patients

Mean age of the participants in each group was 57 (23–75) and 54 (19–74) years, respectively. There were no differences in sex, age, preoperative New York Heart Association (NYHA) functional class, and comorbidities (Table 1).

Outcome measures

The primary endpoint was freedom from moderate or severe mitral regurgitation (MR) recurrence. Secondary endpoints included survival, freedom from reoperations, and freedom from severe MR recurrence. The severity of MR was evaluated and defined in accordance with the recommendations [9]. Valve-related complications were evaluated and defined in accordance with the guidelines [10].

Surgical techniques

Real-time two-dimensional/three-dimensional transesophageal echocardiography (TEE, Phillips iE33, Philips Ultrasound Inc., PA, USA) was performed after the induction of anesthesia for MV lesion estimation. Cold crystalloid

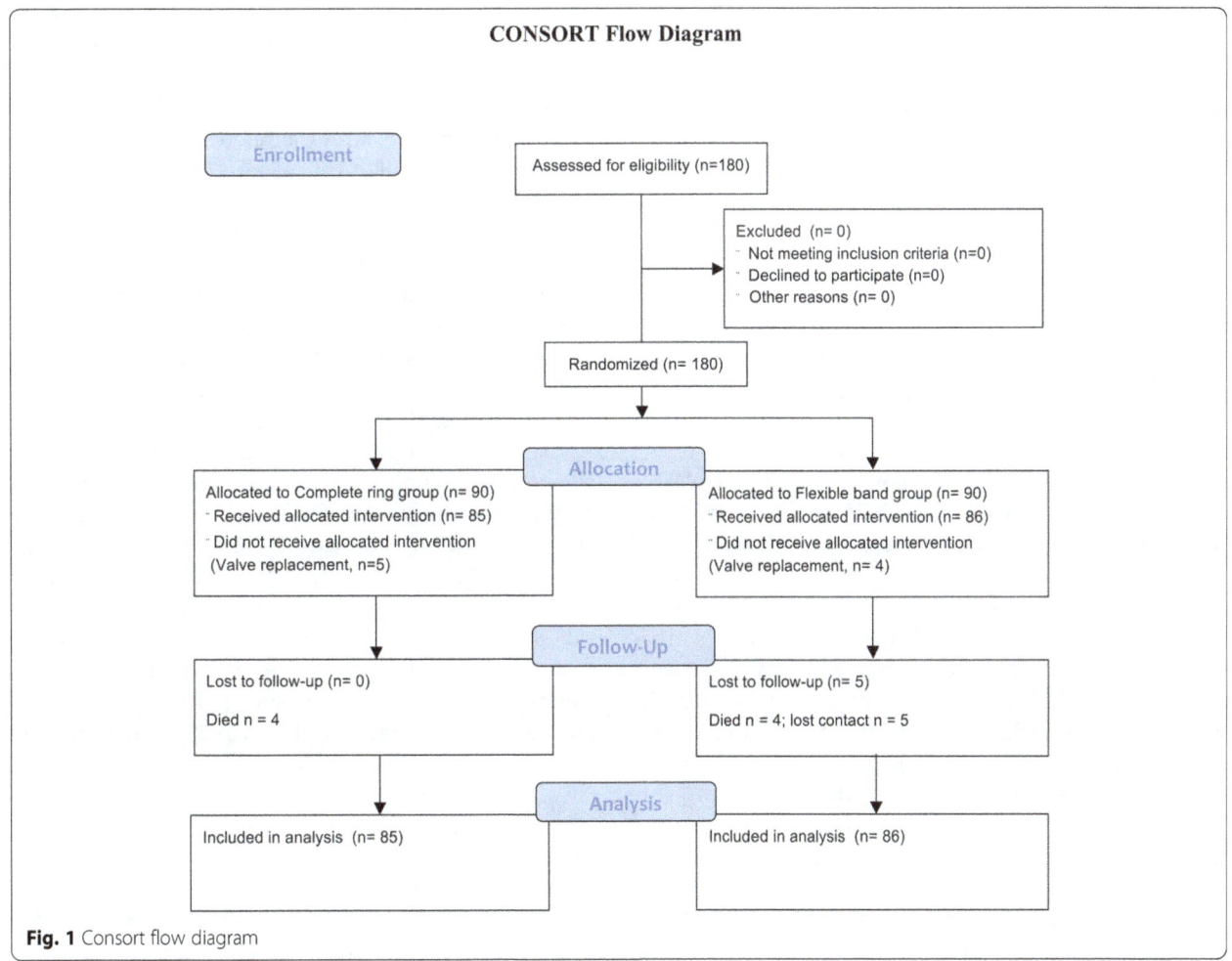

CONSORT Flow Diagram

Enrollment

Assessed for eligibility (n=180)

Excluded (n= 0)
- Not meeting inclusion criteria (n=0)
- Declined to participate (n=0)
- Other reasons (n= 0)

Randomized (n= 180)

Allocation

Allocated to Complete ring group (n= 90)
- Received allocated intervention (n= 85)
- Did not receive allocated intervention (Valve replacement, n=5)

Allocated to Flexible band group (n= 90)
- Received allocated intervention (n= 86)
- Did not receive allocated intervention (Valve replacement, n= 4)

Follow-Up

Lost to follow-up (n= 0)

Died n = 4

Lost to follow-up (n= 5)

Died n = 4; lost contact n = 5

Analysis

Included in analysis (n= 85)

Included in analysis (n= 86)

Fig. 1 Consort flow diagram

Table 1 Baseline

	SR Group, n = 85	FB Group, n = 86	P value
FED, n (%)	65 (76.5)	56 (65.1)	0.103
Forme fruste, n (%)	12 (14.1)	18 (20.9)	0.241
Barlow, n (%)	8 (9.4)	12 (14.0)	0.355
Male, n (%)	59 (69.4)	58 (67.4)	0.782
Age, years	57 (23–75)	54 (19–74)	0.092
Height, cm	173 (148–192)	175 (151;193)	0.079
Weight, kg	79.1 ± 14.6	77.1 ± 16.4	0.388
BMI, kg/m²	26.9 ± 4.3	25.4 ± 4.6	0.522
BSA, m²	1.94 ± 0.21	1.93 ± 0.24	0.801
NYHA I, n (%)	7 (8.2)	12 (14.0)	0.234
NYHA II, n (%)	22 (25.9)	29 (33.7)	0.263
NYHA III, n (%)	54 (63.5)	43 (50.0)	0.742
NYHA IV, n (%)	2 (2.4)	2 (2.3)	0.991
AF, n (%)	22 (25.9)	16 (18.6)	0.252
Paroxysmal, n (%)	2 (2.4)	2 (2.3)	0.991
Persistent, n (%)	5 (5.9)	3 (3.5)	0.459
Long-standing, n (%)	11 (12.9)	9 (10.5)	0.614
Permanent, n (%)	4 (4.7)	2 (2.3)	0.398
CAD, n (%)	10 (11.8)	4 (4.7)	0.090
Arterial hypertension, n (%)	46 (54.1)	42 (48.8)	0.490
Diabetes mellitus, n (%)	4 (4.7)	5 (5.8)	0.746
Moderate renal impairment, n (%)	1 (1.2)	1 (1.2)	0.993
Peripheral vascular disease, n (%)	5 (5.9)	3 (3.5)	0.459
Cerebrovascular disease, n (%)	5 (5.9)	4 (4.7)	0.719
LV EF, %	65.5 (49–80)	67.0 (51–89)	0.212
PA pressure, mm Hg	48.5 (29–80)	45.0 (29–94)	0.053

SR semirigid ring, *FB* flexible band, *BMI* body mass index, *BSA* body surface area, *NYHA* New York Heart Association functional class, *AF* atrial fibrillation, *CAD* coronary artery disease, *LV EF* left ventricle ejection fraction, *PA* pulmonary artery

cardioplegic solution (Custodiol® HTK Solution, Dr. Franz Köhler Chemie, Alsbach-Hahnlein, Germany) was used for myocardial protection with antegrade root flow.

The two most experienced surgeons in MV repair in our Institute performed the operations in the study. Surgeons were evenly split between the treatment groups. The surgical technique for MV repair was chosen according to the MV lesion (Table 2). The most common techniques were quadrangular ("sliding maneuver") or triangular resection for posterior MV prolapse, and artificial chordal replacement (separate or loop technique) for anterior leaflet pathology. The minimally invasive approach through the right fourth intercostal space with femoral–femoral cannulation for arterial and venous lines was

used in 29.4% (n = 25) and 31.4% (n = 27) of patients in the SR and FB groups, respectively.

All mitral valve repairs were performed with flexible bands ("C Flex", CardiaMed, Penza, Russia) or complete rings ("D Ring", CardiaMed, Penza, Russia), which routinely use since 2005. The ring size was selected according to the size of the anterior leaflet and the inter-trigonal distance. In Barlow's cases, 36–40 mm rings were used. Flexible bands were implanted along the posterior mitral semicircle with an extension to both commissures for 3–5 mm. Valve competence was assessed intraoperatively by saline test and "ink-test" (symmetrical closure line, coaptation depth ≥ 5 mm, absence of leaflet prolapse and regurgitation jet).

After bypass weaning, patients were followed-up with TEE. In cases with residual MR ≥ grade 2, cardiopulmonary bypass was re-established, and the valve was re-repaired or replaced; residual MR grade 1 (mild) was left alone. Intraoperative data and concomitant procedures are shown in Table 2.

Patient follow-up

All patients underwent TTE evaluation before discharge. In total, 170 patients were discharged and followed-up periodically by cardiologists and surgeons. After discharge, examinations were scheduled annually. When annual clinic visits were unavailable, follow-up was performed by contact with the referring cardiologist, the patient or their family. Anticoagulation therapy with an international normalized ratio (INR) target in the range of 2.5–3.0 was prescribed for all patients after surgery. The decision to stop anticoagulation therapy with Coumadin was based on echocardiography (normal left ventricle function, presence of atrial contractility) and Holter data (absence of atrial fibrillation, flutter, tachycardia) after 3 months. Echocardiograms obtained from outside physicians were re-analyzed at our Institute by the most experienced echocardiographers. Clinical follow-up was completed in 165 patients (97.1%), and five patients were lost to follow-up. Follow-up echocardiography was performed 6–12 months after the operation and every year thereafter. Seventy-nine (94.0%) of the 84 discharged patients in the SR group and 78 (90.7%) of the 86 patients in the FB group underwent follow-up TTE. The mean duration from the operation to echocardiographic follow-up was 20.2 (95% confidence interval [CI], 18.6–21.8) months. The mean clinical follow-up period was 24.7 (95% CI, 23.5–27.0) months.

Statistical analysis

Assuming 5% significance (two sided), 80% power, event rates of 20 and 5% in the complete ring and flexible band groups, respectively, and a hazard ratio for

Table 2 Intraoperative data

	SR Group, n = 85	FB Group, n = 86	P value
Approach:			
Conventional, n (%)	60 (70.6)	59 (65.1)	0.778
Minimally invasive, n (%)	25 (29.4)	27 (31.4)	0.778
CPB time, min	140 (110;179.5)	160 (122;206)	0.091
Cross clamp time, min:			
Conventional	92 (73;117)	101 (79;125)	0.230
Minimally invasive	116 (101;129)	123 (106;156)	0.171
Mitral valve analyze and intervention in certain patients			
A₁ prolapse, n (%)	9 (10.6)	11 (12.8)	0.654
A₂ prolapse, n (%)	23 (27.1)	33 (38.4)	0.115
A₃ prolapse, n (%)	13 (15.3)	19 (22.1)	0.254
P₁ prolapse, n (%)	6 (7.1)	12 (13.9)	0.142
P₂ prolapse, n (%)	59 (69.4)	68 (79.1)	0.119
P₃ prolapse, n (%)	17 (20.0)	27 (31.4)	0.088
AMVL prolapse, n (%)	31 (36.5)	40 (46.5)	0.183
PMVL prolapse, n (%)	73 (85.9)	74 (86.1)	0.975
DMVL prolapse, n (%)	19 (22.4)	28 (32.5)	0.135
Chordae rupture, n (%)	64 (75.3)	53 (61.6)	0.055
AMVL resection, n (%)	1 (1.2)	4 (4.7)	0.178
PMVL resection, n (%)	37 (43.5)	49 (56.9)	0.079
AMVL neochordae, n (%)	22 (25.9)	29 (33.7)	0.263
PMVL neochordae, n (%)	30 (35.3)	27 (31.4)	0.589
Ring size, mm	32 (30;32)	34 (30;34)	0.456
Concomitant procedure			
Maze IV procedure, n (%)	18 (21.2)	14 (16.3)	0.412
CABG, n (%)	10 (11.8)	4 (4.7)	0.090
TV repair, n (%)	32 (37.6)	24 (27.9)	0.175
SAM-syndrome, n (%)	0	1 (1.2)	0.319
Intraoperative TEE			
Depth of coaptation, mm	9 (7;11)	6 (5;8)	0.006
Peak MV gradient, mm Hg	8.0 (6.7;10.9)	6.4 (4;9)	<0.001
Mean MV gradient, mm Hg	3 (2.4;4)	2 (2;3.9)	<0.001

SR semirigid ring, *FB* flexile band, *AMVL* anterior mitral valve leaflet, *PMVL* posterior mitral valve leaflet, *DMVL prolapse* dual (anterior and posterior) mitral valve leaflet prolapse, *CABG* coronary artery bypass grafting, *TV* tricuspid valve, *CPB* cardiopulmonary bypass, *TEE* transesophageal echocardiography

significant MR recurrence of 0.23 and expected 5% withdrawal rate, the sample size (total n = 170 in both groups) was calculated using log-rank test (Freedman method) of freedom from MR recurrences in two groups. Data are presented as mean ± SD or median with range. The variables of the two groups were compared using the unpaired t test for continuous variables with normal distribution or the Mann-Whitney U test for other distributions. To analyze the risk factors of early postoperative complications, we reviewed preoperative

and intraoperative variables (Tables 1, 2, 3); a multivariate logistic regression model was used to calculate odds ratios (ORs). Estimates of survival and event-free survival for reoperation and the recurrence of significant MR were calculated using the Kaplan-Meier method and are reported with 95% CIs. Patients were censored at the time of reoperation or at the time of death. Estimates are reported with their standard errors. Comparison of the curves was established by using the log-rank test for mid-term results. To analyze risk factors of late mortality, reoperation, and MR recurrence, we reviewed preoperative and intraoperative variables (Tables 1, 2, 3); multivariable Cox proportional hazard regression models were used to calculate HRs. HRs and 95% CIs were calculated. The inclusion criterion for the multivariable model was P value ≤0.2) in the univariable analysis. The significance level in the final "multivariable" model assessed as the 0.05. Stata/MP for Windows v. 13.0 (StataCorp. 2013. *Stata Statistical Software: Release 13*. College Station, TX: StataCorp LP.) was used for the statistical analysis.

Results

Overall repair rate was 95%. The mean (median) cross clamp time did not differ between the SR and FB groups. The subgroup analysis of variances by the surgical approach revealed no differences in cross clamp time between the minimally invasive (25 and 27 patients, respectively, p = 0.171) and median sternotomy subgroups (60 and 59 patients, respectively, p = 0.230).

The incidence of systolic anterior motion (SAM) syndrome was observed in 1 patient in the FB group. Conservative management was not effective and SAM was successfully treated using posterior MV leaflet folding technique. Two patients from SR group were re-repaired due to residual moderate MR revealed by intraoperative TEE.

Intraoperative TEE control revealed that MV coaptation depth was significantly higher in the SR group than the FB group (9 [7–11] vs. 6 [5–8] mm; p = 0.006); however, the FB group had a lower rate of peak and mean transmitral pressure gradients (p < 0.001; Table 2).

There were no early (at 30/60/90 days) deaths. One 65 years old man with p3 prolapse and coronary artery

Table 3 Echocardiography data

	SR Group, n = 85					FB Group, n = 86					Group comparison, P value		
	Baseline	At discharge	P value at discharge	Follow up, n = 79	P value	Baseline	At discharge	P value at discharge	Follow up, n = 78	P value	Baseline	At discharge	Follow up
RA, cm	5.4 (4.1–8.9)	4.9 (4.0–7.9)	<0.001	4.8 (3.6–7.8)	0.499	5.3 (3.3–8.5)	4.8 (3.7–6.8)	<0.001	4.8 (3.0–7.5)	0.805	0.155	0.187	0.204
LA, cm	6.1 (4.3–9.6)	5.2 (4.4–8.2)	<0.001	5.1 (3.5–7.9)	0.460	5.7 (4.4–9.5)	5.1 (4.0–7.2)	<0.001	4.9 (3.2–7.2)	0.070	0.070	0.067	0.291
S MO (Doppler) cm^2	3.8 (2.6–6.9)	3.3 (2.4;7.6)	<0.001	3.2 (1.9–5.7)	0.806	4.1 (2.8–9.8)	3.3 (2.6–4.9)	<0.001	3.3 (1.8–4.8)	0.054	0.062	0.202	0.699
Peak MV pressure gradient, mm Hg	8.7 (3–24)	8.8 (2.7–17.0)	0.684	8.5 (3.9–17)	0.206	7.9 (3.0–22.0)	7.0 (2.1–15.2)	0.027	6 (2.1–18.0)	0.212	0.680	<0.001	<0.001
Mean MV pressure gradient, mm Hg	2.8 (1–8)	3.0 (1.0–8.0)	0.236	3.7 (1.3–8.0)	0.288	2.6 (1.0–7.0)	2.7 (0.9–5.7)	0.872	2.8 (0.6–6.8)	0.232	0.985	0.002	0.001
Severe MR, n (%)	85 (100)	0	<0.001	7 (8.9)	0.023	86 (100)	0	<0.001	1 (1.3)	1.0	1.0	1.0	0.031
Total moderate or severe MR, n (%)	85 (100)	5 (5.9)	<0.001	12 (15.2)	0.023	86 (100)	4 (4.6)	<0.001	7 (9.0)	0.248	1.0	0.719	0.343
LV EDD, cm	5.78 ± 0.59	5.03 ± 0.53	<0.001	4.82 ± 0.67	0.135	5.78 ± 0.74	5.04 ± 0.52	<0.001	4.83 ± 0.47	0.017	0.962	0.874	0.908
LV ESD, cm	3.49 ± 0.55	3.36 ± 0.49	0.055	3.3 ± 0.7	0.731	3.51 ± 0.71	3.35 ± 0.58	0.783	3.15 ± 0.46	<0.001	0.815	0.891	0.263
LV EDV, ml	172.5 ± 42.0	120.9 ± 32.6	<0.001	111.2 ± 42.7	0.487	169.0 ± 50.0	123.4 ± 32.3	<0.001	105 ± 23.1	0.001	0.624	0.618	0.375
LV ESV, ml	53.0 (19–145)	44.5 (22–135)	<0.001	35 (18–102)	0.130	50.5 (16–146)	45 (20–140)	0.165	38 (18–154)	<0.001	0.127	0.360	0.808
LV EF, %	65.5 (49–80)	61 (35–76)	<0.001	61 (35–87)	0.518	67.0 (51–89)	59 (35–78)	<0.001	65 (36–78)	<0.001	0.212	0.247	0.043
PA systolic pressure, mm Hg	48.5 (42;56)	36 (29–46)	0.003	34.5 (20–68)	0.080	45 (39;54.5)	36.5 (25–49)	<0.001	29.5 (8–48)	0.833	0.0n3	0.416	<0.001

SR semirigid ring, *FB* flexible band, *RA* size of right atrium, *LA* size of left atrium, *S MO* mitral orifice area, *MV* mitral valve, *MR* mitral regurgitation, *LV* left ventricle, *EDD* end diastolic diameter, *ESD* end systolic diameter, *EDV* end diastolic volume, *ESV* end systolic volume, *EF* ejection fraction, *PA* pulmonary artery

disease who was underwent triangular posterior leaflet resection and concomitant CABG in the SR group died after 6 months of hospital stay because of severe multiple organ failure. Two patients (one from each group) with severe LV systolic dysfunction in early postoperative period required extracorporeal life support with complete recovering after 7 days.

The mean intensive care unit stay was 2 days in both groups (*p* = 0.453). Ventilation and inotropic support time also did not differ between the groups (Table 4). There were no significant differences in terms of heart failure, prolonged ventilation or requirement of extracorporeal life support. Electrical cardioversion for atrial fibrillation paroxysm was required in 7 (8.2%) and 3 (3.5%) cases in the SR and FB groups, respectively (*p* = 0.186). Five patients (SR group, 4 vs. FB group, 1; *p* = 0.169) were re-explored for bleeding on the first postoperative day. Pacemaker implantation rates were 5.9% (due to sinus node dysfunction, 3 patients; complete AV-conductance disturbances, 2 patients) and 4.7% (due to sinus node dysfunction, 3 patients; complete AV-conductance disturbances, 1 patient) in the SR and FB groups, respectively (*p* = 0.719).

There were no significant between-group differences in major valve-related complications. There were no cases of thromboembolic events, leakage, or structural dysfunction. There were 4 cases of transient ischemic attack with reversible neurologic deficits in the SR group versus none in the FB group (*p* = 0.042).

The median length of hospital stay after MV repair in the SR and FB groups was 17 (9–178) and 17 (7–36) days, respectively (*p* = 0.455, Table 4). The preoperative independent predictor of heart failure was left ventricular ejection fraction (LVEF) (OR, 0.94; 95% CI, 0.9–0.98); of myocardial infarction – cardiopulmonary bypass time with 1-min step (OR, 1.03; 95% CI, 1.01–1.1); and prolonged ventilation – preoperative NYHA functional class (OR, 2.6; 95% CI, 1.2–5.7).

Echocardiographic results
All echocardiographic parameters significantly changed from the preoperative to immediate postoperative period at discharge, except transmitral pressure gradients and LV end-systolic diameter (LVESD) (Table 3). There were no significant between-group differences in changes in LV function and left and right atria remodeling; however, transmitral peak and mean pressure gradients were

significantly lower in the FB group. The mitral orifice area did not differ between the groups. The TTE before discharge revealed that 5 (5.9%) and 4 (4.7%) patients in the SR and FB groups, respectively, had grade 2 residual MR ($p = 0.719$). Follow-up echocardiography data at 24 months are shown in Table 3. The repeated-measures analysis of variance in the FB group revealed significant changes in LV end-diastolic diameter (LVEDD), LV end-diastolic volume (LVEDV), and LV end-systolic volume (LVESV) at discharge; moreover, these parameters and LVESD were also decreased at 24 months of follow up. Meanwhile, the LVEF significantly decreased at discharge; however, it significantly increased during the follow-up. In the SR group, there were no significant differences in LV function changes at serial examinations. We also revealed higher transmitral pressure gradients in the SR group, including significant differences in systolic pulmonary artery pressure among patients with sinus rhythm, with favorable results in the FB group.

Survival analysis

At the latest follow-up, 158 patients were alive. There were 3 late deaths among the 84 patients in the SR group (mortality 3.6%), and 4 late deaths among the 81 patients in the FB group (mortality 4.9%). The causes of death in the SR group were endocarditis (1 case), malignancy (1 case), and unknown cause (1 case); two of them were regarded as cardiac-related deaths. The causes of death in the FB group were ischemic stroke (2 cases), acute myocardial infarction (1 case), and pulmonary edema (1 case), all of which were cardiac-related. The Kaplan-Meier survival rates at 2 years were 96.0 ± 2.3% (95% CI, 88.6–98.7%) and 94.3 ± 2.8% (95% CI, 85.5–97.9%) in the SR and FB groups, respectively (Figure 2) (log-rank, $p = 0.899$).

The Kaplan-Meier freedom from cardiac-related death at 2 years was 97.7 ± 2.0% (95% CI, 89.1–99.3%) and 94.3 ± 2.8% (95% CI, 85.5–97.9%) in the SR and FB groups, respectively (Additional file 1: Figure S1) (log-rank, $p = 0.411$). The multivariable Cox regression hazard model did not identify independent risk factors of late death.

Clinical status

Before surgery, 65.9% and 52.3% of patients in the SR and FB groups, respectively, had an NYHA functional classification of III and IV. Most patients demonstrated significant improvement of functional capacity at the last follow-up (43.2% and 34.6% of 81 SR patients and 44.1% and 40.3% of 77 FB patients had an NYHA functional classification of I and II, respectively). A total of 57 (75%) and 61 (84.7%) patients presented with sinus rhythm in the SR and FB groups, respectively ($p = 0.201$).

Thromboembolism and anticoagulation-related hemorrhage

There was no major bleeding case during follow-up. Two patients form each group had transient ischemic attack. In the FB group, 2 out of 3 patients who had stroke died. Two patients had atrial fibrillation and were kept on anticoagulation therapy, and another one was in sinus rhythm at the last follow up and was not anticoagulated. Central retina occlusion occurred in 1 case in each group. The overall freedom from thromboembolic events at 3 years after MV repair in the SR and FB groups was 94.7 ± 3.6% (95% CI, 80.6–98.7%) and

Table 4 Early (30-days) results

	SR Group, $n = 85$	FB Group, $n = 86$	P value
Hospital mortality[a], n (%)	1 (1.2)	0	0.313
ICU stay, days	2 (1–14)	2 (1–14)	0.453
Ventilation time, h	7 (0–49)	5 (1–41)	0.068
Inotropic support, h	10 (0–151)	14 (0–105)	0.591
Heart failure, n (%)	23 (27.1)	19 (22.1)	0.451
Prolonged ventilation, n (%)	14 (16.5)	15 (17.4)	0.866
ECLS, n (%)	1 (1.2)	1 (1.2)	0.993
AF Early paroxysm, n (%),	39 (45.9)	30 (34.9)	0.143
Electrical cardioversion, n (%)	7 (8.2)	3 (3.5)	0.186
Valve-related complications, n (%):			
MI, n (%)	5 (5.9)	3 (3.5)	0.459
TIA, n (%)	4 (4.7)	0	0.042
Stroke, n (%)	0	1 (1.2)	0.319
AKF, n (%)	5 (5.9)	4 (4.7)	0.719
IE, n (%)	1 (1.2)	1 (1.2)	0.993
Ring dehiscence, n (%)	1 (1.2)	0	0.313
Leak, n (%)	0	0	–
Thrombosis, n (%)	0	0	–
Other embolic events, n (%)	0	0	–
Structural dysfunction, n (%)	0	0	–
Bleeding, n (%);	9 (10.6)	6 (7.0)	0.404
Re-exploration for bleeding, n (%)	4 (4.7)	1 (1.2)	0.169
Lymphorrhea, n (%)	0	1 (1.2)	0.319
Pacemaker implantation, n (%)	5 (5.9)	4 (4.7)	0.719
Pleural effusion, n (%)	14 (16.5)	20 (23.2)	0.266
Deep sternal infection, n (%)	0	0	–
Superficial infection, n (%)	1 (1.2)	1 (1.2)	0.993
Hospital stay, days	17 (9–178)	17 (7–36)	0.455

SR semirigid ring, *FB* flexible band, *ICU* intensive care unit, *ECLS* extracorporeal life support, *AF* atrial fibrillation, *MI* myocardial infarction, *TIA* transient ischemic attack, *AKF* acute kidney failure, *IE* infective endocarditis
[a]hospital death occurred 6 months after surgery

90.8 ± 3.7% (95% CI, 80.4–95.9%), respectively (log-rank, p = 0.416).

Infective endocarditis

Three patients had infective endocarditis. Two of them were in the SR group, and one of them died because of pacemaker lead endocarditis and heart failure. The 2 patients who survived were treated with antibiotics alone. Freedom from infective endocarditis at 3 years was 97.3 ± 1.9% (95% CI, 89.4–99.3%) and 98.5 ± 1.5% (95% CI, 89.9–99.8%) in the SR and FB groups, respectively (log-rank, p = 0.573).

Recurrence of mitral regurgitation

Moderate or severe MR was observed in 12 (15.2%) of 79 patients and 7 (9.0%) of 78 patients in the SR and FB groups, respectively (p = 0.343). Among them, 3 patients in the SR group underwent redo MV surgery. The Kaplan-Meier estimate for freedom from recurrence of moderate or severe MR at 2 years was 85.3 ± 5.0% (95% CI, 71.9–92.6%) and 95.3 ± 2.7% (95% CI, 85.9–98.5%) in the SR and FB groups, respectively, (log-rank test, p = 0.011) (Figure 3A). The multivariable Cox proportional hazard model identified residual MR before discharge as an independent risk factor of late recurrence of significant MR (HR, 4.1; 95% CI, 1.5–11.5) (Additional file 2: Table S1).

Among them, severe MR was observed in 7 (9.7%) and 1 (1.3%) patient(s) in the SR and FB groups, respectively. The Kaplan-Meier estimate for freedom from severe MR at 2 years was 84.8 ± 6.8% (95% CI, 65.1–93.8%) and 98.7 ± 1.3% (95% CI, 90.8–99.8%) in the SR and FB groups, respectively (log-rank test, p = 0.006) (Figure 3B). The multivariable Cox proportional hazard model identified residual MR before discharge as an independent risk factor of late recurrence of severe MR (HR, 8.4; 95% CI, 1.6–43.3).

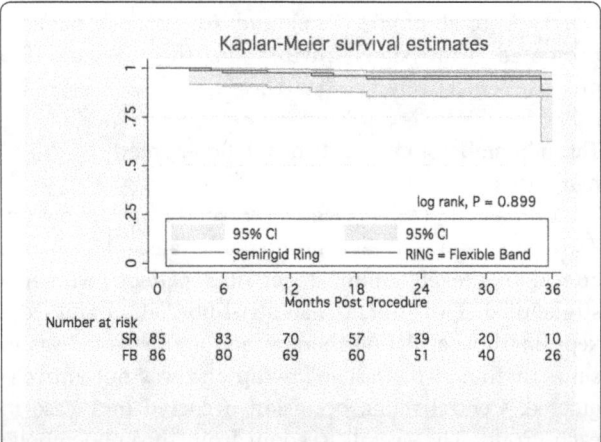

Fig. 2 Kaplan-Meier survival estimates. Abbreviation: SR – semirigid ring; CI, confidence interval

Reoperations

Reoperations were required in 3 patients in the SR group for partial ring dehiscence in all cases. The MV was re-repaired in 2 patients and replaced in 1 case. The Kaplan-Meier estimate for freedom from reoperation at 2 years of follow-up was 97.0 ± 2.1% (95% CI, 88.4–99.3%) and 100% in the SR and FB groups, respectively (Figure 4) (log-rank, p = 0.044). The Cox regression hazard model did not identify any preoperative or intraoperative risk factor of late reoperations.

Discussion

In the late 1960's, Carpentier developed annuloplasty rings, considered the "gold standard" for the surgical treatment of MR [11]. Subsequent studies showed that the MV annulus continually changes size and shape during the cardiac cycle [12–14]. This led to the development of a flexible ring that could conform to the physiologic changing annular shape [15, 16]. However, there is controversy regarding the optimal mechanical characteristics of annuloplasty rings and the use of rigid rings or flexible bands in degenerative MV disease [5, 17].

David et al. [18] conducted one of the first randomized studies comparing the rigid ring (13 patients) and flexible ring (12 patients). The results showed significantly better LV systolic function and stroke volume/LVEDV index in the flexible group and no significant reduction in LVESV and LVESD in the rigid ring group. However, the clinical outcomes of these 2 ring types have not been reported. In the present study, there were similar results in LV changes with no significant differences between the SR and FB groups intermediately and 2 years post-surgery. However, only the FB group showed a significant reduction in LVEDD, LVESD, LVEDV, and LVESV (when comparing postoperative values and those 2 years postsurgery).

Chang et al. conducted the largest randomized trial (363 patients) comparing the Carpentier-Edwards rigid ring and flexible Duran annuloplasty ring [19]. The mean duration from the operation to follow-up echocardiography was 26.7 ± 24.1 months. LVEF, LVESD, and LVEDD parameters changed significantly at serial examinations in both groups with no significant difference between the two ring types. There were no significant differences in survival, reoperation rates, and recurrences of significant MR at a mean follow-up of 46.6 ± 32.6 months. However, their study was limited by the heterogeneous MR etiology, the long recruitment period, and the fact that the echocardiography parameters were not presented at separate time points, which may have caused bias.

Shahin et al. [20] conducted a randomized study comparing the Carpentier-Edwards rigid Classic and

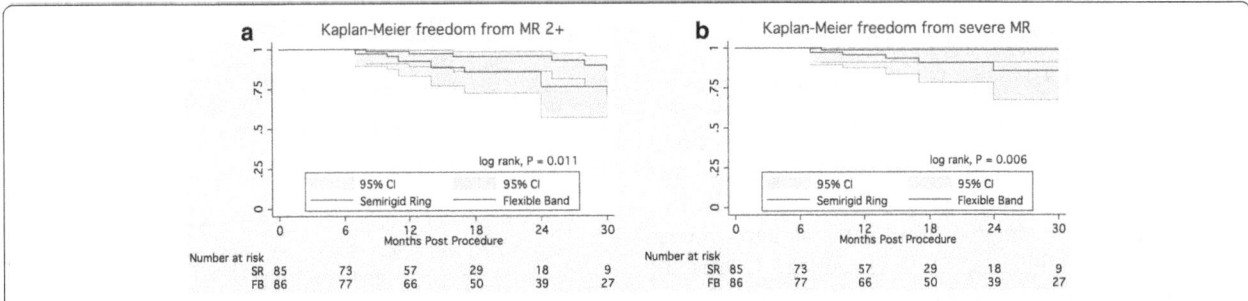

Fig. 3 a. Kaplan-Meier freedom from moderate and severe mitral regurgitation. **b**. Kaplan-Meier freedom from severe mitral regurgitation. Abbreviation: MR, mitral regurgitation; SR – semirigid ring; CI, confidence interval

semi-flexible Physio rings (mean follow up, 5.1 years). There were no between-groups differences in terms of mortality, morbidity, and LV function. However, an unexplained 16% difference in mortality was considered clinically important.

At least 3 randomized studies did not demonstrate the clinical benefits of flexible or rigid types of annuloplasty devices [18–20]. However, one of them [18] suggested better LV systolic function with flexible rings. Similar results were reported by Okada et al. [21], and concern that rigid rings could restrict LV wall motion was raised.

In a prospective echocardiographic study by Unger-Graeber et al. [22], no significant difference was shown between the Carpentier rigid ring and flexible Duran ring in terms of transmitral velocity and pressure gradient. In contrast, our study showed higher transmitral pressure gradients in the SR group.

After David et al. criticized the rigid ring for impaired LV function [18] and Kreindel et al. [23] reported the potential risk of SAM syndrome after rigid ring annuloplasty, Carpentier et al. introduced a new concept of mitral annuloplasty with the semirigid prosthetic ring, which combines remodeling and flexibility [24]. At mid-term follow-up between 6 and 18 months, 93.2% of 94 followed-up patients were free from MR

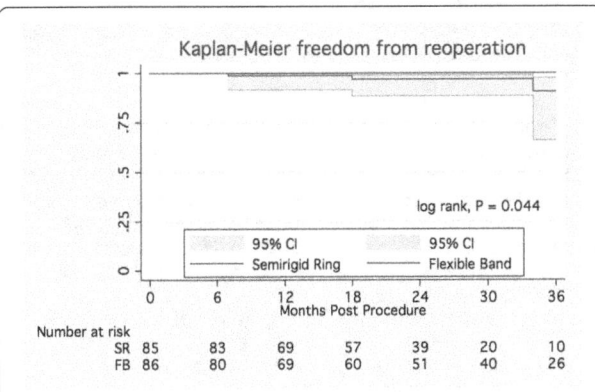

Fig. 4 Kaplan-Meier freedom from reoperations. Abbreviation: SR – semirigid ring; CI, confidence interval

recurrence with a transmitral pressure gradient at 3.55 ± 1.93 mmHg. Thereafter, excellent mid-term results with semirigid rings have been reported by other investigators [25, 26]. Since then, the concept of a semirigid ring has gained popularity, and the semirigid ring (instead of the rigid ring) has been successfully adopted in mitral annuloplasty for degenerative MV disease. Flexible posterior annuloplasty bands have also shown high effectiveness in preserving mitral annulus flexibility and provide good mid-term and long-term durability [4, 27, 28].

The semirigid ring and flexible ring have not been sufficiently compared. An animal randomized study [29] showed that LV function was not altered with either flexible or semirigid ring annuloplasty. A Japanese, retrospective, propensity score matched study [30] evaluated intermediate echocardiography results only. The overall cohort's LVEF decreased during the first week after surgery and then recovered gradually at 6 months and 1 year; LVEDD abruptly decreased and LVESD minimally decreased at the first week postoperatively, then gradually decreased at 6 months and later stabilized. There were no significant between-group differences in LVEF, LVEDD, and LVESD. They suggested that the semirigid ring might prevent LV impairment compared with the rigid ring. However, their study was limited by the retrospective design, low rate of followed-up patients, and difference in annuloplasty devices used in the flexible group.

Previously was shown that experience in mitral valve repair is an important determinant of operative efficiency and late survival [31], in our study both surgeons are well experienced and evenly split between groups. However, our results seem different to Castillo JG report [32]. We assume that limited experience in Barlow valves disease was influenced for our results. In this view complex mitral valve cases should be consolidated and addressed to one surgeon. It might be helpful to use scoring system [33] to allow stratification of complexity for degenerative mitral valve repair for improving results and develop local expertise.

We examined the immediate and mid-term results of patients with degenerative MV disease who underwent primary MV repair with a complete semirigid ring or flexible posterior annuloplasty band. Both groups had comparable early clinical results; however, the SR group had better coaptation depth, while the FB group demonstrated significantly lower transmitral pressure gradients. At serial echocardiographic examinations, only the FB group showed significant LV remodeling. Consistent with previous studies, there were no between-group differences in overall survival, freedom from cardiac-related death, and follow-up LV remodeling. Our study is the first to show the superiority of the flexible posterior band over the semirigid complete ring in terms of freedom from recurrences of significant and/or severe MR and risk of MV reoperation.

Conclusion

The present study is limited by the 2-year follow-up period and single-center design. Important limitation is low number of patients at late risk. Further study with a longer follow-up is warranted. In conclusion, patients with degenerative MV disease may benefit from valve repair with flexible bands. Residual MR is an independent risk factor of late insufficiency recurrence.

Abbreviations

CI: Confidence interval; HR: Hazard ratio; ITT: Intention-to-treat; LV: Left ventricle; LVEDD: Left ventricle end-diastolic diameter; LVEDV: Left ventricle end-diastolic volume; LVEF: Left ventricular ejection fraction; LVESD: Left ventricle end-systolic diameter; LVESV: Left ventricle end-systolic volume; MR: Mitral regurgitation; MV: Mitral valve; NYHA: New York Heart Association; OR: Odds ratio; SAM: Systolic anterior motion; TEE: Transesophageal echocardiography

Acknowledgements

We would like to thank Editage for their editorial support.

Funding

This research received no specific grant from any funding agency in the public, commercial, or not-for-profit sectors.

Authors' contributions

Please contact author for data requests. All authors read and approved the final manuscript.

Competing interests

The authors declare that they have no competing interests.

References

1. Lillehei CW, Gott VL, Dewall RA, Varco RL. Surgical correction of pure mitral insufficiency by annuloplasty under direct vision. J Lancet. 1957;77:446–9.
2. Carpentier A. Cardiac valve surgery–the "French correction". J Thorac Cardiovasc Surg. 1983;86:323–37.
3. Filsoufi F, Carpentier A. Principles of reconstructive surgery in degenerative mitral valve disease. Semin Thorac Cardiovasc Surg. 2007;19:103–10.
4. Brown ML, Schaff HV, Li Z, Suri RM, Daly RC, Orszulak TA. Results of mitral valve annuloplasty with a standard-sized posterior band: is measuring important? J Thorac Cardiovasc Surg. 2009;138:886–91.
5. Hu X, Zhao Q. Systematic evaluation of the flexible and rigid annuloplasty ring after mitral valve repair for mitral regurgitation. Eur J Cardiothorac Surg. 2011;40:480–7.
6. Wan S, Lee AP, Jin CN, Wong RH, Chan HH, Ng CS, et al. The choice of mitral annuloplastic ring-beyond "surgeon's preference". Ann Cardiothorac Surg. 2015;4:261–5.
7. Adams DH, Rosenhek R, Falk V. Degenerative mitral valve regurgitation: best practice revolution. Eur Heart J. 2010;31:1958–67.
8. Bonow RO, Carabello BA, Chatterjee K, de Leon AC Jr, Faxon DP, Freed MD, et al. 2008 Focused update incorporated into the ACC/AHA 2006 guidelines for the management of patients with valvular heart disease: a report of the American College of Cardiology/American Heart Association task force on practice guidelines (writing committee to revise the 1998 guidelines for the Management of Patients with Valvular Heart Disease): endorsed by the Society of Cardiovascular Anesthesiologists, Society for Cardiovascular Angiography and Interventions, and Society of Thoracic Surgeons. Circulation. 2008;118:e523–661.
9. Lancellotti P, Moura L, Pierard LA, Agricola E, Popescu BA, Tribouilloy C, et al. European Association of Echocardiography recommendations for the assessment of valvular regurgitation. Part 2. Mitral and tricuspid regurgitation (native disease). Eur J Echocardiogr. 2010;11:307–32.
10. Akins CW, Miller DC, Turina MI, Kouchoukos NT, Blackstone EH, Grukemeier GL, et al. Guidelines for reporting mortality and morbidity after cardiac valve interventions. Ann Thorac Surg. 2008;85(4):1490–5.
11. Carpentier A. Reconstructive valvuloplasty. A new technique of mitral valvuloplasty. Presse Med. 1969;77:251–3.
12. Glasson JR, Komeda M, Daughters GT, Niczyporuk MA, Bolger AF, Ingels NB, et al. Three-dimensional regional dynamics of the normal mitral anulus during left ventricular ejection. J Thorac Cardiovasc Surg. 1996;111:574–85.
13. Grewal J, Suri R, Mankad S, Tanaka A, Mahoney DW, Schaff HV, et al. Mitral annular dynamics in myxomatous valve disease: new insights with real-time 3-dimensional echocardiography. Circulation. 2010;121:1423–31.
14. Lansac E, Lim KH, Shomura Y, Goetz WA, Lim HS, Rice NT, et al. Dynamic balance of the aortomitral junction. J Thorac Cardiovasc Surg. 2002;123:911–8.
15. Cosgrove DM, Arcidi JM, Rodriguez L, Stewart WJ, Powell K, Thomas JD. Initial experience with the Cosgrove-Edwards Annuloplasty system. Ann Thorac Surg. 1995;60:499–503. discussion 503-4
16. Dagum P, Timek T, Green GR, Daughters GT, Liang D, Ingels NB Jr, et al. Three-dimensional geometric comparison of partial and complete flexible mitral annuloplasty rings. J Thorac Cardiovasc Surg. 2001;122:665–73.
17. Chee T, Haston R, Togo A, Raja SG. Is a flexible mitral annuloplasty ring superior to a semi-rigid or rigid ring in terms of improvement in symptoms and survival? Interact Cardiovasc Thorac Surg. 2008;7:477–84.
18. David TE, Komeda M, Pollick C, Burns RJ. Mitral valve annuloplasty: the effect of the type on left ventricular function. Ann Thorac Surg. 1989;47:524–7. discussion 527-8
19. Chang B, Youn Y, Ha J, Lim S, Hong Y, Chung N. Long-term clinical results of mitral valvuloplasty using flexible and rigid rings: a prospective and randomized study. J Thorac Cardiovasc Surg. 2007;133(4):995–1003.
20. Shahin GM, van der Heijden GJ, Bots ML, Cramer MJ, Jaarsma W, Gadellaa JC, et al. The Carpentier-Edwards classic and Physio mitral annuloplasty rings: a randomized trial. Heart Surg Forum. 2005;8:E389–94. discussion E394-5
21. Okada Y, Shomura T, Yamaura Y, Yoshikawa J. Comparison of the Carpentier and Duran prosthetic rings used in mitral reconstruction. Ann Thorac Surg. 1995;59:658–62. discussion 662-3
22. Unger-Graeber B, Lee RT, Sutton MS, Plappert M, Collins JJ, Cohn LH. Doppler echocardiographic comparison of the Carpentier and Duran anuloplasty rings versus no ring after mitral valve repair for mitral regurgitation. Am J Cardiol. 1991;67:517–9.

23. Kreindel MS, Schiavone WA, Lever HM, Cosgrove D. Systolic anterior motion of the mitral valve after Carpentier ring valvuloplasty for mitral valve prolapse. Am J Cardiol. 1986;57:408–12.

24. Carpentier AF, Lessana A, Relland JY, Belli E, Mihaileanu S, Berrebi AJ, et al. The "physio-ring": an advanced concept in mitral valve annuloplasty. Ann Thorac Surg. 1995;60:1177–85. discussion 1185-6

25. Raffoul R, Uva MS, Rescigno G, Belli E, Scorsin M, Pouillart F, et al. Clinical evaluation of the Physio annuloplasty ring. Chest. 1998;113:1296–301.

26. Accola KD, Scott ML, Thompson PA, Palmer GJ, Sand ME, Ebra G. Midterm outcomes using the physio ring in mitral valve reconstruction: experience in 492 patients. Ann Thorac Surg. 2005;79:1276–83. discussion 1276-83

27. Gillinov AM, Cosgrove DM 3rd, Shiota T, Qin J, Tsujino H, Stewart WJ, et al. Cosgrove-Edwards Annuloplasty system: midterm results. Ann Thorac Surg. 2000;69:717–21.

28. Chitwood WR, Rodriguez E, Chu MW, Hassan A, Ferguson TB, Vos PW, et al. Robotic mitral valve repairs in 300 patients: a single-center experience. J Thorac Cardiovasc Surg. 2008;136:436–41.

29. Green GR, Dagum P, Glasson JR, Daughters GT, Bolger AF, Foppiano LE, et al. Semirigid or flexible mitral annuloplasty rings do not affect global or basal regional left ventricular systolic function. Circulation. 1998;98:II128–35. discussion II135-6

30. Manabe S, Kasegawa H, Fukui T, Tabata M, Shinozaki T, Shimokawa T, et al. Do semi-rigid prosthetic rings affect left ventricular function after mitral valve repair? Circ J. 2013;77:2038–42.

31. Burt BM, ElBardissi AW, Huckman RS, Cohn LH, Cevasco MW, Rawn JD, et al. Influence of experience and the surgical learning curve on long-term patient outcomes in cardiac surgery. J Thorac Cardiovasc Surg. 2015;150:1061–68.e3.

32. Castillo JG, Anyanwu AC, Fuster V, Adams DH. A near 100% repair rate for mitral valve prolapse is achievable in a reference center: implications for future guidelines. J Thorac Cardiovasc Surg. 2012;144:308–12.

33. Anyanwu AC, Itagaki S, Chikwe J, El-Eshmawi A, Adams DH. A complexity scoring system for degenerative mitral valve repair. J Thorac Cardiovasc Surg. 2016;151:1661–70.

14

Assessment of the prognostic role of neutrophil-to-lymphocyte ratio following complete resection of thymoma

Piergiorgio Muriana*[iD], Angelo Carretta, Paola Ciriaco, Alessandro Bandiera and Giampiero Negri

Abstract

Background: The introduction of the new TNM staging system for thymic epithelial malignancies produced a significant increase in the proportion of patients with stage I disease. The identification of new prognostic factors could help to select patients for adjuvant therapies based on their risk of recurrence. Neutrophil-to-lymphocyte ratio (NLR) has recently gained popularity as reliable prognostic biomarker in many different solid tumors. The aim of this study is to assess the utility of NLR evaluation as a prognostic marker in patients with surgically-treated thymoma.

Methods: A retrospective analysis was conducted among patients who underwent resection for thymoma in a single center. Patients were divided in two groups, under (low-NLR-Group = 47 patients, 60%) and above (high-NLR-Group = 32 patients, 40%) a ROC-derived NLR cut-off (2.27). Associations with clinical-pathological variables were analyzed; disease-free survival (DFS) was identified as the primary endpoint.

Results: Between 2007 and 2017, 79 patients had surgery for thymoma. Overall 5-year DFS was 80%. Univariate survival analysis demonstrated that NLR was significantly related to DFS when patients were stratified for TNM stage ($p = 0.043$). Five-year DFS in the low-NLR-Group and in the high-NLR-Group were respectively 100 and 84% in stage I-II, and 66 and 0% in stage III. TNM stage resulted as the only independent prognostic factor at multivariate analysis, with hazard ratio of 3.986 (95% CI 1.644–9.665, $p = 0.002$).

Conclusions: High preoperative NLR seems to be associated to a shorter DFS in patients submitted to surgery for thymoma and stratified for TNM stage.

Keywords: Neutrophil-to-lymphocyte ratio, Thymoma, Surgery, Prognostic markers, TNM staging

Background

Thymoma is the most common primary tumor of the anterior mediastinum, with a reported incidence of 1.7 cases per million per year in Europe [1]. Complete surgical resection is the mainstay of treatment [1, 2], and is associated with favorable survival results. Nevertheless, recurrence after surgery is observed in up to 50% of patients with locally-advanced disease [2] and can occur even many years after initial treatment due to the indolent nature of these slowly-progressive tumors. Recurrence has been related to many prognostic factors, such as age, tumor stage, size, World Health Organization (WHO) histological classification, completeness of resection, presence of paraneoplastic syndromes, local invasion and presence of lymph-nodes metastasis [1, 2]. Furthermore, genomic factors may also influence prognosis in patients with thymoma [3].

Following the proposals of a working group of the International Thymic Malignancies Interest Group (ITMIG) and the International Association for the Study of Lung Cancer (IASLC), a new staging system for thymic epithelial tumors has been included in the last TNM cancer staging system revision [4, 5]. TNM staging has been shown to have a stronger correlation with disease-free survival (DFS) analysis in comparison with the Masaoka-Koga staging system [6]. However, following further analysis, the

* Correspondence: muriana.piergiorgio@hsr.it
Department of Thoracic Surgery, San Raffaele Scientific Institute, Milan, Italy

introduction of the new TNM staging system for thymic epithelial malignancies produced a significant imbalance of tumors toward stage I [6]. The identification of new prognostic factors may therefore be useful to obtain an additional stratification of early-stage tumors according to the risk of recurrence to define the indications for adjuvant treatments.

Recently, a growing number of studies examined the role of tumor-induced systemic inflammation. Neutrophils cover an important role in the tumor microenvironment. These cells are able to produce cytokines and oxidative stress derivatives, and may favor tumor promotion, progression and distant spread by inhibiting the antitumor activity of the immune system [7, 8]. Among inflammatory markers, the prognostic significance of neutrophil-to-lymphocyte ratio (NLR) has been extensively investigated in the very last few years. Many studies demonstrated that high NLR value is predictive of reduced overall survival (OS), cancer-related survival, DFS, progression-free survival, and enhanced resistance to therapies in a multitude of solid neoplasms [7, 9]. NLR could therefore represent an easily available and cost-effective indicator of tumor-related inflammatory response for therapeutic planning and follow-up.

The aim of our study is to investigate the prognostic role of NLR and its association to clinical and pathological characteristics in patients with thymoma who underwent surgical resection at our Department.

Methods

The data of patients who underwent complete surgical resection for pathologically proven thymic epithelial tumor at our Department of Thoracic Surgery of the San Raffaele Scientific Institute, Milan, between January 2007 and April 2017 were retrospectively analyzed. Exclusion criteria included thymic carcinoma and incomplete resection (R1 or R2).

The following data were entered in a prospective database: age, gender, presence of myasthenia gravis (MG) and MGFA classification, neoadjuvant or adjuvant therapy, surgical approach, tumor histology according to the current WHO classification [10], Masaoka-Koga staging [11], DFS, OS, and cause of death. Histopathologic reports were retrospectively reviewed, and all the cases were reclassified according to the 8th edition of TNM staging [5].

Patients were followed up at intervals of 3 months for the first year after surgery, then every 6 months for the next 2 years, and annually thereafter. Recurrence was defined either in case of histologically proven disease relapse, or in case of radiological evidence of recurrence followed by response to treatment. OS was defined as the time

from the date of surgery to death from any cause or the last follow-up. DFS was defined as the time from the date of surgery to recurrence or the last follow-up.

For each patient, a peripheral blood sample was collected between 72 and 24 h before surgery. Complete blood cell count was performed: total white blood cell (WBC), neutrophil, and lymphocyte counts were entered in the database. MG cases who received specific preoperative pharmacologic treatment and patients who underwent induction treatment were not excluded from the analysis. In fact, NLR mean value in these patients did not significantly differ from patients without MG history and patients who did not receive neoadjuvant therapies ($p = 0.13$ and $p = 0.35$, respectively).

Optimal cut-off level for NLR (2.27, sensitivity = 83.3%, specificity = 93.2%) was determined by receiver-operating curve (ROC) analysis (AUC = 0.83, 95% CI 0.73–0.91, Fig. 1); population was divided in 2 groups (above and under the cut-off level), in order to evaluate association with clinical and pathological features, and prognostic value.

Preoperative work-up included routine physical examination, contrast-enhanced chest CT scan, and total body 18-FDG positron emission tomography (PET) scan. The patients who were not already known to be myasthenic before admission underwent a neurological evaluation in order to rule-out the presence of MG.

Preoperative histological diagnosis was obtained in case of indication to neoadjuvant therapy or when differential diagnosis with lymphoproliferative disorder or other anterior mediastinal neoplasms was needed.

Surgery was performed by 5 experienced surgeons by means of either median sternotomy, muscle-sparing thoracotomy or VATS based on size, local extension and location of the tumor. VATS thymectomy has been performed since 2011 in case of small encapsulated tumors (< 2 cm) in non-myasthenic patients. Complete thymectomy (removal of the thymus with surrounding adipose tissue) or extended thymectomy (additional removal of all the mediastinal and pericardiophrenic fat between bilateral mediastinal pleura) was carried out according to MG status, as previously described [12].

Statistical analysis

Analysis was performed by SAS v9 software (SPSS, v. 18, INC. Chicago, IL, USA). Values are expressed as means ± standard deviation unless otherwise stated. Categorical variables among the groups of patients were compared by means of either Chi-square test or Fisher Exact test as appropriate. Student's t-test was used to determine the significance of the differences between continuous variables.

Survival curves were estimated by the Kaplan and Meier method. Cox regression analysis was used to assess the

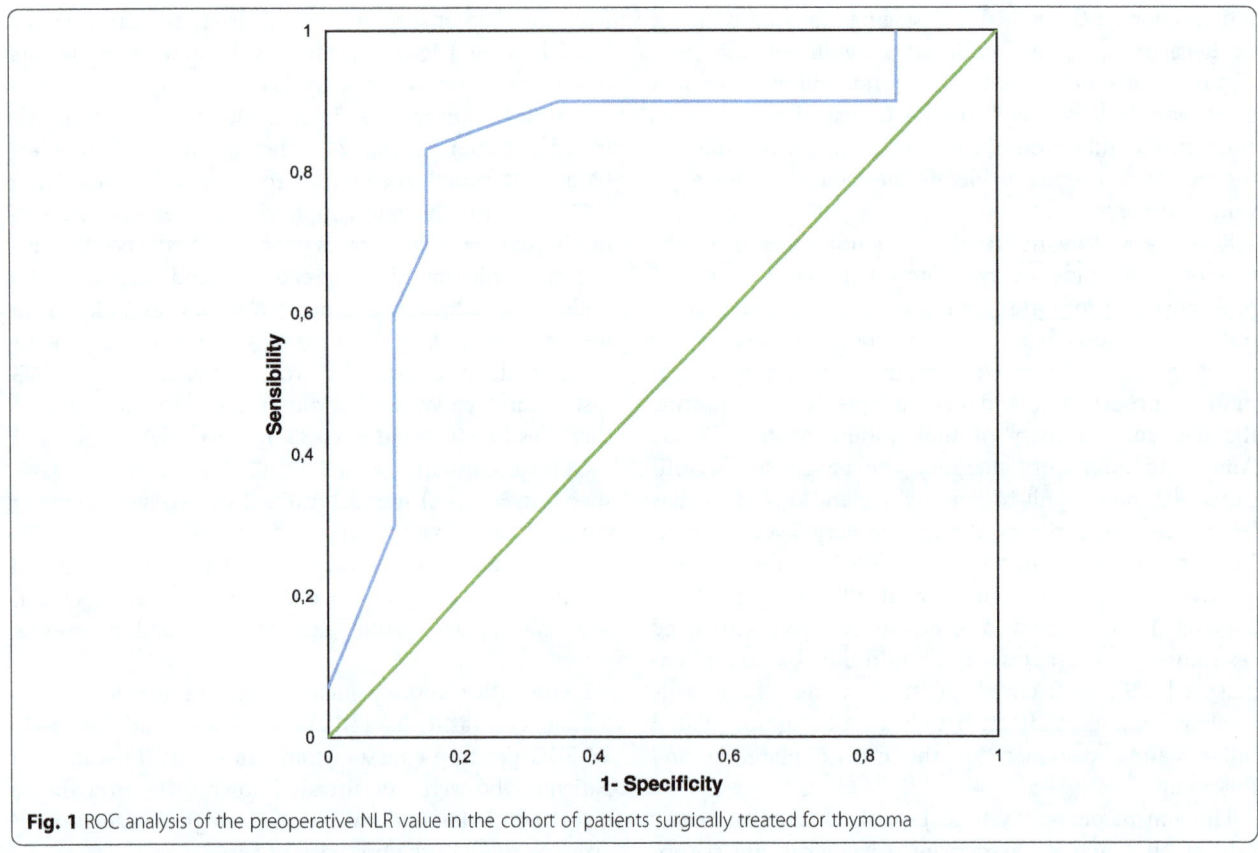

Fig. 1 ROC analysis of the preoperative NLR value in the cohort of patients surgically treated for thymoma

risks of the variables. Survival rates of patients grouped according to selected variables were compared by means of the log-rank test. According to the indolent nature of the disease, DFS (i.e. the interval between the date of surgery and the first recurrence) was identified as primary endpoint.

On the univariate survival analysis basis, in order to evaluate the independent contribution of the variables on DFS and OS, a multivariate analysis was performed using the Cox regression method.

Hazard Ratio (HR) and 95% Confidence Interval (95% CI) are shown; a p-value < 0.05 was considered statistically significant.

Results

Between 2007 and 2017, 79 patients underwent complete surgical treatment for pathologically proven thymoma (Table 1). The median follow-up was 29 months (range 1–99 months). At the time of last follow-up, 67 patients (85%) were alive with no evidence of disease, 5 (6%) were alive with disease recurrence (Table 2), and 6 (8%) died of causes other than thymoma relapse (one of acute coronary disease, 4 of metastatic spread of other malignancies not present at the time of surgery, and one for unknown reasons with last follow-up CT scan negative for recurrence).

One patient showed disease recurrence 24 months after surgery, and eventually died for pulmonary thromboembolism 75 months after surgery.

According to the IASLC/ITMIG TNM staging, all Masaoka-Koga stage I and II patients and three stage III patients were re-classified as TNM stage I (82% of total patients), and 11 (14%) were classified in TNM stage IIIA. Fifty-two out of 65 patients (80%) in TNM stage I had WHO type A to B1 thymoma, while 10 out of 11 patients (91%) in stage IIIA had WHO type B2 or B3 tumors ($p < 0.001$).

All the three patients who received neoadjuvant therapy before surgery had TNM stage IIIA disease ($p < 0.001$). Forty-seven patients (60%) with locally-advanced disease underwent adjuvant radiotherapy after surgery (45–50 Gy); 96% of them had stage II and III tumors according to the Masaoka-Koga staging system (p < 0.001). No correlation was found between indication to adjuvant treatment and TNM staging ($p = 0.16$).

Overall 1-, 2- and 5-year survival rates for the entire cohort were 100, 94 and 87%, respectively. DFS at 1, 2 and 5 years was respectively 100, 96 and 80%.

Patients were divided in two groups according to the NLR cut-off value (Table 3). Forty-seven patients (60%) had a NLR < 2.27 (low-NLR-Group), and other 32 patients (40%) had a NLR ≥ 2.27 (high-NLR-Group).

Table 1 Patients' characteristics

Total	79
Age (years)	
Mean ± SD; range	58.9 ± 13.4; 27–84
Median	61
Gender (male)	47 (60%)
Myasthenia gravis	15 (19%)
MGFA class I	13
MGFA class IIa	1
MGFA class IIb	1
Neoadjuvant therapy	3 (4%)
Chemotherapy	2
Chemo-radiotherapy	1
Adjuvant radiotherapy	47 (60%)
Surgical approach	
Median sternotomy	65 (82%)
Thoracotomy	4 (5%)
VATS	10 (13%)
Surgical procedure	
Complete thymectomy	64 (81%)
Extended thymectomy	15 (19%)
WHO classification	
A	5 (6%)
AB	32 (41%)
B1	16 (20%)
B2	11 (14%)
B3	15 (19%)
Masaoka-Koga stage	
I	21 (27%)
II	41 (52%)
III	16 (20%)
IV	1 (1%)
TNM stage	
I	65 (82%)
II	2 (3%)
IIIA	11 (14%)
IIIB	1 (1%)

The proportion of patients older than the median age (61 years) was significantly higher ($p = 0.021$) in the high-NLR-Group (69%) than in the low-NLR-Group (40%). There were no differences between the two groups regarding sex, presence of MG, preoperative WBC count, indication to neoadjuvant and adjuvant therapies, histology and Masaoka-Koga staging.

A significant imbalance emerged in the distribution of patients among TNM stages. In particular, 21% of the low-NLR-Group patients had IIIA/B stage disease; on the other hand, only two patients (6%) in the high-NLR-Group had a thymoma in these stages of the disease ($p = 0.028$).

Total WBC and neutrophil mean counts (Fig. 2a-b) did not differ between TNM stages I-II and stages IIIA/B patients ($p = 0.074$ and $p = 0.36$, respectively). Conversely, mean lymphocyte count in stages I-II and in stages IIIA/B (Fig. 2c) were respectively $2.1 \times 10^9/L$ and $3.1 \times 10^9/L$ ($p = 0.036$), a point which could justify lower NLR values in a higher proportion of stage III tumors.

At univariate survival analysis, WHO classification was the only variable significantly associated with both OS and DFS. AB type thymomas showed the worst 5-year OS (84%, $p = 0.042$), while patients affected by B2 type disease had 40% 5-year DFS ($p = 0.011$). History of neo-adjuvant or adjuvant therapy, higher Masaoka-Koga and TNM staging were all significantly associated with a lower DFS ($p = 0.047$, $p = 0.043$, $p = 0.013$, and $p < 0.001$, respectively).

1, 2- and 5-year DFS (Fig. 3) was respectively 100, 100 and 88% in the low-NLR-Group, and 100, 92 and 73% in the high-NLR-Group, but these data failed to reach statistical significance ($p = 0.34$). OS was also not significantly different between the low-NLR-Group and the high-NLR-Group ($p = 0.29$). However, following stratification of the patients according to TNM stage, DFS rates for patients in the low-NLR-Group were significantly higher (p = 0.043) than those in the high-NLR-Group both in I-II stages (Fig. 4) and in IIIA/B stages.

At multivariate analysis (Table 4), only TNM staging was an independent prognostic factor for DFS, with a HR of 3.986 (95% CI 1.644–9.665, $p = 0.002$), while NLR approached but failed to reach statistical significance ($p = 0.066$).

Discussion

In this study, we analyzed the prognostic value of NLR in a group of 79 patients with surgically-treated thymomas. Factors as gender, presence of MG, total WBC count, neo- and adjuvant therapies, WHO classification and Masaoka-Koga staging did not correlate with NLR.

It is noteworthy that a lower proportion of patients with locally-advanced disease (TNM stages IIIA/B) showed a NLR higher than the cut-off value than those in stages I and II (6% vs 21%, $p = 0.028$). At first glance, this result appears in contrast with the data of the literature, since previous reports show that NLR values usually increase along with the invasiveness of the tumor [9]. However, we found that while mean neutrophil count was homogeneously distributed among different stages of the disease, TNM stages IIIA/B patients exhibited a higher mean lymphocyte count ($p = 0.036$), a point which could explain a mean lower NLR in stage III tumors. In detail, since NLR is the quotient between the peripheral neutrophil

Table 2 Clinical and pathological features of the patients who experienced recurrence

Pt #	Age	Sex	MG	NLR	NT	WHO	Masaoka	TNM	AT	DFS	Site	OS	LFU
14	36	M	yes	2.16	no	B3	III	IIIA	yes	27	LR	31	AL
15	63	M	no	5.85	no	B3	III	IIIB	yes	16	LR	47	AL
32	50	M	no	1.68	yes	B2	IV	IIIA	yes	48	LR	61	AL
39	36	M	no	2.27	no	B2	III	I	yes	48	LR	99	AL
50	72	M	no	2.46	no	B3	II	I	yes	24	LR	75	D
66	52	F	no	2.61	yes	B2	III	IIIA	yes	57	LR	59	AL

Legend: *NT* Neoadjuvant therapy, *AT* Adjuvant therapy, *LR* Loco-regional recurrence, *LFU* Status at the time of the last follow up, *AL* Alive, *D* Deceased

and lymphocyte counts, a lower NLR value in locally advanced disease could be due to a relative increase of lymphocyte count rather than by a reduction of the neutrophil count.

In fact, thymomas generate autoreactive T-lymphocytes that are responsible for the development of associated paraneoplastic autoimmune diseases [1, 2]. Most of these cells undergo apoptosis before relapse in the systemic blood flow, thus patients affected by thymoma usually show normal peripheral lymphocyte count when compared to healthy controls [13]. However, some authors [14–20] described sporadic patients affected by aggressive thymic malignancies showing absolute peripheral polyclonal lymphocytosis. The distinctive feature of these tumors was an invasive pattern, with local extracapsular infiltration of mediastinal fat, pleura, and pericardium, with distant pleural or pulmonary metastasis, but also to bone and liver.

The prognostic role of NLR in patients with thymic epithelial tumors has been investigated only in an extremely limited number of studies and has still to be completely assessed.

Yuan et al. [21] evaluated the value of NLR in 79 patients who underwent resection of thymic carcinoma over an 11-year period. According to the aggressive nature of the disease, a cut-off value of 4.1 was identified. High NLR resulted associated to tumor dimensions, Masaoka-Koga stage, worse DFS and OS. However, the marker did not result to be an independent prognostic factor of death or recurrence at multivariate analysis.

In 2017, Yanagiya et al. [22] analyzed preoperative NLR in 159 patients completely resected for thymoma between 1976 and 2015. Patients with NLR ≥1.96 had significantly shorter OS, recurrence-free survival, disease-specific survival, disease-related survival, and showed higher cumulative incidence of recurrence. Moreover, NLR resulted independently prognostic for recurrence in early-stage disease.

Recently, Janik et al. [23] reported about the prognostic value of NLR and other inflammatory markers in 122 patients affected by thymic epithelial tumors (75% thymoma, 25% thymic carcinoma). Higher preoperative values of NLR resulted predictive of lower freedom from recurrence at survival analysis, but not at multivariate analysis. Interestingly, this study included a longitudinal analysis of NLR variation on repeated measurements acquired during the follow-up, and association to the incidence of recurrence.

In our study, univariate survival analysis showed that, when the patients were stratified according to TNM stage, DFS was significantly lower in the group with higher NLR values. NLR could therefore be a useful tool

Table 3 Classification of patients grouped by NLR < 2.27 (low-NLR-Group) and NLR ≥2.27 (high-NLR-Group)

	Low-NLR-Group (n = 47)	High-NLR-Group (n = 32)	P-value
Age (years)			
< 61	28 (60%)	10 (31%)	0.021*
≥ 61	19 (40%)	22 (69%)	
Gender (male)	26 (55%)	21 (66%)	0.48
Myasthenia gravis	8 (17%)	7 (22%)	0.77
WBC (× 10⁹/L)	7.0	8.1	0.09
Neoadjuvant therapy	2 (4%)	1 (3%)	0.79
Adjuvant radiotherapy	29 (62%)	18 (56%)	0.65
WHO classification			
A	3 (6%)	2 (6%)	0.39
AB	15 (32%)	17 (53%)	
B1	12 (26%)	4 (13%)	
B2	7 (15%)	4 (13%)	
B3	10 (21%)	5 (15%)	
Masaoka-Koga stage			
I	12 (26%)	9 (28%)	0.68
II	23 (49%)	18 (56%)	
III	11 (23%)	5 (16%)	
IV	1 (2%)	0 (0%)	
TNM stage			
I	37 (79%)	28 (88%)	0.028*
II	0 (0%)	2 (6%)	
IIIA	10 (21%)	1 (3%)	
IIIB	0 (0%)	1 (3%)	

Significant data are marked (*)

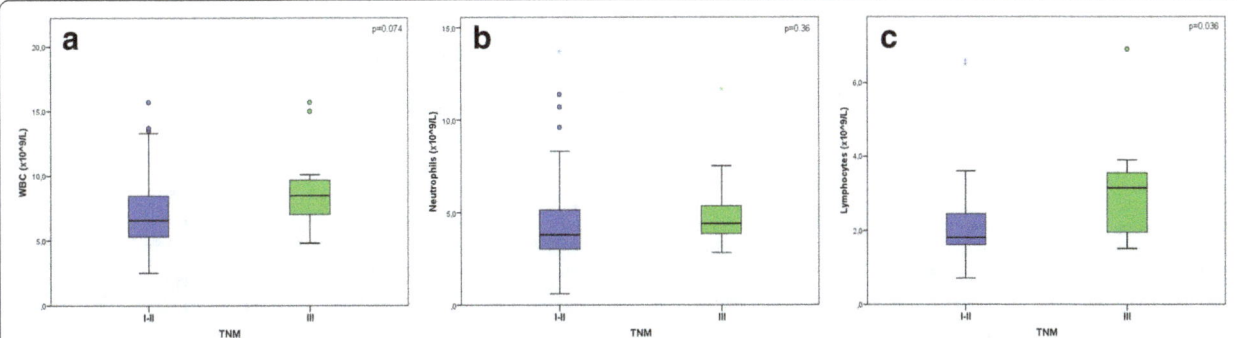

Fig. 2 Boxplots reporting WBC, neutrophil and lymphocyte values according to TNM stage. Total WBC (**a**) and neutrophil (**b**) count means did not significantly differ between patients in stages I-II and those in stages IIIA/B (7.2 vs 9.1 × 10^9/L and 4.4 vs 5.1 × 10^9/L, $p = 0.074$ and $p = 0.36$, respectively). By contrast, lymphocyte count mean (**c**) resulted higher in stages IIIA/B compared to stages I-II (3.1 vs 2.1 × 10^9/L, $p = 0.036$)

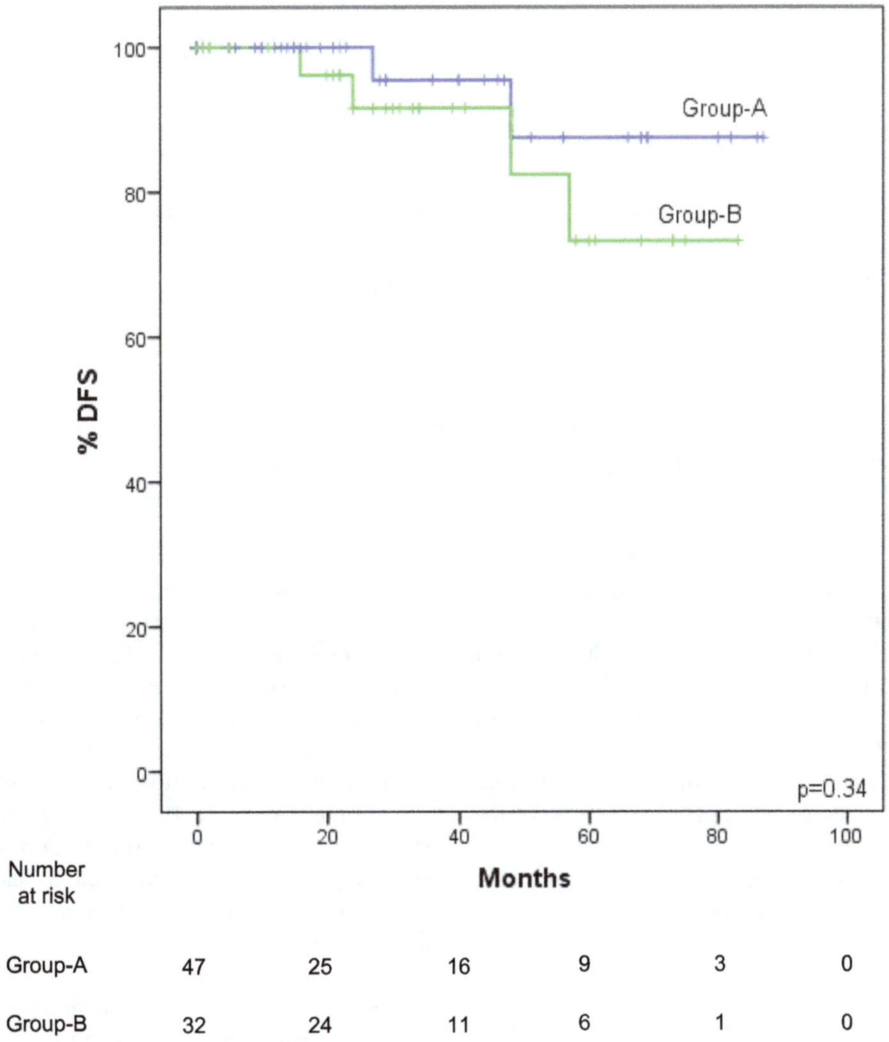

Number at risk					
Group-A	47	25	16	9	3	0
Group-B	32	24	11	6	1	0

Fig. 3 Kaplan-Meier DFS curves for the low-NLR-Group (NLR < 2.27) and the high-NLR-Group (NLR ≥2.27). DFS is lower in the high-NLR-Group patients, but does not reach statistical significance ($p = 0.34$)

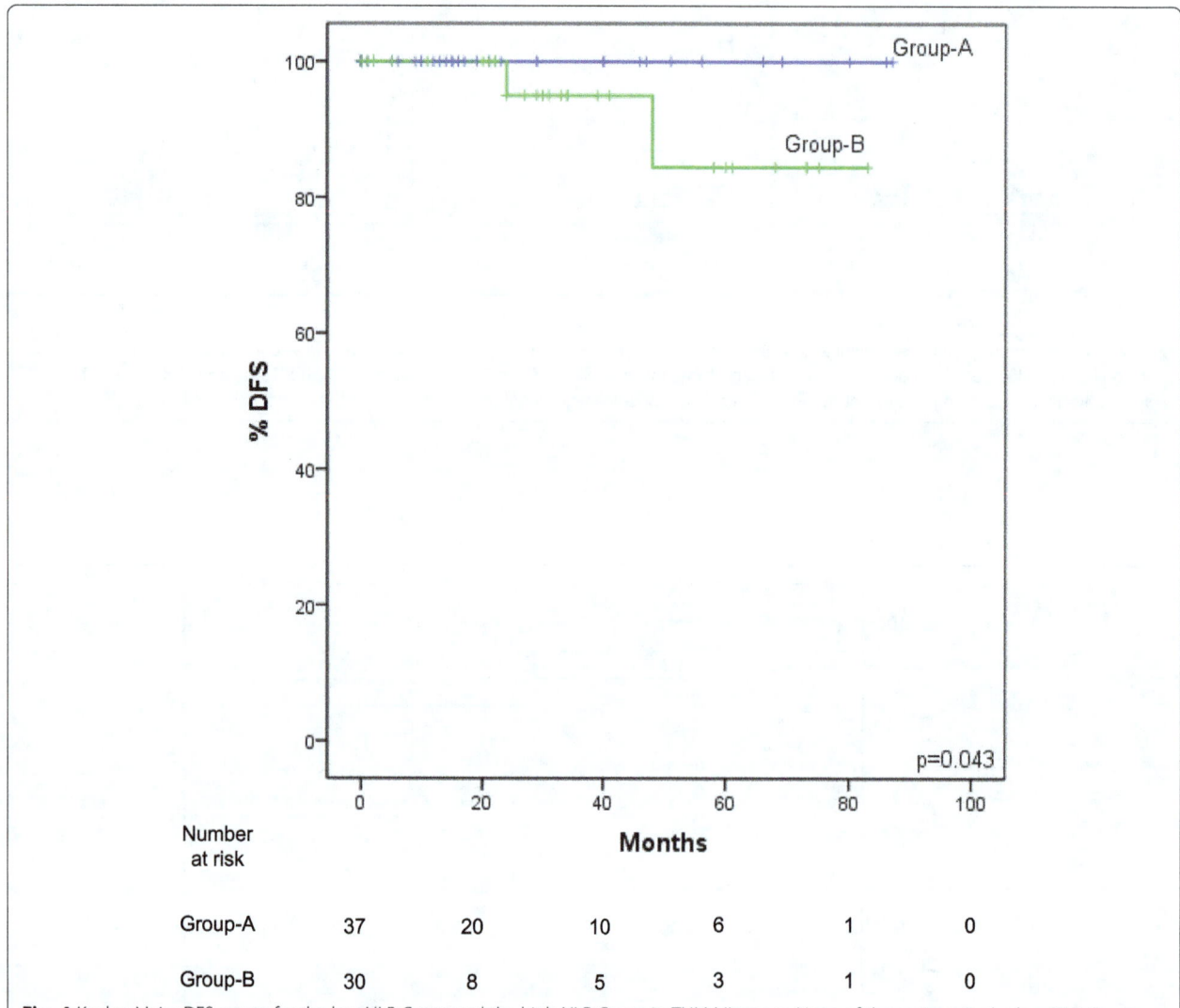

Fig. 4 Kaplan-Meier DFS curves for the low-NLR-Group and the high-NLR-Group in TNM I-II stages. None of the patients in the low-NLR-Group had disease relapse. One-, 2- and 5-year DFS in the high-NLR-Group were 100, 95 and 84%, respectively (*p* = 0.043)

to identify patients with surgically-treated thymoma at higher risk of relapse among the different stages of the disease. Nevertheless, with regard to locally-advanced disease, it is important to notice that such result may be conditioned by the small sample size of patients with TNM stage IIIA/B tumors.

A point which has to be taken into due consideration when selecting patients for adjuvant treatments is the fact

Table 4 Cox regression multivariate analysis of predictors of DFS

	HR (95% CI)	*P*-value
WHO classification	5.315 (0.812–34.788)	0.081
Masaoka-Koga stage	4.040 (0.366–44.596)	0.254
TNM stage	3.986 (1.644–9.665)	0.002*
NLR	5.272 (0.897–30.995)	0.066

Significant data are marked (*)

that in the new TNM classification system for thymic malignancies [5] the percentage of patients with stage I disease is considerably higher (approximating to 80%) than that of other stages [6]. Local invasion of the mediastinal pleura is indeed considered to have negligible influence on prognosis [4], a point which causes downstaging of almost all previously Masaoka-Koga stage II as well as a significant number of stage III tumors, as confirmed by our study. However, further stratification of patients with early-stage disease seems advisable to select those patients who may benefit from adjuvant treatments in order to reduce the risk of recurrence [24].

Beyond the radiological assessment [25, 26], a number of markers, such as C-reactive protein, have been suggested as possible tools to improve the accuracy of follow-up [27]. If our results will be confirmed by larger studies, preoperative NLR could be used to identify patients with early stage thymoma at higher risk of relapse. Moreover, a few studies are currently in progress focusing on different steps of neutrophils-mediated cancer progression [7]. The introduction of new specific drugs may cover in the future a key role in targeted post-operative therapy of thymoma patients according to their NLR status.

The current indications to adjuvant therapy in early-stage thymoma are still a matter of debate. ESMO [25] and NCCN [26] guidelines recommend to consider post-operative radiotherapy in case of tumoral extension beyond the capsule, and state a clear indication in case of more invasive disease. Wu et al. [28] suggest irradiation following surgery for all Masaoka-Koga stages II and III, but advocate randomized clinical trials to assess its utility in stage I disease. The administration of fractioned radiotherapy with a total dose of 45 to 50 Gy is widely accepted, as it is able to reduce significantly the risk of recurrence. Moreover, the use of advanced techniques, such as intensity-modulated radiotherapy, is advocated to minimize the toxicity over the irradiated field [29].

Chemotherapy has seldom been adopted alone as adjuvant treatment in thymoma patients. Platinum-based regimens concomitant with radiotherapy are usually administered as first-line treatment [30]. Recently, Carillo et al. [31] demonstrated that adjuvant chemo-radiotherapy is able to improve survival in Masaoka-Koga stage II disease in case of WHO type B thymomas.

New parameters to identify early-stage tumors at higher risk of recurrence, such as NLR, could therefore be useful in the development of future strategies for adjuvant treatments.

The major limitations of this study are the retrospective design, the relatively small size of the cohort and the relatively short follow-up considering the indolent nature of the disease, which may present recurrences up to 10 years after surgery [2]. At multivariate analysis, NLR did not result an independent prognostic factor of relapse. In fact, other factors, such as the higher proportion of younger patients in the low-NLR-Group, may be responsible for their favorable DFS. Moreover, the limited number of TNM stage IIIA/B patients does not allow to establish significant conclusions about the prognostic role of NLR in locally-advanced thymoma. Further research with a multi-center prospective study is therefore needed to validate the use of this easily accessible and inexpensive tool in the selection process of candidates to adjuvant therapies and follow-up.

Conclusions

Following the introduction of the 8th edition of TNM staging for thymic epithelial tumors, a large number of patients resected for thymoma will show early-stage disease. Therefore, further analysis to assess the risk of recurrence is essential.

Our analysis demonstrates that higher preoperative NLR seems to be associated to a worst outcome with regard to DFS in patients submitted to surgery for thymoma and stratified for TNM stage. In our opinion, this easy-available and cost-effective biomarker could therefore be of help for a better prognostic stratification among TNM stages, with particular notice to early-stage disease, to guide clinicians both for selection of candidates to adjuvant treatments and follow-up.

Abbreviations
AUC: Area under curve; CI: Confidence interval; DFS: Disease-free survival; HR: Hazard ratio; IASLC: International Association for the Study of Lung Cancer; ITMIG: International Thymic Malignancies Interest Group; MG: Myasthenia gravis; MGFA: Myasthenia Gravis Foundation of America classification; NLR: Neutrophil-to-lymphocyte ratio; OS: Overall survival; PET: Positron emission tomography; ROC: Receiver-operating curve; TNM: Tumor – Node – Metastasis Staging System; VATS: Video-assisted thoracic surgery; WBC: White blood cell; WHO: World Health Organization

Acknowledgements
Not applicable.

Funding
Not applicable.

Authors' contributions
PM and AC concepted and designed the study and prepared the manuscript. PM, PC and AB collected, analyzed and interpreted the data. AC and GN overviewed the quality of data and algorithms and reviewed the manuscript. All authors read and approved the final manuscript.

Competing interests
The authors declare that they have no competing interests.

References
1. Scorsetti M, Leo F, Trama A, et al. Thymoma and thymic carcinomas. Crit Rev Oncol Hematol. 2016;99:332–50.
2. Venuta F, Rendina EA, Anile M, et al. Thymoma and thymic carcinoma. Gen Thorac Cardiovasc Surg. 2012;60:1–12.
3. Feng Y, Lei Y, Wu X, et al. GTF2I mutation frequently occurs in more indolent thymic epithelial tumors and predicts better prognosis. Lung Cancer. 2017;110:48–52.
4. Detterbeck FC, Stratton K, Giroux D, et al. The IASLC/ITMIG thymic epithelial tumors staging project: proposal for an evidence-based stage classification system for the forthcoming (8th) edition of the TNM classification of malignant tumors. J Thorac Oncol. 2014;9:S65–72.
5. Asamura H. Lung, pleural and thymic tumours. In: Brierley JD, Gospodarowicz MK, Wittekind C, editors. UICC TNM classification of malignant tumours, 8th ed. Oxford-Hoboken: Wiley; 2017. p. 115–118.
6. Fukui T, Fukumoto K, Okasaka T, et al. Clinical evaluation of a new tumour-node-metastasis staging system for thymic malignancies proposed by the International Association for the Study of Lung Cancer staging and prognostic factors committee and the international Thymic malignancy interest group. Eur J Cardiothorac Surg. 2016;49:574–9.

7. Ocana A, Nieto-Jiménez C, Pandiella A, et al. Neutrophils in cancer: prognostic role and therapeutic strategies. Mol Cancer. 2017;16:137.

8. Corrêa LH, Corrêa R, Farinasso CM, et al. Adipocytes and macrophages interplay in the orchestration of tumor microenvironment: new implications in cancer progression. Front Immunol. 2017;8:1129.

9. Templeton AJ, McNamara MG, Šeruga B, et al. Prognostic role of neutrophil-to-lymphocyte ratio in solid tumors: a systematic review and meta-analysis. J Natl Cancer Inst. 2014;106:dju124.

10. Tumours of the thymus. In: Travis WD, Brambilla E, Burke AP, et al, editors. WHO classification of tumours of the lung, pleura, thymus and heart, 4th ed. Lyon: IARC Press; 2015. 183–298.

11. Koga K, Matsuno Y, Noguchi M, et al. A review of 79 thymomas: modification of staging system and reappraisal of conventional division into invasive and non-invasive thymoma. Pathol Int. 1994;44:359–67.

12. Toker A, Sonett J, Zielinski M, et al. Standard terms, definitions, and policies for minimally invasive resection of thymoma. J Thorac Oncol. 2011;6:S1739–42.

13. Buckley C, Douek D, Newsom-Davis J, et al. Mature, long-lived CD4+ and CD8+ T cells are generated by the thymoma in myasthenia gravis. Ann Neurol. 2001;50:64–72.

14. Pedraza MA. Thymoma immunological and ultrastructural characterization. Cancer. 1977;39:1455–61.

15. Smith GP, Perkins SL, Segal GH, et al. T-cell lymphocytosis associated with invasive thymomas. Am J Clin Pathol. 1994;102:447–53.

16. de Jong D, Richel DJ, Schenkeveld C, et al. Oligoclonal peripheral T-cell lymphocytosis as a result of aberrant T-cell development in a cortical thymoma. Diagn Mol Pathol. 1997;6:244–8.

17. Barton AD. T-cell lymphocytosis associated with lymphocyte-rich thymoma. Cancer. 1997;80:1409–17.

18. Otton SH, Standen GR, Ormerod IE. T cell lymphocytosis associated with polymyositis, myasthenia gravis and thymoma. Clin Lab Haematol. 2000;22:307–8.

19. Puljiz Z, Karin Z, Bratanic A, et al. Late distant metastases of malignant thymoma associated with peripheral T-cell lymphocytosis. Pathol Int. 2013;63:516–8.

20. Zhao L, Zhou X, Li Z, et al. Bone metastasis of malignant thymomas associated with peripheral T-cell lymphocytosis. BMC Surg. 2016;16:58.

21. Yuan Z, Gao S, Mu J, et al. Prognostic value of preoperative neutrophil-lymphocyte ratio is superior to platelet-lymphocyte ratio for survival in patients who underwent complete resection of thymic carcinoma. J Thorac Dis. 2016;8:1487–96.

22. Yanagiya M, Nitadori J, Nagayama K, et al. Prognostic significance of the preoperative neutrophil-to-lymphocyte ratio for complete resection of thymoma. Surg Today. 2018;48:422–30.

23. Janik S, Raunegger T, Hacker P, et al. Prognostic and diagnostic impact of fibrinogen, neutrophil-to-lymphocyte ratio, and platelet-to-lymphocyte ratio on thymic epithelial tumors outcome. Oncotarget. 2018;9:21861–75.

24. Basse C, Merveilleux du Vignaux C, Girard N. Postoperative radiotherapy in completely resected stage II and III thymoma: how to translate the potential survival benefit in the setting of the future adoption of the IASLC-ITMIG TNM-based staging system. J Thorac Oncol. 2017;12:e8–9.

25. Girard N, Ruffini E, Marx A, et al. Thymic epithelial tumours: ESMO clinical practice guidelines for diagnosis, treatment and follow-up. Ann Oncol. 2015;26:v40–55.

26. NCCN guidelines for thymomas and thymic carcinomas. 2016. https://www.nccn.org/store/login/login.aspx?ReturnURL https://www.nccn.org/professionals/physician_gls/pdf/thymic.pdf. Accessed 9 Nov 2017.

27. Janik S, Bekos C, Hacker P, et al. Elevated CRP levels predict poor outcome and tumor recurrence in patients with thymic epithelial tumors: a pro- and retrospective analysis. Oncotarget. 2017;8:47090–102.

28. Wu KL, Mao JF, Chen GY, et al. Prognostic predictors and long-term outcome of postoperative irradiation in thymoma: a study of 241 patients. Cancer Investig. 2009;27:1008–15.

29. Lombe DC, Jeremic B. A review of the place and role of radiotherapy in thymoma. Clin Lung Cancer. 2015;16:406–12.

30. Hamaji M. The role of adjuvant chemotherapy following resection of early stage thymoma. Ann Cardiothorac Surg. 2016;5:45–50.

31. Carillo C, Diso D, Mantovani S, et al. Multimodality treatment of stage II thymic tumours. J Thorac Dis. 2017;9:2369–74.

15

Salvage thoracic surgery in patients with lung cancer: potential indications and benefits

Erkan Kaba[1]* ⓘ, Mehmet Oguzhan Ozyurtkan[1], Kemal Ayalp[2], Tugba Cosgun[1], Mazen Rasmi Alomari[2] and Alper Toker[2]

Abstract

Background: To investigate the feasibility and efficacy of salvage lung resection and describe the possible indications and contraindications in patients with primary lung cancer.

Methods: Thirty patients undergoing anatomical salvage lung resection were classified into three groups: GI, patients with progressive lung tumor despite definitive chemo- and/or radiotherapy; GII, patients who underwent emergency resection; and GIII, patients in whom neoadjuvant or definitive chemo- and/or radiotherapy was contraindicated because of severe comorbidities. The groups were compared based on, peri- and postoperative factors, and survival rates.

Results: The morbidity rate was 70%. Revision surgery was required in 23% of patients. Morbidity was affected by lower hematocrit and hemoglobin levels ($P = 0.05$). Mean hospital stay was 11 ± 4 days, which was longer in patients in whom complications developed ($P = 0.0003$). The in-hospital or 30-day mortality rate was 3%. Mean relapse-free survival and overall survivals were 14 ± 12 and 19 ± 13 months.

Conclusion: Patients with progression of the persistent primary tumor after definitive chemo- and/or radiotherapy can undergo salvage lung resection with acceptable mortality and high morbidity rates, if the tumor is considered resectable. Other indications may be considered for salvage lung resection based on each patient's specific evaluation.

Keywords: Non-small-cell lung cancer, Salvage surgery, Pulmonary resection, Survival

Background

Lung cancer is a leading cause of death worldwide. Although surgery is the standard of care for patients with operable early-stage lung cancer, definitive chemoradiation has been introduced for resectable tumors in high-risk patients or for unresectable locally advanced tumors [1]. Local relapses have been reported to develop within 2 years after definitive chemoradiotherapy in >30% of patients [2]. In such a situation, treatment options are repeat irradiation, chemotherapy, cryo- and radiofrequency ablation, and observation only [3].

Salvage operations are occasionally performed in selected patients with advanced colon and esophageal cancer and malignant mediastinal tumors, such as thymoma [4].

Recently, this term has been adopted for lung cancer. Some retrospective studies demonstrated that salvage lung resection (SLR) can improve survival with acceptable surgical adverse events [5–7]. However, the experiences are limited. The impact of SLR on the early and long-term effects and the indications for SLR remain unclear.

In this single-institution study, we reported patients undergoing SLR and investigated the feasibility and efficacy of the procedure. We also described the possible indications and contraindications for SLR.

Methods

This study was approved by the institutional review board of Istanbul Bilim University, and the need for individual patient consent was waived. Among 496 patients who underwent anatomical pulmonary resections because of primary lung cancer at our institution between January 2011 and

* Correspondence: erkankaba@hotmail.com
[1]Department of Thoracic Surgery, Istanbul Bilim University Medical Faculty, 34381 Sisli, Istanbul, Turkey
Full list of author information is available at the end of the article

December 2016, we retrospectively evaluated 30 (6%) who underwent SLR. SLR was defined as anatomical resection in patients who had progression of the persistent primary lung tumor after definitive chemo- and/or radiotherapy (GI, 22 patients); in those who underwent resection due to an emergency situation that could not be treated with other major therapeutic modalities, such as hemoptysis, broncho-oesophageal or bronchopleural fistula, and severe infectious situations, including lung abscess or empyema (GII, three patients); and in those who should have undergone neoad-juvant or definitive chemo- and/or radiotherapy, but these were contraindicated because of severe comorbidities des-pite the clinical diagnosis of stage IIIA, IIIB, or IV disease, as previously described (GIII, five patients) [4, 8].

Patients had been discussed during our weekly multi-disciplinary tumor board, in which thoracic surgeons, chest physicians, pulmonary oncologists, radiation on-cologists, radiologists, and nuclear medicine specialists took part. Patients were chosen as candidates for SLR when their physical status and cardiopulmonary func-tions, as determined using lung function tests, exercise tests, and cardiac evaluation, were sufficient for them to undergo resection, and when complete resection of all suspicious or proven disease was technically feasible. However, patients in GIII were accepted to have border-line pulmonary or cardiac levels at the time of evalu-ation. For patients in GI, the operation was performed at least 6 months after definitive chemo- and/or radiother-apy. SLR entailed appropriate anatomical lung resection and mediastinal lymph node dissection. All patients in GI and selected patients in the other groups underwent reinforcement of the bronchial stump using any of the following: intercostal muscle flap, diaphragm, pleura, and thymus. In the postoperative period, all patients re-ceived similar drug regiments including bronchodilators, analgesics, expectorants and antibiotics (ampicillin-sul-bactam and ciprofloxacin).

Data retrieved from the database included age, sex, co-morbidity, postoperative pathology, N- and T-stages of the tumor, indication for operation, type of operation, preoperative levels of hemoglobin, hematocrit (%) and albumin, respiratory function tests [forced expiratory volume in one second (FEV1) and diffusion capacity of the lung for carbon monoxide (DLCO) values], pulmon-ary arterial pressure and ejection fraction values, length of hospital stay, mortality, morbidity, and follow-up re-cords. Surgical complications were classified based on the proposal made by Dindo et al. [9]

The date of surgery was used for follow-up measures. The patients underwent a chest and abdomen physical examination. The initial computed tomography (CT) scan was performed 3 months postoperatively, and chest and upper abdomen CTs were performed every 6 months for the first 2 years and once yearly thereafter for 5 years.

Overall survival was calculated from the time of surgery. Relapse-free survival rate was calculated from the date of surgery to the date of recurrence.

The three groups were compared based on the aforemen-tioned parameters. The data were collected and analyzed using Excel software (Microsoft Corp., Seattle, WA, USA). Descriptive statistics were used to report the means and standard deviations of the continuous variables and the number and percent of categorical variables. Categorical data were compared using the Fisher's exact test and t-tests, as appropriate. To test significant differences between the groups, one-way analysis of variance followed by Tukey's test was used for normally distributed variables and the Kruskal–Wallis test was used for non-normally distributed variables. $P \leq 0.05$ was considered statistically significant.

Results

Table 1 demonstrates the characteristics of the patients. Mean patient age at resection was 63 ± 7 years. Most were male patients ($n = 26$, 87%). A total of 18 patients (60%) had comorbidities, including chronic obstructive pulmon-ary disease in eight, coronary artery disease in seven, pres-ence of cancer other than lung cancer in three, severe hyperthyroidism in one, and severe liver insufficiency in

Table 1 Characteristics of the patients*

	Total ($n = 30$)	Group 1 ($n = 22$)	Group 2 ($n = 3$)	Group 3 ($n = 5$)
Age (years, ± SD)	63 ± 7	63 ± 8	64 ± 3	62 ± 8
Male/Female	26/4	21/1	3/0	2/3
Presence of comorbidity (n, %)	18 (60%)	11 (50%)	2 (67%)	5 (100%)
Operation type (n)				
Lobectomy	14	11	0	3
Greater resection	11[a]	8[b]	2[c]	1[d]
Segmentectomy	5	3	1	1
Extended resection (n, %)**	16 (53%)	13 (59%)	1 (33%)	2 (40%)
Length of hospital stay (mean days ± SD)	11 ± 4	10 ± 4	14 ± 2	13 ± 9
Mortality (n, %)	1 (3%)	0	0	1 (20%)
Morbidity (n, %)	21 (70%)	14 (64%)	3 (100%)	4 (80%)
Overall survival (mean months ± SD)	19 ± 13	22 ± 13	13 ± 5	6 ± 2
Relapse-free survival (mean months ± SD)	14 ± 12	16 ± 13	9 ± 4	6 ± 2

[a]Pneumonectomy, 8; bilobectomy, 2; lobectomy + segmentectomy, 1
[b]Pneumonectomy, 6; bilobectomy, 1 lobectomy +segmentectomy, 1
[c]Pneumonectomy, 1; bilobectomy, 1
[d]Pneumonectomy, 1
SD: Standart Deviation
*$P > 0.05$ for all parameters
**Including sleeve resection (bronchial or arterial), chest wall resection, pericardial resection and reconstruction, right atrial resection, and diaphragmatic resection and reconstruction

one. There were no significant differences between the groups in terms of age, sex, and presence of comorbidities.

A total of 22 patients (73%) underwent SLR because of either progression of the primary lung tumors after previous chemotherapy (7 patients) and/or definitive radiotherapy with concurrent chemotherapy (10 patients) or recurrent primary lung tumor after previous pulmonary resections and adjuvant treatment (5 patients). Five patients (17%) underwent SLR, because they were considered unsuitable to undergo chemotherapy or radiotherapy because of severe comorbidities. SLR was performed as palliative intent in three patients (10%; two had septic pulmonary abscess and one had severe empyema).

Of the 30 operations, three were performed in 2013, seven in 2014, five in 2015, and 15 in 2016, and they included 14 lobar resections, 11 greater resections (eight pneumonectomies, two bilobectomies, and one lobectomy combined with segmentectomy), and five segmentectomies. A total of 16 patients (53%) required extended surgery (bronchial and/or arterial sleeve in six, chest wall resection in four, pericardial resection and reconstruction in three, right atrial resection in two, and diaphragmatic resection and reconstruction in one). Although most patients in GI required extended resections compared with the other groups, the difference was insignificant.

Overall, 18 patients (60%) had squamous cell carcinoma, 11 (37%) had adenocarcinoma, and one (3%) had adenosquamous cell carcinoma. R0 resections of bronchial and/or vascular margins were performed in 28 patients (93%). Only two patients (7%) had incomplete resections, and they both had positive arterial vascular margins. Final pathological examination demonstrated viable tumor cells in 27 patients (90%). T-stage was T1 in four patients, T2 in six, T3 in 12, and T4 in five. N-stage was N0 in 16 patients, N1 in five, and N2 in six.

Morbidity occurred in 21 patients (70%). According to the Clavien–Dindo classification, the rates of grades 1, 2, and 3 complications were 6.7%, 36.6%, and 26.7%, respectively. Pneumonia was the most common complication (40%), followed by arrhythmia (20%). Among seven patients (23.3%) who underwent revision surgery, five had intrathoracic hematoma and underwent exploration via thoracotomy, which did not reveal major vascular or active bleeding. One patient who had undergone an emergency right upper bilobectomy because of septic pulmonary abscess required revision surgery because of a bronchopleural fistula. One patient in GI who underwent right lower bilobectomy with pericardial resection and reconstruction suffered pericardial graft infection requiring reoperation. Morbidity was not related to age, indication for surgery, type of surgery, presence of comorbidities, requirement of extended resections, results of respiratory function tests, or echocardiographic parameters. Patients who suffered complications had significantly lower hematocrit (34% vs. 37%, $P = 0.04$) and hemoglobin (11 vs. 12 g/dL, $P = 0.05$) levels.

There were no intraoperative deaths. One patient (3%) died of pneumonia 28 days postoperatively. This patient had lower respiratory functions [DLCO, 34%; FEV1, 41%; and maximum volume of oxygen (VO2 max), 13.2 mL/kg/min]. She was considered unsuitable to undergo chemotherapy. She also had a history of lymphoma and treatment, including radiotherapy, which compromised pulmonary function. She underwent double-sleeve left upper lobectomy, and she was one of the aforementioned patients who required revision surgery because of intrathoracic hematoma.

Mean hospital stay was 11 ± 4 days, which was significantly longer in patients in whom a complication developed (12 vs. 7 days, $P = 0.0003$). The hospital stay was not significantly longer in patients with grade 3 compared with those with grade 1 or 2 complications according to the Clavien–Dindo classification (16 vs. 12 days, $P = 0.06$).

Median postoperative follow-up for the surviving 29 patients was 15 (range, 2–50) months. A total of 15 patients (50%) were alive without disease at the end of the study. In 12 patients (40%), locoregional recurrence and/or distant metastasis developed at a median of 10 (range, 6–19) months. Among these patients, five had local recurrence in the ipsilateral thoracic cavity within a median of 6 (range, 6–18) months, whereas seven had metastasis to the brain (three), bones (two), and multiorgan systems (two) at a median of 11 (range, 6–19) months. These patients received further chemotherapy and/or radiotherapy when appropriate, and nine of them died at a median of 24 (range, 8–30) months. Two patients (7%) without evidence of recurrence or distant metastasis died of cardiac failure 2 and 3 months postoperatively. These patients had undergone right upper lobectomy with chest wall resection and reconstruction and partial vertebral corpus resection, and left upper lobe bronchial sleeve lobectomy, respectively. Mean relapse-free and overall survivals were 14 ± 12 months and 19 ± 13 months. Survival rates were not affected by factors analyzed in this study.

Among two patients with positive arterial resection margins (both had negative bronchial margins), one had a recurrence at 6 months, and died of metastasis at 26 months postoperatively, whereas the other had a recurrence at 18 months, and died of metastasis at 30 months. Although patients in GI had longer overall and relapse-free survivals compared with the other groups, the results were insignificant (22 vs. 13 and 6 months; 16 vs. 9 and 6 months, respectively, $P > 0.05$).

Discussion

We evaluated the feasibility and efficacy of SLR in patients with primary lung cancer and compared our results to those of previous reports. SLR in the field of lung cancer treatment is not yet a commonly accepted treatment modality, and the definition of SLR varies among several investigators. The term SLR is generally used when the operation is performed after stereotactic radiotherapy [10, 11] or chemotherapy [12, 13]. A review of the literature mostly reveals cohorts of patients undergoing SLR after local recurrence or persistent tumor following chemoradiotherapy [3, 14–16], radiotherapy, or steretotactic radiotherapy [7, 17, 18]. Table 2 demonstrates several studies published since 2014, including the current study.

The clinical significance of SLR remains controversial, and comparing the results of the aforementioned studies to each other may not be reliable. This is because of the differences in the definition of SLR among investigators and in the patient selection [4]. Therefore, it was proposed that performing SLR might be feasible with appropriate patient selection because the median survival after other treatment modalities generally is <1 year for patients with recurrent local lung cancer [19].

Most of our patients (n = 22) underwent SLR because of progresion of the persistent primary lung tumor after previous chemo and/or definitive radiotherapy and because of local recurrence of primary lung tumor after previous surgery and adjuvant treatment. Our study also included patients in whom chemo- or radiotherapy was considered to be contraindicated (n = 5) and those requiring palliative resection because of complications of the tumor or treatment (n = 3). Similar patient selection criteria were applied in the study reported by Uramoto et al. [12]

There is no exact timing for performing SLR after chemo- and/or radiotherapy. Patients underwent SLR at an interval of 18–96 weeks after completion of the previous treatment (Table 2). Bauman et al. [5] recommended not delaying the operation further because the increased time between completion of radiotherapy and surgery theoretically may cause the development of more fibrosis. Operating on a fibrotic lung, which has brittle and devascularized tissue and obliterated planes, may result in increased risks of fistulae and impaired wound healing. Increasing the duration may cause more difficult identification, manipulation, and dissection of tissues, leading to increased blood loss compared towith standard procedures [20]. However, further delaying SLR after definitive radiotherapy was reported to result in comparable outcomes in terms of complication rates [7]. Shimada et al. [15] reported a large volume of intraoperative blood loss (399 mL) and considerably longer operative duration (5 h).

In our study, SLR was performed at least 24 weeks following the previous definitive chemo- and/or radiotherapy

Table 2 Recent studies concerning SLR

Authors	Years	N	Indication	Timing of surgery in weeks (range)	Mortality (%)	Morbidity (%)	Follow-up (months)	Overall survival (months)	Relapse-free survival (months)
Uramoto et al. [12]	2014	8	Mixed	n.g	0	25	14	n.g.	5.9
Yang et al. [7]	2015	31	Recurrent or persistent tumor after radiotherapy	18 (8–111)	0l	48	n.g.	32	10
Dickhoff et al. [14]	2016	15	Local recurrence and persistent tumor after chemo-, radiotherapy	21 (3–95)	6.7	40	12.1	46	43.6
Schreiner et al. [3]	2016	9	Local recurrence after chemo-, radiotherapy	30 (12–165)	11	22	30	23	21
Verstegen et al. [17]	2016	9	Recurrent or persistent tumor after stereotactic radiotherapy	n.g.	0	33	19	26	n.g.
Shimada et al. [15]	2016	18	Local recurrence and persistent tumor after chemo-, radiotherapy	38 (3–282)	0	28	47	n.g.	n.g.
Mizobuchi et al. [18]	2016	12	Recurrent or persistent tumor after radiotherapy	96 (36–312)	0	n.s.	18	n.g.	n.g.
Sawada et al. [16]	2017	8	Local recurrence and persistent tumor after chemo-, radiotherapy	n.g.	0	38	48	n.g.	n.g
This study	2017	30	Mixed	n.g.	3	70	15	15	11
Only GI patients		22	Recurrent or persistent tumor after definitive chemo-, radiotherapy, or previous surgery and ajduvant treatment	24	0	64	22	22	16

n.g.: not given

in all patients in GI. There was no mortality in this subgroup, whereas the complication rate was higher (64%) than that in previous reports (Table 2). Another important retrospective study by Bauman et al. [5] demonstrated that patients undergoing SLR had a mortality rate of 4% and a high complication rate of 58%. Concerning the whole study population, our mortality and morbidity rates were 3% and 70%, respectively. We demonstrated that the lower hematocrit and hemoglobin levels were related to the development of complications. No other factors were related to morbidity. The complication rate was insignificantly higher in patients who underwent extended resections (44% vs. 57%). As seen in Table 1, all patients who underwent an emergency operation and 80% of the patients in GIII suffered morbidities compared with GI (64%), but the result was insignificant.

To minimize perioperative complications, Yang et al. [7] proposed that pneumonectomy should be avoided, if possible, and the bronchial stump should be covered using appropriate tissues. Dickhoff et al. [14] reported that the survival rate in patients undergoing lobectomy was higher. They also favored coverage of the bronchial stump, especially in patients undergoing pneumonectomy, none of whom had a postoperative bronchopleural fistula in their series. In our series, we routinely reinforced the bronchial stump. We also performed pneumonectomy in only eight patients, five of whom suffered a complication (three had pneumonia and two had atrial fibrillation). As we previously described, morbidity was not related to the type of operation. As pneumonia is the most common complication in our study population, we would like to suggest to obtain preoperative sputum culture the day before operation these subset of patients due to possible colonization of microorganisms during oncological treatment process or preoperatively defined abscess condition.

Follow-up outcomes of several studies are shown in Table 2. Overall and relapse-free survivals were 23–46 and 5.9–43.6 months, respectively. Similar results have been reported in the study by Bauman et al. [5], wherein the survivals were 30 and 5 months, respectively. They concluded that early SLR in patients with abnormal fludeoxyglucose positron emission tomography scans resulted in higher survival rates than in patients with obvious relapse as seen using CT. Yang et al. [7] reported a median overall survival of 32.5 months. Patients with complete resection lived significantly longer compared with those with incomplete resection (60 vs. 20 months). Contrary to these encouraging results, Kuzmik et al. [6] reported a worse overall survival of 9 months.

We demonstrated that the mean overall survival was 19 ± 13 months, slightly lower than that reported in previous reports, and mean relapse-free survival was 14 ± 12 months, similar to that reported in previous studies. However, based on GI only, in which studies include only these patients, we had better results in agreement with the literature (22 and 16 months, respectively). There was no correlation with the survival rates and T- and N-stages of the tumor.

Conclusion

Clinical experience with SLR remains limited, but the reports suggest that SLR is a worthwhile treatment with acceptable morbidity and low mortality rates. Identification of appropriate candidates for SLR has not been clarified and is challenging. We demonstrated that SLR is technically feasible when indicated and can be performed with acceptable mortality, morbidity, and long-term outcomes, even when anatomical resections greater than a lobectomy or extended resections are required. Patients with lower hematocrit and hemoglobin levels may suffer complications.

Based on our results, we suggest that surgery should be performed in patients with progression of the persistent primary tumor after definitive chemo- and/or radiotherapy. Despite the disappointing survival, other indications may be considered for SLR surgery based on the specific evaluation of each patient.

Abbreviations
CT: computed tomography; DLCO: diffusion capacity of the lung for carbon monoxide; FEV1: forced expiratory volume in one second; GI: group 1; GII: group 2; GIII: group 3; SD: standart deviation; SLR: salvage lung surgery; VO2max: maximum volume of oxygen

Acknowledgements
Not applicable.

Funding
This study was not supported.

Authors' contributions
EK designed the study. EK, KA and AT performed surgical procedures. MOO analysed the patienets data. MRA, EK and TC writing the manuscript. All authors read and approved the final manuscript.

Competing interests
The authors declare that they have no competing interests.

Author details
[1]Department of Thoracic Surgery, Istanbul Bilim University Medical Faculty, 34381 Sisli, Istanbul, Turkey. [2]Department of Thoracic Surgery, Group Florence Nightingale Hospitals, Istanbul, Turkey.

References

1. Aupérin A, Le Péchoux C, Rolland E, Curran WJ, Furuse K, Fournel P, et al. Meta-analysis of concomitant versus sequential radiochemotherapy in locally advanced non-small cell lung cancer. J Clin Oncol. 2010;28(13):2181–90.

2. Bradley JD, Paulus R, Komaki R, Masters G, Blumenschein G, Schild S, et al. Standard-dose versus high-dose conformal radiotherapy with concurrent and consolidation carboplatin plus paclitaxel with or without cetuximab for patients with stage IIIA or IIIB non-small-cell lung cancer (RTOG 0617): a randomised, two-by-two factorial phase 3 study. Lancet Oncol. 2015;16(2): 187–99.

3. Schreiner W, Dudek W, Lettmaier S, Fietkau R, Sirbu H. Should salvage surgery be considered for local recurrence after definitive chemoradiation in locally advanced non-small cell lung cancer. J Cardiothorac Surg. 2016. https://doi.org/10.1186/s13019-016-0396-0.

4. Uramoto H. Current topics on salvage thoracic surgery in patients with primary lung cancer. Ann Thorac Cardiovasc Surg. 2016. https://doi.org/10. 5761/atcs.ra.16-00019.

5. Bauman JE, Mulligan MS, Martins RG, Kurland BF, Eaton KD, Wood DE. Salvage lung resection after definitive radiation (>59 Gy) for non-small cell lung cancer: surgical and oncologic outcomes. Ann Thorac Surg. 2008;86(5): 1632–8.

6. Kuzmik GA, Detterbeck FC, Decker RH, Boffa DJ, Wang Z, Oliva IB, et al. Pulmonary resections following prior definitive chemoradiation therapy are associated with acceptable survival. Eur J Cardiothorac Surg. 2013. https:// doi.org/10.1093/ejcts/ezt184.

7. Yang CJ, Meyerhoff RR, Stephens SJ, Singhapricha T, Toomey CB, Anderson KL, et al. Long-term outcomes of lobectomy for non-small cell lung cancer after definitive radiation treatment. Ann Thorac Surg. 2015;99(6):1914–20.

8. Maguire MF, Berry CB, Gellett L, Berrisford RG. Catastrophic haemoptysis during rigid bronchoscopy: a discussion of treatment options to salvage patients during catastrophic haemoptysis at rigid bronchoscopy. Interact Cardiovasc Thorac Surg. 2004;3(2):222–5.

9. Dindo D, Demartines N, Clavien PA. Classification of surgical complications: a new proposal with evaluation in a cohort of 6336 patients and results of a survey. Ann Surg. 2004;240(2):205–13.

10. Chen F, Matsuo Y, Yoshizawa A, Sato T, Sakai H, Bando T, et al. Salvage lung resection for non-small cell lung cancer after stereotactic body radiotherapy in initially operable patients. J Thorac Oncol. 2010;5(12): 1999–2002.

11. Van Schill PE. Salvage surgery after stereotactic radiotherapy: a new challenge for thoracic surgeons. J Thorac Oncol. 2010;5(12):1881–2.

12. Uramoto H, Tanaka F. Salvage thoracic surgery in patients with primary lung cancer. Lung Cancer. 2014;84(2):151–5.

13. Hishida T, Nagai K, Mitsudomi T, Yokoi K, Kondo H, Horinouchi H, et al. Salvage surgery for advanced non-small cell lung cancer after response to gefitinib. J Thorac Cardiovasc Surg. 2010. https://doi.org/10.1016/j.jtcvs.2010. 06.035.

14. Dickhoff C, Dahele M, Paul MA, van de Ven PM, de Langen AJ, Senan S, et al. Salvage surgery for locoregional recurrence or persistent tumor after high döşe chemoradiotherapy for locally advanced non-small cell lung cancer. Lung Cancer. 2016;94:108–13.

15. Shimada Y, Suzuki K, Okada M, Nakayama H, Ito H, Mitsudomi T, et al. Feasibility and efficacy of salvage lung resection after definitive chemoradiation therapy for stage III non-small-cell lung cancer. Interact Cardiovasc Thorac Surg. 2016;23(6):895–901.

16. Sawada S, Suehisa H, Ueno T, Yamashita M. Eight cases of salvage pulmonary resection for residual disease or isolated local recurrence detected after definitive chemoradiotherapy for N2 stage-IIIA lung cancer. Asian J Surg. 2017;40(2):95–9.

17. Verstegen NE, Maat APWM, Lagerwaard FJ, Paul MA, Versteegh MI, Joosten JJ, et al. Salvage surgery for local failures after stereotactic ablative radiotherapy for early stage non-small cell lung cancer. Radiat Oncol. 2016;11(1):131.

18. Mizobuchi T, Yamamoto N, Nakajima M, Baba M, Miyoshi K, Nakayama H, et al. Salvage surgery for local recurrence after carbon ion radiotherapy for patients with lung cancer. Eur J Cardiothorac Surg. 2016;49(5):1503–9.

19. Noble J, Ellis PM, Mackay JA, Evans WK. Second-line or subsequent systemic therapy for recurrent or progressive non-small cell lung cancer: a systematic review and practice guideline. J Thorac Oncol. 2006;1(9): 1042–58.

20. Van Breussegem A, Hendriks JM, Lauwers P, Van Schill PE. Salvage surgery after high-dose radiotherapy. J Thorac Dis. 2017;9(3):193–200.

16

Patients want more information after surgery: a prospective audit of satisfaction with perioperative information in lung cancer surgery

Nicola Oswald[1], John Hardman[2], Amy Kerr[2], Ehab Bishay[2], Richard Steyn[2], Pala Rajesh[2], Maninder Kalkat[2] and Babu Naidu[1*]

Abstract

Background: Receiving information about their disease and treatment is very important to patients with cancer. There is an association between feeling appropriately informed and better quality of life. This audit aimed to estimate patient satisfaction with perioperative information in those undergoing surgery for lung cancer and any change in satisfaction over time.

Methods: A questionnaire (EORTC-Info-25) was administered prospectively to patients preoperatively and up to six months postoperatively. The preoperative questionnaire was completed by 292 patients and 88 free text comments were completed. Intrapersonal responses were compared over time.

Results: Patients were highly satisfied with information prior to surgery. The overall helpfulness of information did not change over time but satisfaction with the amount of information decreased. Patients who received more information about 'the disease' and 'things you can do to help yourself get well' were less likely to report a drop in satisfaction (Odds Ratio 0.858, 95% Confidence interval 0.765 to 0.961, $p = 0.008$ and OR 0.102, 95% CI 0.018 to 0. 590, $p = 0.011$ respectively). Free text responses revealed patients most frequently wanted more information on the disease, aftercare and self-care. Suffering complications from surgery was not associated with a change in satisfaction with information postoperatively.

Conclusions: Patients want to know more about their diagnosis, but also how to recover and cope with issues once they have gone home after surgery. Postoperative satisfaction with information may improve if patients are given more information on these topics.

Keywords: Education, Patient, Lung neoplasm, Assessment, Patient outcome, Patient satisfaction, Thoracic surgery

Background

Cancer patients want to know as much as possible about their illness [1]. Appropriate provision of information is associated with superior health related quality of life, lower levels of anxiety and lower levels of depression amongst cancer survivors [2, 3]. Appropriate information has also been shown to have benefits with regards to pain and preparedness for surgery [3–5]. However, clinic appointments are time limited and there is often a short interval between this appointment and surgery being undertaken [1, 6]. The aim of this audit was to record patient satisfaction with perioperative information and to identify unmet informational needs in patients undergoing lung cancer resection in order to benchmark and then improve our service.

Methods

A prospective single centre audit was undertaken at a tertiary thoracic surgical unit after registration with

* Correspondence: b.naidu@bham.ac.uk
[1]Institute of Inflammation and Ageing, University of Birmingham Laboratories, University of Birmingham, Queen Elizabeth Hospital Birmingham, Edgbaston, Birmingham B15 2TT, UK
Full list of author information is available at the end of the article

the local Audit and Governance department. Consecutive patients attending the preoperative assessment clinic in preparation for any lung resection, pleural procedures or lung cancer staging procedures under general anaesthetic were invited to complete questionnaires. As part of routine care prior to undergoing surgery patients receive information from their Cancer Specialist Nurse, Respiratory Physician, Thoracic Surgeon and Preoperative Assessment Nurse. The audit institution routinely provides a lung surgery handbook and DVD to patients via their Cancer Specialist Nurse.

Preoperative questionnaires were completed in the preoperative assessment clinic. Follow up questionnaires were posted to patients between at six weeks postoperatively, and again at five months postoperatively to assess the performance of the department throughout the surgical pathway. Data on postoperative complications were collected prospectively including the occurrence of atrial fibrillation, wound infection, discharge with a drain in situ, discharge with a urinary catheter in situ, chest infection, the need to have a chest drain reinserted postoperatively, unplanned admission to the Intensive Care Unit, return to theatre and readmission to hospital within 30 days of discharge.

Satisfaction was assessed via administration of the European Organisation for Research and Treatment of Cancer Quality of Life Questionnaire – Information Module (EORTC-QLQ-Info25), which has been validated internationally among cancer patients [7]. The questionnaire multi-item scales are organised across four groups—information about the disease, medical tests, treatment and other services, and eight single items. Scaling of responses between 0% and 100% was performed as per EORTC guidance [8]. Questions about the amount of information (question 52) and helpfulness of information (question 55) were used to assess overall satisfaction.

Data were not normally distributed and so non parametric tests were employed. Comparison of ordinal data before and after surgery was performed using a Wilcoxon signed rank test. Binary logistic regression was performed with the presence of a drop in overall satisfaction as the dependent variable and satisfaction with each topic of information as the independent variables. Analysis was performed using IBM SPSS version 22 (IBM Corp. Armonk, NY). A p value of less than 0.05 was deemed statistically significant. Missing data were handled as per the EORTC scoring manual; if more than half of the data points for a group were present a mean was calculated [7, 8]. Free text responses were grouped into themes according to broad categories after review by two individuals.

Results

Over 27 months 292 patients filled in a response to the preoperative questionnaire, the response rate was 36.5%. Postoperative follow up questionnaires were completed by 85 patients at five months; seven patients did not undergo surgery and 36 died prior to completing a postoperative questionnaire giving a follow up rate of 34.1%. Individual preoperative questionnaires were 95.5% complete, individual postoperative questionnaires were 94.6% complete. The baseline characteristics of the patients included within the study are listed in Table 1. The overall incidence of complications was 34%.

Amongst preoperative questionnaires the highest score was obtained for information about medical tests (median 77.8%, Inter Quartile Range 66.7%–100.0%); the lowest score was recorded for information about other services (median 25.0%, IQR 8.3–50.5%).

Overall helpfulness of information did not change over time (median 66.7% and IQR 66.7–100% at each time point, $p = 0.108$), however satisfaction with the amount of information was significantly lower postoperatively ($p = 0.043$). Preoperatively the median satisfaction with amount of information was 100% (IQR 66.7–100%), and five months postoperatively the median satisfaction was 66.7% (IQR 33.3–100%). The trends over time are illustrated in Figs. 1 and 2.

The factors underlying the decline in satisfaction postoperatively were investigated further using binary logistic regression and a significant model was found, correctly classifying 84.0% of cases (X^2 35.635, $p < 0.001$, Nagelkerke R^2 0.683). Patients who received more information about 'the disease' and 'things you can do to help yourself get well' were less likely to report a drop in satisfaction (Odds Ratio 0.858, 95%

Table 1 Baseline patient characteristics

	Total sample ($n = 292$)
Mean age (range)	67 (24–88)
Gender % male	55.5% (162)
Operative procedure	
Cervical mediastinoscopy	4.1% (12)
Wedge resection, segment	18.2% (53)
Metastasectomy	5.5% (16)
Lobectomy/bilobectomy	59.2% (173)
Pneumonectomy	3.4% (10)
Open and close	2.4% (7)
None[a]	2.4% (7)
Other	4.8% (14)
Incision	
VATS	37.3% (109)

[a]Patients did not proceed to surgery for medical reasons

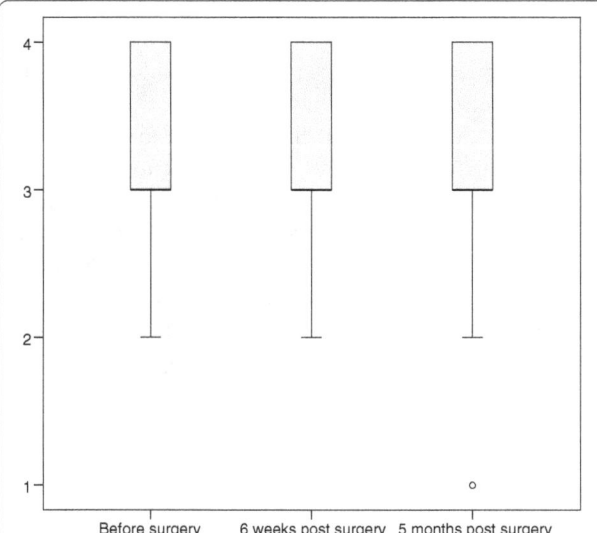

Fig. 1 Box plot displaying satisfaction reported in question 55 over time 'Overall has the information you have received been helpful?': 1 = not at all, 2 = a little, 3 = quite a bit, 4 = very much

Confidence interval 0.765 to 0.961, $p = 0.008$ and OR 0.102, 95% CI 0.018 to 0.590, $p = 0.011$ respectively). Patients who received more information about 'medical tests' were more likely to report a drop in satisfaction postoperatively, although this had smaller effect (OR 1.072, 95% CI 1.003–1.146, $p = 0.041$). The presence of a complication did not significantly change satisfaction with information (OR 0.636, 95% CI 0.055 to 7.324, $p = 0.717$).

A total of 88 free text responses were completed by 65 individuals. General comments about information or

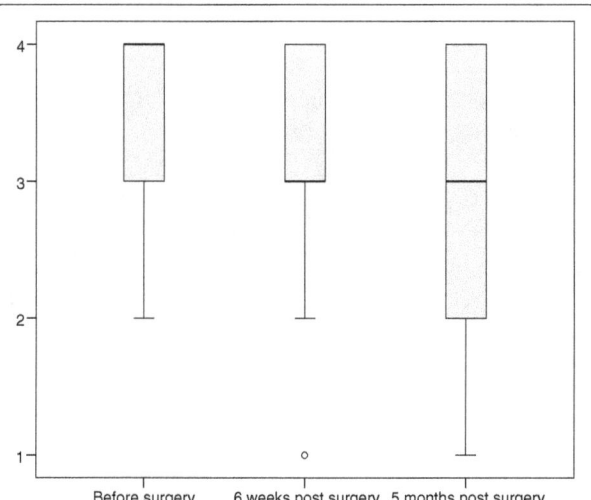

Fig. 2 Box plot displaying satisfaction reported in question 52 over time 'Were you satisfied with the amount of information you received?': 1 = not at all, 2 = a little, 3 = quite a bit, 4 = very much

clinical care were frequent. For example, 'Cancer Nurse Specialist information was invaluable'. The topics that patients wished to know more about are shown in Table 2. The most commonly desired topics (the disease, aftercare and self-care) match the topics that were associated with a decline in postoperative satisfaction.

The underlying theme of self-care encapsulates what the patient can do to help himself or herself. The underlying theme of aftercare is what healthcare professionals can do to help the patient. There is of course extensive crossover between the two categories with a dynamic interaction between patient and healthcare professional. Within 'the disease', four patients wanted to know more about mycobacterium tuberculosis (TB). This is an important consideration for patients undergoing surgery with a diagnostic element because the medical treatment of TB is intensive and may come as a shock to patients. One patient commented that information 'made me scared'.

Discussion

This report of the findings from a prospective audit of patient satisfaction with perioperative information before and after thoracic surgery is the first to use the EORTC-QLQ-Info25 questionnaire specifically in those undergoing surgery for lung cancer. Satisfaction with information preoperatively was high amongst our patients and compares favourably with published scores [7]. The fall in satisfaction postoperatively may mean patients are less well prepared for surgery than they had thought. This would be consistent with qualitative research in which patients felt prepared for lung cancer surgery preoperatively, but felt less well prepared postoperatively [9]. The qualitative report included follow up limited to five days after surgery, thus our audit covering the weeks and months following discharge provides important additional information that this effect is not limited to the immediate inpatient period. In addition, the quantitative questionnaire used can be completed in any surgical centre to compare and reflect upon the services being provided locally. The decline postoperatively may indicate patients thought they were well informed but with the benefit of hindsight they needed more information preoperatively. Alternatively patients may be well informed before surgery but less well informed during the weeks and months following surgery as they recover. Both interpretations indicate that patients want more information about recovery and carrying on with life after surgery. Research should seek to describe the experience of patients in recovering from surgery after discharge, including the return to normal life, and then the impact of including this information in patient information.

Our finding that complications had no effect on satisfaction with information supports the concept that

Table 2 Topics that patient would like to know more about

Topic	Responses % (n)	Equivalent Info 25 question
Aftercare	17.0% (15)	44, 45, 46, 47
The disease	12.5% (11)	31, 32, 33, 34
Self-care	10.2% (9)	49
Chemo/radiotherapy	6.8% (6)	38
Specific information about their case	6.8% (6)	No question
Prognosis & outcome of surgery	6.8% (6)	32, 34, 39
Everything	5.7% (5)	52
Finances	3.4% (3)	No question
Pain	2.3% (2)	40
The surgery	2.3% (2)	38
Other	26.1% (23)	

Patient Reported Outcome Measures (PROMs) measure a different aspect of care to traditional measures such as morbidity and mortality. This is in agreement with a published case-matched analysis that found complications did not impact upon patients' satisfaction with the quality of care they received [10, 11]. Assessment of quality in surgical lung cancer care currently relates to mortality and resection rate. This audit supports the stance that PROMs are not a surrogate marker of conventional outcomes, but they represent complementary measures with value in their own right.

The consequences of receiving insufficient information may go beyond low patient satisfaction. Patients may have a decreased quality of life for many years following surgery for lung cancer, the reasons for this are currently uncertain [12]. In patients with head and neck cancer, satisfaction with information has been shown to predict postoperative depression and psychological components of quality of life [13]. A variety of formats of information are effective for patient education, resulting in reduced anxiety and increased satisfaction [14, 15]. Patients report wanting to talk with healthcare professionals prior to surgery and then read information independently postoperatively [9]. Patients undergoing thoracic surgery and their carers also frequently use the internet to seek more information [9, 16]. Websites allow the provision of written and audiovisual information that is readily accessible, accurate websites could be a valuable addition to preoperative information.

Our audit findings are subject to some limitations, most importantly the number of missing postoperative questionnaires. However, the patients who did or did not return postoperative questionnaires had similar baseline characteristics and the distribution of operative procedures was similar to national figures [17]. Patients commented upon the large number of questions in each questionnaire during the audit, this may well have contributed to our loss to follow up. A PROM tool which has fewer questions may be more acceptable to patients.

Confounding factors may be present among our patientd including personality types and educational level. Distressed personality types report lower satisfaction and that they have been given less information and those with higher educational levels report lower satisfaction [18, 19]. Intrapersonal comparison should reduce the impact of these in comparing responses across time; in addition the fact that free text responses and binary regression analysis identified similar topics of importance supports the findings being real and not due to a statistical phenomenon.

Conclusions

Patients feel well informed before lung cancer resection. In the weeks and months following surgery patients feel less well informed and want to know more about the disease they have, recovery and how to cope with issues once they have gone home after surgery. Improving the information given to patients may have additional benefits in terms of quality of life outcomes so research into the patient experience of recovery from lung cancer resection and the impact of including this information in patient information literature is desirable. The findings of this audit were used to develop content for a patient information website available at http://www.thoracicsurgery.co.uk.

Acknowledgements
We would like to thank Dr. Sarah Flanagan at the University of Birmingham for her advice in categorising free text responses to questionnaires and second review of these responses.

Funding
The authors have no funding source to declare.

Authors' contributions
BN is the principal investigator and designed and registered the study. JH and AK collected patient data, distributed and collected questionnaires, collected data on postoperative complications and input data into electronic spreadsheets. RS, EB, MK and PR assisted in data collection. NO collected any missing data points, performed and interpreted the statistical analysis, and wrote the manuscript. All authors have read, critically reviewed, and approved the manuscript.

Competing interests
The authors declare that they have no competing interests.

Author details
[1]Institute of Inflammation and Ageing, University of Birmingham Laboratories, University of Birmingham, Queen Elizabeth Hospital Birmingham, Edgbaston, Birmingham B15 2TT, UK. [2]Department of Thoracic Surgery, Heart of England NHS Foundation Trust, Bordesley Green East, Birmingham Heartlands Hospital, Birmingham B9 5SS, UK.

References

1. Jenkins V, Fallowfield L, Saul J. Information needs of patients with cancer: results from a large study in UK cancer centres. Br J Cancer. 2001;84:48–51. https://doi.org/10.1054/bjoc.2000.1573.

2. Husson O, Mols F, van de Poll-franse LV. The relation between information provision and health-related quality of life, anxiety and depression among cancer survivors: a systematic review. Ann Oncol. 2011;22:761–72. https://doi.org/10.1093/annonc/mdq413.

3. Annunziata MA, Foladore S, Magri MD, Crivellari D, Feltrin A, Bidoli E, et al. Does the information level of cancer patients correlate with quality of life? A prospective study. Tumori. 1998;84:619–23.

4. Crabtree TD, Puri V, Bell JM, Bontumasi N, Patterson GA, Kreisel D, et al. Outcomes and perception of lung surgery with implementation of a patient video education module: a prospective cohort study. J Am Coll Surg. 2012; 214:816–821.e2. https://doi.org/10.1016/j.jamcollsurg.2012.01.047.

5. Barlési F, Barrau K, Loundou A, Doddoli C, Simeoni M-C, Auquier P, et al. Impact of information on quality of life and satisfaction of non-small cell lung cancer patients: a randomized study of standardized versus individualized information before thoracic surgery. J Thorac Oncol Off Publ Int Assoc Study Lung Cancer. 2008;3:1146–52. https://doi.org/10.1097/JTO. 0b013e3181874637.

6. Pimentel FL, Ferreira JS, Vila Real M, Mesquita NF, Maia-Gonçalves JP. Quantity and quality of information desired by Portuguese cancer patients. Support Care Cancer Off J Multinatl Assoc Support Care Cancer. 1999;7:407–12.

7. Arraras JI, Greimel E, Sezer O, Chie WC, Bergenmar M, Costantini A, et al. An international validation study of the EORTC QLQ-INFO25 questionnaire: an instrument to assess the information given to cancer patients. Eur J Cancer Oxf Engl. 2010;46:2726–38. https://doi.org/10.1016/j.ejca.2010.06.118.

8. Fayers P, Aaronson N, Bjordal K, et al. EORTC QLQ-C30. Scoring manual. 2002.

9. King J, Chamberland P, Rawji A, Ager A, Léger R, Michaels R, et al. Patient educational needs of patients undergoing surgery for lung cancer. J Cancer Educ. 2014;29:802–7. https://doi.org/10.1007/s13187-014-0658-2.

10. Pompili C, Tiberi M, Salati M, Refai M, Xiumé F, Brunelli A. Patient satisfaction with health-care professionals and structure is not affected by longer hospital stay and complications after lung resection: a case-matched analysis. Interact Cardiovasc Thorac Surg. 2015;20:236–41. https://doi.org/10.1093/icvts/ivu371.

11. Barlési F, Boyer L, Doddoli C, Antoniotti S, Thomas P, Auquier P. THe place of patient satisfaction in quality assessment of lung cancer thoracic surgery*. Chest. 2005;128:3475–81. https://doi.org/10.1378/chest.128.5.3475.

12. Rauma V, Sintonen H, Räsänen JV, Salo JA, Ilonen IK. Long-term lung cancer survivors have permanently decreased quality of life after surgery. Clin Lung Cancer. 2015;16:40–5. https://doi.org/10.1016/j.cllc.2014.08.004.

13. Llewellyn CD, McGurk M, Weinman J. How satisfied are head and neck cancer (HNC) patients with the information they receive pre-treatment? Results from the satisfaction with cancer information profile (SCIP). Oral Oncol. 2006;42:726–34. https://doi.org/10.1016/j.oraloncology.2005.11.013.

14. Wallace LM. Surgical patients' preferences for pre-operative information. Patient Educ Couns. 1985;7:377–87.

15. Friedman AJ, Cosby R, Boyko S, Hatton-Bauer J, Turnbull G. Effective teaching strategies and methods of delivery for patient education: a systematic review and practice guideline recommendations. J Cancer Educ Off J Am Assoc Cancer Educ. 2011;26:12–21. https://doi.org/10.1007/s13187-010-0183-x.

16. Lussiez AD, Burdick S, Kodali S, Rubio G, Mack JA, Lin J, et al. Internet usage trends in thoracic surgery patients and their caregivers. J Cancer Educ Off J Am Assoc Cancer Educ. 2017;32:91–6. https://doi.org/10.1007/s13187-015-0934-9.

17. West D, Dunning J, Lim E, Asif M, McManus K, Healey D, et al. SCTS thoracic registry brief report: 2011–12 to 2013–14 n.d.

18. Husson O, Denollet J, Oerlemans S, Mols F. Satisfaction with information provision in cancer patients and the moderating effect of type D personality. Psychooncology. 2013;22:2124–32. https://doi.org/10.1002/pon.3267.

19. Pompili C, Brunelli A, Rocco G, Salvi R, Xiumé F, La Rocca A, et al. Patient satisfaction after pulmonary resection for lung cancer: a multicenter comparative analysis. Respir Int Rev Thorac Dis. 2013;85: 106–11. https://doi.org/10.1159/000337262.

SIRT1 overexpression is an independent prognosticator for patients with esophageal squamous cell carcinoma

Ming-Chun Ma[1], Tai-Jan Chiu[1], Hung-I Lu[2], Wan-Ting Huang[3], Chien-Ming Lo[2], Wan-Yu Tien[1], Ya-Chun Lan[1], Yen-Yang Chen[1], Chang-Han Chen[4,5,6] and Shau-Hsuan Li[1*]

Abstract

Background: Sirtuin 1 (SIRT1) regulates DNA repair and metabolism by deacetylating target proteins. SIRT1 may be oncogenic because its overexpression has been detected in many cancers. The aim of the present study was to clarify the prognostic role of SIRT1 in patients with esophageal squamous cell carcinoma (ESCC) and evaluate the effect of SIRT1 inhibitor in vitro.

Methods: The expression of SIRT1 was evaluated immunohistochemically in 155 surgically resected ESCC and the staining results were evaluated semiquantitatively by the Immunoreactive Scoring System. The clinical features and treatment outcome were analyzed. The effect of SIRT1 inhibitor, SIRT 1 inhibitor IV, (S)-35, was investigated in vitro on ESCC cell lines.

Results: The expression of SIRT1 on ESCC did not correlate with age, gender, tumor location, stage, T classification, N classification, surgical margin or histology. Univariate analysis showed that SIRT1 overexpression was associated with inferior overall survival ($P = 0.004$) and disease-free survival ($P = 0.004$). In multivariate comparison, SIRT1 overexpression remained independently associated with worse overall survival ($P = 0.009$, hazard ratio = 1.776) and disease-free survival ($P = 0.017$, hazard ratio = 1.642). In cell lines, SIRT1 inhibitor inhibited ESCC growth.

Conclusions: Our study suggests that SIRT1 overexpression is an independent prognosticator for patients with ESCC and the SIRT1 inhibitor suppressed cell proliferation of ESCC cell lines. Our findings suggest that inhibition of SIRT1 signaling may be a promising novel target for ESCC.

Keywords: Esophageal squamous cell carcinoma, SIRT1, Overexpression

Background

The standard therapy for patients with esophageal squamous cell carcinoma (ESCC) is surgery and concurrent chemoradiothrapy [1–3]. Much improvement was achieved during the past decades. However, the tumor recurs despite of extensive surgery, and the prognosis was still unsatisfactory [1, 4, 5]. Identification of prognostic biomarkers for ESCC is crucial for clinicians to make risk-adapted treatment plans and the potential for novel target therapy.

Mammalian sirtuins deacetylases consist of seven family members (SIRT1–7) that have been shown to be critical regulators of cell signaling pathways [6, 7]. SIRT1 is a NAD + –dependent deacetylase that plays important roles in many biological processes, including stress response, apoptosis, cellular metabolism, adaptation to calorie restriction, aging, and tumorigenesis.

Because some members of the various classes of histone deacetylases (HDACs) have been shown to be overexpressed in diverse cancers, current views suggest that perturbed acetylation patterns on proteins may contribute to cellular transformation and tumor progression [6, 8, 9]. SIRT1 can activate stress defense and DNA repair mechanisms, and therefore aids in the preservation of genomic integrity [10, 11]. SIRT1 also functions in the regulation of

* Correspondence: lee.a0928@msa.hinet.net
[1]Department of Hematology-Oncology, Kaohsiung Chang Gung Memorial Hospital and Chang Gung University College of Medicine, 123 Ta-Pei Road, Niaosong Dist, Kaohsiung, Taiwan, Republic of China
Full list of author information is available at the end of the article

metabolism and maintaining the integrity of the genome, and thus has been described as a potential tumor suppressor [11]. For example, both breast cancer and hepatocellular carcinoma exhibit reduced SIRT1 levels compared with normal tissues [12]. Wang et al. [12] demonstrated that Sirt1(+/−); p53(+/−) mice develop tumors in multiple tissues, whereas activation of SIRT1 by resveratrol treatment reduces tumorigenesis, and thus suggested that SIRT1 may act as a tumor suppressor through its role in DNA damage response and genome integrity. Previous study [11] also showed that SIRT1 activity is required for suppressing survivin transcription, and reduction of survivin via SIRT1 activity may play an important role in breast cancer susceptibility gene 1 (BRCA1)-associated mammary tumor formation. Conversely, other studies showed that overexpression of SIRT1 caused the suppression of DNA damage repair proteins and factors involved in tumor suppression, and thus led to increased tumor growth and cell survival [11, 13]. Previous studies [11] revealed that SIRT1-mediated deacetylation suppresses the functions of several tumor suppressors, including p53, p73, and hypermethylated in cancer 1 (HIC1). Upregulation of SIRT1 has been reported in various human malignancies including prostate cancer, breast cancer, lung cancer, lymphoma, leukemia, soft tissue sarcomas, colon cancer, and gastric cancer [11, 14–19]. In recent years, a number of inhibitors have been discovered and characterized. This raises the possibility that SIRT1 inhibition might suppress cancer cell proliferation [11]. However, the role of SIRT1 in ESCC remains largely undefined. Therefore, we conducted the present study to evaluate the prognostic significance of SIRT1 in patients with ESCC by immunohistochemistry and investigate the effect of SIRT1 inhibitor in vitro.

Methods

Patient population

Patients with ESCC who received surgical resection at Kaohsiung Chang Gung Memorial Hospital were reviewed retrospectively. This study was approved by the Institutional Review Board of Chang Gung Memorial Hospital. The approval number of this project was 201800339B0. Patients with second malignancy and who receiving chemotherapy and/or radiotherapy before surgery were excluded. We identified 155 patients with available paraffin blocks and follow-up. Patients underwent a radical esophagectomy with cervical esophagogastric anastomosis (McKeown procedure) or an Ivor Lewis esophagectomy with intrathoracic anastomosis, reconstruction of the digestive tract with gastric tube, and pylorus drainage procedures. Two-field lymph node dissection was performed in all patients. The pathologic TNM stage was determined according to the 7th American Joint Committee on Cancer (AJCC) staging system. After surgery, patients were followed at 3-month intervals for 2 years, 6-month

intervals up to year 5, and annually thereafter. Disease-free survival (DFS) was calculated from the time of operation to the recurrence or death from any cause without evidence of recurrence. Overall survival (OS) was calculated from the time of operation to death as a result of all causes.

Immunohistochemistry

Immunohistochemistry was used to evaluate the expression of SIRT1. Formalin-fixed and paraffin-embedded 4-μm thick tumor tissue slices were dewaxed and rehydrated before antigen retrieval. The microwave antigen retrieval method was then utilized, and the slides were immersed in EDTA antigen retrieval solution (pH 9.0) for 15 min. Subsequently, we added 3% hydrogen peroxide to the slides to inhibit endogenous peroxidase activity. Subsequently, SIRT1 (1:150; Abcam, Cambridge, UK) was applied to the sections that were later incubated at 4 °C overnight. On the second day, biotinylated antibody and streptavidinperoxidase reagent were successively applied for 15 min each at 37 °C. Finally, 3,3′-diaminobenzidine tetrahydrochloride (DAB) was used for visualization, and hematoxylin was added as a counterstain. The positive controls were human non-small cell lung cancer tissues expressing SIRT1. Sections that were incubated with PBS instead of primary antibodies were used as negative controls. Both the positive and negative controls were used to evaluate the reliability of staining and exclude nonspecific reactions. The expression level of SIRT1 protein was calculated utilizing a semiquantitative scoring system. The staining score was classified as 0 (negative staining), 1 (weak staining), 2 (moderate staining) and 3 (strong staining). The quantity score, which represented the percentage of cancer cells that were positively stained, was calculated as follows: 0 (0–5%), 1 (6–25%), 2 (26–50%), 3 (51–75%), and 4 (≥76%). By multiplying the staining score by the quantity score of each slide, the final semiquantitative score was obtained (ranging from 0 to 12). Scores that ranged from 4 to 12 were considered to represent overexpression.

Cell culture and 3-(4.5-dimethylthiazol-2-yl)-2,5-diphenyltetrazolium bromide assay

Human esophageal squamous cell carcinoma cell line KYSE 270 and KYSE 70 were obtained from the European Collection of Authenticated Cell Cultures (ECACC). The KYSE 270 cell line was maintained in RPMI 1640 (Invitrogen, Carlsbad, CA) and Ham's F12 (Nissui Pharmaceutical, Tokyo, Japan) mixed (1:1) medium containing 2% fetal bovine serum. The KYSE 70 cell line was maintained in RPMI 1640 medium (Invitrogen, Carlsbad, CA) medium containing 10% fetal bovine serum. To test the effects of cell proliferation of SIRT1 inhibitor, SIRT 1 inhibitor IV, (S)-35 (Calbiochem, Merck Millipore, Darmstadt, Germany), cells were plated into 96-well, flat bottomed plates at 3×10^3 cells per 100 mL per well in the recommended medium containing 10% fetal bovine serum. After overnight incubation, triplicate wells were treated with different concentrations of SIRT1 inhibitor (0, 5, 10 and 20 µM) for 24 h. The relative percentages of metabolically active cells compared with untreated controls were then determined on the basis of mitochondrial conversion of 3- (4.5-dimethylthiazol-2-yl)-2,5-diphenyltetrazolium bromide (MTT) to formazine. In brief, after incubation, 10 mL of MTT (Sigma, St Louis, MO) solution (5 mg/mL) was added to each well for 3 h, and the medium was then replaced with 150 mL of dimethylsulfoxide per well. Results were assessed in a 96-well format plate reader by measuring the absorbance at a wavelength of 540 nm using a Titertek Multiscan (Thermo, Vantaa, Finland).

Statistical analysis

The SPSS software package (18.0; SPSS, Chicago, IL, USA) was used for statistical analysis. Correlations among SIRT1 and various clinicopathologic characteristics were compared using the chi-square test. Survival curves were constructed using the Kaplan-Meier method, and the significance of differences in the survival of subgroups was examined with the log rank test. Independent prognostic factors were determined by multivariate Cox regression analysis. P values less than 0.05 were considered significant.

Results

Patient characteristics

The median age for the 155 patients (150 men and 5 women) was 55 years (range, 29–77). The 7th AJCC stages of 155 patients with ESCC were stage I in 44 patients, stage II in 68, stage III in 39, and stage IV in 4 (Table 1). The histologic grading was grade 1 in 16 patients, grade 2 in 108, and grade 3 in 31. The tumor locations were upper esophagus in 22 patients, middle in 60, and lower in 73. At the time of analysis, the median periods of follow-up were 65.8 months (range, 50.4~ 238 months) for the 50 survivors and 37.6 months (range, 0.9~ 238 months) for all 155 patients. The 3-year OS and DFS rates for these 155 patients were 52% and 43%, respectively. The 5-year OS and DFS rates for these 155 patients were 44% and 37%, respectively.

Correlation between clinicopathologic parameters and SIRT1 expression

Among the 155 patients, SIRT1 overexpression was identified in 77 (55%) patients (Fig. 1). There was no correlation between the clinicopathological factors and the IHC expression of SIRT1 (Table 2).

Table 1 Characteristics of 155 patients with esophageal squamous cell carcinoma receiving esophagectomy

Age	median	55
	mean	56.2
	range	29~ 77
Sex	male	150 (97%)
	female	5 (3%)
Primary tumor location	Upper	22 (14%)
	Middle	60 (39%)
	Lower	73 (47%)
T classification	T1	48 (31%)
	T2	31 (20%)
	T3	61 (39%)
	T4	15 (10%)
N classification	N0	106 (68%)
	N1	30 (19%)
	N2	13 (9%)
	N3	6 (4%)
7th AJCC Stage	IA	7 (5%)
	IB	37 (24%)
	IIA	25 (16%)
	IIB	43 (28%)
	IIIA	15 (9%)
	IIIB	6 (4%)
	IIIC	18 (12%)
	IV	4 (2%)
Histological grading	Grade 1	16 (10%)
	Grade 2	108 (70%)
	Grade 3	31 (20%)
Surgical margin	Negative	135 (87%)
	Positive	20 (13%)
SIRT1 expression	Low expression	78 (50%)
	Overexpression	77 (50%)

AJCC American Joint Committee on Cancer, *SIRT1* Sirtuin1

Survival analyses

Correlations of clinicopathologic parameters and SIRT1 with OS and DFS are shown in Table 3. Univariate analyses demonstrated that 7th AJCC stage III + IV ($P < 0.001$), T3 + 4 disease ($P < 0.001$), positive regional lymph node ($P < 0.001$), histological grading 3 ($P = 0.001$), positive surgical margin ($P = 0.023$), SIRT1 overexpression ($P = 0.004$, Fig. 2a) were associated with inferior OS. Additionally, 7th AJCC stage III + IV, T3 + 4 disease ($P < 0.001$), histological grading 3 ($P = 0.002$), positive regional lymph node ($P < 0.001$), positive surgical margin ($P = 0.046$) and SIRT1 overexpression ($P = 0.004$, Fig. 2b) were associated with inferior DFS. The 3-year OS and DFS rates were 63% and 54% in patients with

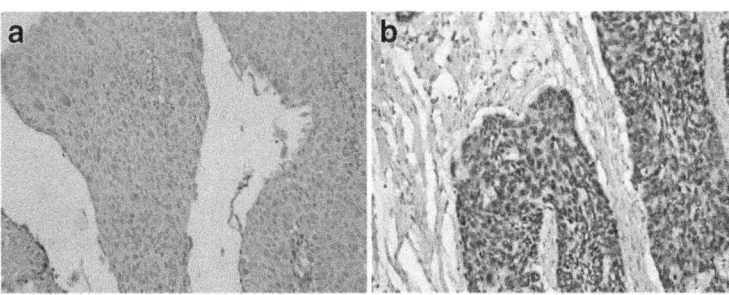

Fig. 1 Immunohistochemical staining of SIRT1. **a** Low expression of SIRT1. **b** Overexpression of SIRT1. Original magnification × 200

low expression of SIRT1 and 39% and 33% in patients with overexpression of SIRT1, respectively. The 5-year OS and DFS rates were 55% and 49% in patients with low expression of SIRT1 and 34% and 26% in patients with overexpression of SIRT1, respectively.

In multivariate comparisons, SIRT1 overexpression ($P = 0.009$, hazard ratio [HR], 1.776, 95% CI, 1.152–2.747) and T3 + 4 disease ($P = 0.002$, hazard ratio [HR], 2.250, 95% CI, 1.339–3.782) remained independently associated with inferior OS (Table 4). For DFS, SIRT1 overexpression ($P = 0.017$; HR, 1.642; 95% CI, 1.093–2.463), T3 + 4 disease ($P = 0.005$, hazard ratio [HR], 2.011, 95% CI, 1.240–3.261), positive regional lymph node ($P = 0.035$; HR, 1.967; 95% CI, 1.048–3.691) represented an independent adverse prognostic factor.

Table 2 Associations between SIRT1 expressions and clinicopathological parameters in 155 patients with esophageal squamous cell carcinoma receiving esophagectomy

Parameters		SIRT1 expression		
		Low	Over	P value
Age	<55y/o	32	37	0.38
	≧55y/o	46	40	
Sex	Male	75	75	1.00
	Female	3	2	
Primary tumor location	U + M	40	42	0.68
	L	38	35	
T classification	T1 + T2	45	34	0.092
	T3 + T4	33	43	
N classification	N0	55	51	0.57
	N1 + 2 + 3	23	26	
7th AJCC Stage	I + II	57	55	0.82
	III + IV	21	22	
Histological grading	Grade 1 + 2	66	58	0.15
	Grade 3	12	19	
Surgical margin	Negative	75	60	0.38
	Positive	9	11	

AJCC American Joint Committee on Cancer, *SIRT1* Sirtuin1, *p-p70S6K* phosphorylated p70 ribosomal S6 protein kinase

The SIRT1 inhibitor suppressed cell proliferation of ESCC cell lines

Results on whether the SIRT1 inhibitor would suppress cell proliferation in ESCC cell line KYSE 270 and KYSE 70 show that the SIRT1 inhibitor, SIRT 1 inhibitor IV, (S)-35, displayed a dose-dependent, growth-inhibitory effect in both ESCC cell lines (Fig. 3a and b).

Discussion

It is well known that advanced stage, higher histologic grade and residual disease after surgery lead to poor prognosis [1, 4, 5], and our study also showed the same result. In our study, we demonstrated that SIRT1 overexpression was an independent poor prognosticator for clinical outcome, and SIRT1 inhibitor suppressed cell proliferation of ESCC cell lines. Previous studies in several types of cancers [20–38] also showed SIRT1 overexpression was correlated with advanced stages or poor prognosis and inhibition of SIRT1 may suppress tumor progression. There are several possible mechanisms involved in SIRT1 mediated tumor progression. First, Liu et al. [18, 20] reported that SIRT1 can maintain silent chromatin via the deacetylation of histone proteins, and thus protect cells from apoptosis. Second, SIRT1 can repress tumor suppressor genes, such as p53, p27^{kip1}, and FOXO family members, either by directly binding and deacetylating these non-histone proteins or by inducing heritable CpG island methylation at the gene promoter [18, 20, 30]. For example, previous studies [18, 20] showed that SIRT1 binds p53 and deacetylates its C-terminal Lys382, resulting in inhibition of p53 induction of cell cycle arrest and apoptosis in response to DNA damage and oxidative stress. Zhu et al. [30] reported that SIRT1 is an important regulator of p27^{kip1} and SIRT inhibition induces senescence and antigrowth potential in lung cancer. Third, Byles et al. [27] also found that SIRT1 can enhance metastatic potential by inducing epithelial-mesenchymal transition in prostate cancer. Fourth, previous studies [29, 31] showed that SIRT1 is involved in chemotherapy resistance. Liang et al. [29] suggest that reduced glucose use and altered mitochondrial metabolism

Table 3 Results of univariate log-rank analysis of prognostic factors for overall survival and disease-free survival in 155 patients with esophageal squamous cell carcinoma receiving esophagectomy

Factors	No. of patients	Overall survival (OS)		Disease-free survival (DFS)	
		5-yr OS rate (%)	P value	5-yr DFS rate (%)	P value
Age					
< 55y/o	69	54%	0.19	48%	0.10
≧55y/o	86	37%		29%	
Location					
U + M	82	45%	0.84	35%	0.46
L	73	44%		40%	
T classification					
T1 + 2	79	64%	< 0.001[a]	52%	< 0.001[a]
T3 + 4	76	24%		22%	
N classification					
N0	106	56%	< 0.001[a]	47%	< 0.001[a]
N1 + 2 + 3	49	20%		16%	
7th AJCC stage					
I + II	112	55%	< 0.001[a]	46%	< 0.001[a]
III + IV	43	16%		16%	
Histological grading					
Grade 1 + 2	124	51%	0.001[a]	43%	0.002[a]
Grade 3	31	19%		16%	
Surgical margin					
Negative	135	47%	0.023[a]	39%	0.046[a]
Positive	20	25%		25%	
SIRT1 expression					
Low expression	78	55%	0.004[a]	49%	0.004[a]
Overexpression	77	34%		26%	

AJCC American Joint Committee on Cancer, *SIRT1* Sirtuin1 [a]Statistically significant

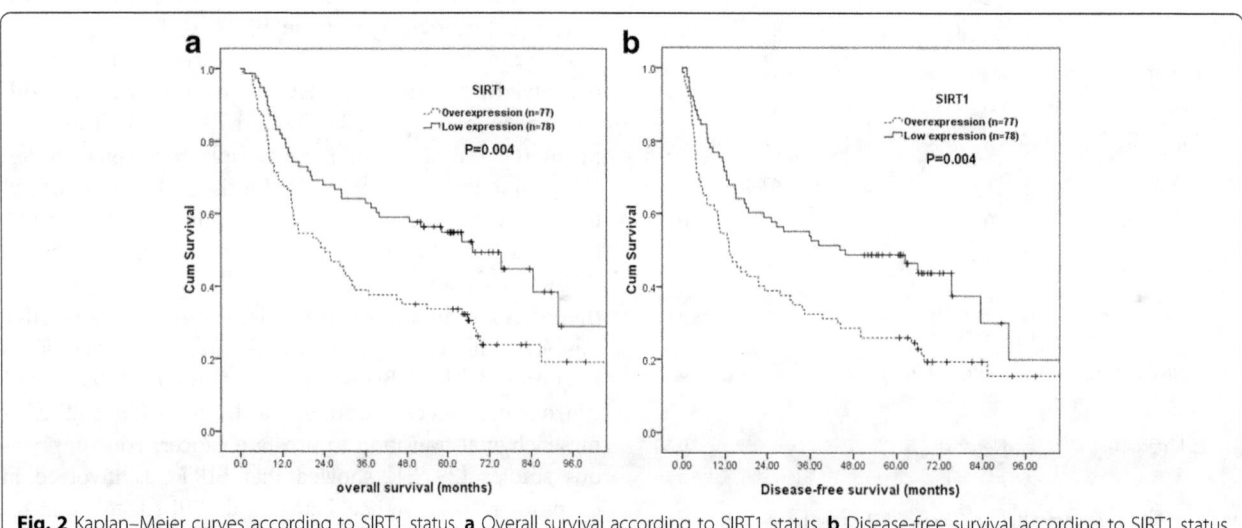

Fig. 2 Kaplan–Meier curves according to SIRT1 status. **a** Overall survival according to SIRT1 status. **b** Disease-free survival according to SIRT1 status

Table 4 Results of multivariate Cox regression analysis for overall survival and disease-free survival in155 patients with esophageal squamous cell carcinoma

Factors	Overall survival		Disease-free survival	
	HR (95% CI)	P value	HR (95% CI)	P value
T3 + 4	2.250 (1.339–3.782)	0.002[a]	2.011 (1.240–3.261)	0.005[a]
SIRT1 expression	1.776 (1.152–2.747)	0.009[a]	1.642 (1.093–2.463)	0.017[a]
N1 + 2 + 3	–	–	1.967 (1.048–3.691)	0.035[a]

HR hazard ratio, *95% CI* 95% confidence interval; [a]Statistically significant

mediated by SIRT1 may contribute to cisplatin resistance. Taken together, the results from our study, together with previous findings, suggest that SIRT1 is not only an adverse prognosticator but also a potential novel therapeutic target.

Despite advance in perioperative management and surgical techniques, the prognosis of patients with ESCC remains poor [1, 2]. Even after radical surgery, patients still develop recurrences and metastases. Over the past decades, several post-operative adjuvant therapy clinical trials were performed to improve unsatisfactory cure rate achieved with surgery alone. Hence, identifying patients at high risk for recurrence who may benefit from post-operative adjuvant therapy is principal. In our study, overexpression of

SIRT1 was highly representative of biological aggressiveness and independently associated with worse disease-free survival. The 5-year disease-free survival rate was only 26% in patients with SIRT1 overexpression, indicating that SIRT1 status may be used to select some patients for adjuvant therapy after esophagectomy.

Conclusions

Higher expression of SIRT1 is an independent prognosticator for patients with ESCC. The SIRT1 inhibitor suppressed cell proliferation of ESCC in vitro. Our findings suggest that Sirtuin inhibitors may be a potential therapy in ESCC patients with SIRT1 overexpression. There were two limitations in our study. First, the patient number was small and was retrospectively analyzed. Second, the effect of SIRT1 inhibitor was analyzed in cell line. The results need further studies to confirm our findings.

Abbreviations
AJCC: American Joint Committee on Cancer; DAB: Diaminobenzidine tetrahydrochloride; DFS: Disease-free survival; DNA: Deoxyribonucleic acid; ECACC: European collection of authenticated cell cultures; EDTA: Ethylene diamine tetraacetie acid; ESCC: Esophageal squamous cell carcinoma; HDAC: Histone deacetylases; HR: Hazard ratio; MTT: diphenyltetrazolium bromide; NDA: Nicotinamide adenine dinucleotide; OS: Overall survival; PBS: Phosphate buffered saline; pH: potential of hydrogen; SIRT1: Sirtuin 1; TNM: Tumor, nodes and metastasis

Acknowledgements
This work was supported in part by grants from the National Science Council, Taiwan (MOST 106-2314-B-182A-159-MY3 and MOST 106-2320-B-182A-015) and Chang Gung Memorial Hospital (CMRPG8E1533 and CMRPG8G0891).

Funding
This work was supported in part by grants from the National Science Council, Taiwan (MOST 106–2314-B-182A-159-MY3 and MOST 106-2320-B-182A-015) and Chang Gung Memorial Hospital (CMRPG8E1533 and CMRPG8G0891).

Authors' contributions
SHL conceptualized the study. CHC contributed to the study design. HIL, CML, WTH, YYC, TJC and SHL acquired the data. WYT and YCL analyzed and interpreted the data. SHL contributed to the statistical analysis. SHL and MCM prepared the manuscript. TJC and YYC edited the manuscript. WTH reviewed the manuscript. All authors read and approved the final manuscript.

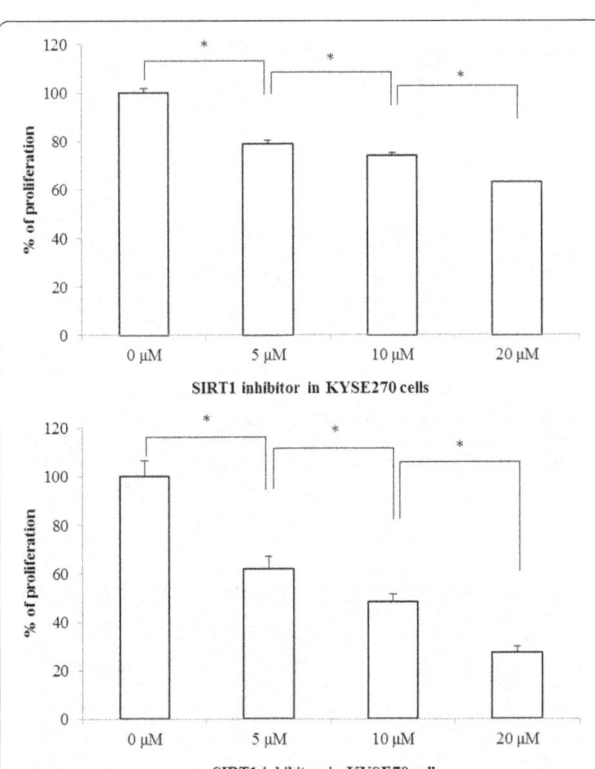

Fig. 3 SIRT1 inhibitor displayed a proliferation-inhibitory effect in a dose-dependent manner in KYSE270 and KYSE70 esophageal squamous cell carcinoma cell lines. *Statistically significant difference in growth inhibition. Any *p* value < 0.05 was considered statistically significant. Columns, mean; bars, SD

Competing interests

The authors declare that they have no competing interests.

Author details

[1]Department of Hematology-Oncology, Kaohsiung Chang Gung Memorial Hospital and Chang Gung University College of Medicine, 123 Ta-Pei Road, Niaosong Dist, Kaohsiung, Taiwan, Republic of China. [2]Department of Thoracic & Cardiovascular Surgery, Kaohsiung Chang Gung Memorial Hospital and Chang Gung University College of Medicine, Kaohsiung, Taiwan, Republic of China. [3]Department of Pathology, Kaohsiung Chang Gung Memorial Hospital and Chang Gung University College of Medicine, Kaohsiung, Taiwan, Republic of China. [4]Institute for Translational Research in Biomedicine, Kaohsiung Chang Gung Memorial Hospital, Kaohsiung, Taiwan, Republic of China. [5]Department of Applied Chemistry, and Graduate Institute of Biomedicine and Biomedical Technology, National Chi Nan University, Nantou, Taiwan, Republic of China. [6]Center for Infectious Disease and Cancer Research, Kaohsiung Medical University, Kaohsiung, Taiwan, Republic of China.

References

1. Li SH, Chen CH, Lu HI, Huang WT, Tien WY, Lan YC, Lee CC, Chen YH, Huang HY, Chang AY, et al. Phosphorylated p70S6K expression is an independent prognosticator for patients with esophageal squamous cell carcinoma. Surgery. 2015;157(3):570–80.
2. Lu HI, Li SH, Huang WT, Rau KM, Fang FM, Wang YM, Lin WC, Tien WY. A comparative study of isolated and metachronous oesophageal squamous cell carcinoma with antecedent upper aerodigestive tract cancer. Eur J Cardiothorac Surg. 2013;44(5):860–5.
3. Li SH, Rau KM, Lu HI, Wang YM, Tien WY, Liang JL, Lin WC. Pre-treatment maximal oesophageal wall thickness is independently associated witeh response to chemoradiotherapy in patients with T3-4 oesophageal squamous cell carcinoma. Eur J Cardiothorac Surg. 2012;42(6):958–64.
4. Rutegard M, Charonis K, Lu Y, Lagergren P, Lagergren J, Rouvelas I. Population-based esophageal cancer survival after resection without neoadjuvant therapy: an update. Surgery. 2012;152(5):903–10.
5. Baba Y, Watanabe M, Shigaki H, Iwagami S, Ishimoto T, Iwatsuki M, Baba H. Negative lymph-node count is associated with survival in patients with resected esophageal squamous cell carcinoma. Surgery. 2013; 153(2):234–41.
6. Simmons GE Jr, Pruitt WM, Pruitt K. Diverse roles of SIRT1 in cancer biology and lipid metabolism. Int J Mol Sci. 2015;16(1):950–65.
7. Haberland M, Montgomery RL, Olson EN. The many roles of histone deacetylases in development and physiology: implications for disease and therapy. Nat Rev Genet. 2009;10(1):32–42.
8. Krusche CA, Wulfing P, Kersting C, Vloet A, Bocker W, Kiesel L, Beier HM, Alfer J. Histone deacetylase-1 and -3 protein expression in human breast cancer: a tissue microarray analysis. Breast Cancer Res Treat. 2005;90(1):15–23.
9. Weichert W, Roske A, Niesporek S, Noske A, Buckendahl AC, Dietel M, Gekeler V, Boehm M, Beckers T, Denkert C. Class I histone deacetylase expression has independent prognostic impact in human colorectal cancer: specific role of class I histone deacetylases in vitro and in vivo. Clin. Cancer Res. 2008;14(6):1669–77.
10. Bordone L, Guarente L. Calorie restriction, SIRT1 and metabolism: understanding longevity. Nat Rev Mol Cell Biol. 2005;6(4):298–305.
11. Kozako T, Suzuki T, Yoshimitsu M, Arima N, Honda S, Soeda S. Anticancer agents targeted to sirtuins. Molecules (Basel, Switzerland). 2014;19(12): 20295–313.
12. Wang RH, Sengupta K, Li C, Kim HS, Cao L, Xiao C, Kim S, Xu X, Zheng Y, Chilton B, et al. Impaired DNA damage response, genome instability, and tumorigenesis in SIRT1 mutant mice. Cancer Cell. 2008;14(4):312–23.
13. Chu F, Chou PM, Zheng X, Mirkin BL, Rebbaa A. Control of multidrug resistance gene mdr1 and cancer resistance to chemotherapy by the longevity gene sirt1. Cancer Res. 2005;65(22):10183–7.
14. Derr RS, van Hoesel AQ, Benard A, Goossens-Beumer IJ, Sajet A, Dekker-Ensink NG, de Kruijf EM, Bastiaannet E, Smit VT, van de Velde CJ, et al. High nuclear expression levels of histone-modifying enzymes LSD1, HDAC2 and SIRT1 in tumor cells correlate with decreased survival and increased relapse in breast cancer patients. BMC Cancer. 2014;14:604.
15. Han L, Liang XH, Chen LX, Bao SM, Yan ZQ. SIRT1 is highly expressed in brain metastasis tissues of non-small cell lung cancer (NSCLC) and in positive regulation of NSCLC cell migration. Int J Clin Exp Pathol. 2013;6(11):2357–65.
16. Chen W, Bhatia R. Roles of SIRT1 in leukemogenesis. Curr Opin Hematol. 2013;20(4):308–13.
17. Huffman DM, Grizzle WE, Bamman MM, Kim JS, Eltoum IA, Elgavish A, Nagy TR. SIRT1 is significantly elevated in mouse and human prostate cancer. Cancer Res. 2007;67(14):6612–8.
18. Liu T, Liu PY, Marshall GM. The critical role of the class III histone deacetylase SIRT1 in cancer. Cancer Res. 2009;69(5):1702–5.
19. Kozako T, Aikawa A, Shoji T, Fujimoto T, Yoshimitsu M, Shirasawa S, Tanaka H, Honda S, Shimeno H, Arima N, et al. High expression of the longevity gene product SIRT1 and apoptosis induction by sirtinol in adult T-cell leukemia cells. Int J Cancer. 2012;131(9):2044–55.
20. Li K, Luo J. The role of SIRT1 in tumorigenesis. N. Am. J. Med. Sci. 2011;4(2):104–6.
21. Jang KY, Hwang SH, Kwon KS, Kim KR, Choi HN, Lee NR, Kwak JY, Park BH, Park HS, Chung MJ, et al. SIRT1 expression is associated with poor prognosis of diffuse large B-cell lymphoma. Am J Surg Pathol. 2008;32(10):1523–31.
22. Lovaas JD, Zhu L, Chiao CY, Byles V, Faller DV, Dai Y. SIRT1 enhances matrix metalloproteinase-2 expression and tumor cell invasion in prostate cancer cells. Prostate. 2013;73(5):522–30.
23. Kriegl L, Vieth M, Kirchner T, Menssen A. Up-regulation of c-MYC and SIRT1 expression correlates with malignant transformation in the serrated route to colorectal cancer. Oncotarget. 2012;3(10):1182–93.
24. Suzuki K, Hayashi R, Ichikawa T, Imanishi S, Yamada T, Inomata M, Miwa T, Matsui S, Usui I, Urakaze M, et al. SRT1720, a SIRT1 activator, promotes tumor cell migration, and lung metastasis of breast cancer in mice. Oncol Rep. 2012;27(6):1726–32.
25. Marshall GM, Liu PY, Gherardi S, Scarlett CJ, Bedalov A, Xu N, Iraci N, Valli E, Ling D, Thomas W, et al. SIRT1 promotes N-Myc oncogenesis through a positive feedback loop involving the effects of MKP3 and ERK on N-Myc protein stability. PLoS Genet. 2011;7(6):e1002135.
26. Saxena M, Dykes SS, Malyarchuk S, Wang AE, Cardelli JA, Pruitt K. The sirtuins promote Dishevelled-1 scaffolding of TIAM1, Rac activation and cell migration. Oncogene. 2015;34(2):188–98.
27. Byles V, Zhu L, Lovaas JD, Chmilewski LK, Wang J, Faller DV, Dai Y. SIRT1 induces EMT by cooperating with EMT transcription factors and enhances prostate cancer cell migration and metastasis. Oncogene. 2012;31(43):4619–29.
28. Nihal M, Ahmad N, Wood GS. SIRT1 is upregulated in cutaneous T-cell lymphoma, and its inhibition induces growth arrest and apoptosis. Cell Cycle. 2014;13(4):632–40.
29. Liang XJ, Finkel T, Shen DW, Yin JJ, Aszalos A, Gottesman MM. SIRT1 contributes in part to cisplatin resistance in cancer cells by altering mitochondrial metabolism. Mol. Cancer Res. 2008;6(9):1499–506.
30. Zhu L, Chiao CY, Enzer KG, Stankiewicz AJ, Faller DV, Dai Y. SIRT1 inactivation evokes antitumor activities in NSCLC through the tumor suppressor p27. Mol. Cancer Res. 2015;13(1):41–9.
31. Chen HC, Jeng YM, Yuan RH, Hsu HC, Chen YL. SIRT1 promotes tumorigenesis and resistance to chemotherapy in hepatocellular carcinoma and its expression predicts poor prognosis. Ann Surg Oncol. 2012;19(6):2011–9.
32. Cha EJ, Noh SJ, Kwon KS, Kim CY, Park BH, Park HS, Lee H, Chung MJ, Kang MJ, Lee DG, et al. Expression of DBC1 and SIRT1 is associated with poor prognosis of gastric carcinoma. Clin. Cancer Res. 2009;15(13):4453–9.
33. Noguchi A, Kikuchi K, Zheng H, Takahashi H, Miyagi Y, Aoki I, Takano Y. SIRT1 expression is associated with a poor prognosis, whereas DBC1 is associated with favorable outcomes in gastric cancer. Cancer Med. 2014;3(6):1553–61.
34. Lee H, Kim KR, Noh SJ, Park HS, Kwon KS, Park BH, Jung SH, Youn HJ, Lee BK, Chung MJ, et al. Expression of DBC1 and SIRT1 is associated with poor prognosis for breast carcinoma. Hum Pathol. 2011;42(2):204–13.
35. Wu M, Wei W, Xiao X, Guo J, Xie X, Li L, Kong Y, Lv N, Jia W, Zhang Y, et al. Expression of SIRT1 is associated with lymph node metastasis and poor prognosis in both operable triple-negative and non-triple-negative breast cancer. Med. Oncol. 2012;29(5):3240–9.
36. Kim JR, Moon YJ, Kwon KS, Bae JS, Wagle S, Yu TK, Kim KM, Park HS, Lee JH, Moon WS, et al. Expression of SIRT1 and DBC1 is associated with poor prognosis of soft tissue sarcomas. PLoS One. 2013;8(9):e74738.
37. Chen X, Sun K, Jiao S, Cai N, Zhao X, Zou H, Xie Y, Wang Z, Zhong M, Wei L. High levels of SIRT1 expression enhance tumorigenesis and associate with a poor prognosis of colorectal carcinoma patients. Sci Rep. 2014;4:7481.

18

The surgical management of non-malignant aerodigestive fistula

Yassar A. Qureshi[1]*[iD], M. Muntzer Mughal[1], Sheraz R. Markar[2], Borzoueh Mohammadi[1], Jeremy George[3], Martin Hayward[4] and David Lawrence[4]

Abstract

Background: Acquired aerodigestive fistula (ADF) are rare, but associated with significant morbidity. Surgery affords the best prospect of cure. We present our experience of the surgical management of ADFs at a specialist unit, highlighting operative techniques, challenges and assess clinical outcomes following intervention. We also illustrate findings of a Hospital Episodes Statistics search for ADFs.

Methods: A prospectively-maintained database was searched to identify all patients diagnosed with an ADF who were managed at our institution. Of 48 patients with an ADF, eight underwent surgical intervention.

Results: Four patients underwent an exploration of the ADF with primary repair of the defect. Two of these patients had proximal ADFs, amenable to repair through a neck incision, and two required a thoracotomy. Two patients suffered fistulae secondary to endoscopic therapy and underwent oesophageal exclusion surgery, with subsequent staged reconstruction. Two patients with previous Tuberculosis had a lung segmentectomy and lobectomy respectively, and a further patient in remission after treatment for lymphoma underwent oesophageal resection with synchronous reconstruction. Three patients suffered a complication, with one post-operative mortality. The remaining seven patients all achieved normal oral alimentation, with no evidence of ADF recurrence at a median follow-up of 32 months.

Conclusions: Surgery to manage ADFs is effective in restoring normal alimentation and alleviates soiling of the airway, with a very low risk of recurrence. Several operative techniques can be utilised dependent on the features of the ADF. Early referral to specialist units is advocated, where the expertise to facilitate the complete management of patients is present, within a multi-disciplinary setting.

Keywords: Aerodigestive fistula, Tracheo-oesophageal fistula, Oesophageal cancer, Oesophageal surgery

Background

Surgical intervention affords the best prospect of long-term cure of aerodigestive fistulae (ADF). Although several operative techniques can be used to treat this debilitating condition, they can only be utilised in selected patients owing to both the underlying diagnosis and the risks associated with such surgery [1–4]. However, with ADFs becoming an increasing health problem, with improving diagnosis and evolving peri-operative care, it is likely that surgery will play a more important role in the management of ADFs.

The choice of operative technique to treat ADFs is dependent on several factors. However, the most important facet relates to the underlying oesophageal or airway disease, which determines the state of tissue and its amenability to repair and future surveillance, if required [1, 2, 5, 6]. Patients often present in a physiologically challenged state owing to the nature of the disease, and many will not be candidates for surgery. However, focused pre-operative intervention and nutritional support may enable some patients to proceed to surgery. For these reasons, a multi-disciplinary (MDT) approach is necessary, and underscores why these patients should be managed in dedicated centralised units. The range of operations include resection and reconstruction, exclusion and bypass of the affected segment of oesophagus, and exploration and repair of the ADF. The expertise of head

* Correspondence: yassar.qureshi.17@ucl.ac.uk
[1]Department of Oesophago-Gastric Surgery, University College London Hospital, 250 Euston Road, London NW1 2BU, UK
Full list of author information is available at the end of the article

and neck, thoracic and oesophago-gastric surgeons is required to manage these patients.

In this study, we present our experience of surgical intervention in patients diagnosed with an ADF. We explore the background leading to the development of an ADF, and relate how this can impact on the nature of surgery performed. Furthermore, we describe the operative technique, challenges and outcomes following intervention. We review the pertinent literature to enable an evidence-based approach to the surgical management of ADFs. We also illustrate findings of a Hospital Episodes Statistics (HES) search for ADFs, highlighting the challenges of diagnosis, management and reporting in contemporary practise.

Methods

We interrogated a prospectively-maintained database to identify patients diagnosed with an ADF and managed at our institution between January 2005 and January 2017. A total of 48 patients with an ADF were identified, of whom eight patients have undergone surgery to treat their fistula. All patients were discussed at a specialist MDT where a consensus on optimal management was reached. Of the 40 patients managed non-surgically, 31 were treated with endoscopic intervention (oesophageal or tracheal stent), mostly owing to the presence of advanced malignancy not amenable to curative treatment. Endoscopic treatment facilitated an alleviation of respiratory soiling, whilst allowing oncological treatment to be commenced. A further seven patients were managed in palliative setting after presenting *in extremis*, and two patients with very small asymptomatic ADFs were managed conservatively with regular surveillance. Follow-up refers to time from diagnosis of ADF (or underlying disease where specified) to last clinical engagement or death. Median follow-up was 32 months. Local ethical approval for retrieval and use of clinical data for this study was granted.

Operative technique

When considering surgery as treatment for ADF, several factors should be specifically assessed for. It is imperative that a careful search for malignancy is performed prior to surgery, particularly as many patients will have a preceding history of proximal oesophageal squamous cell carcinoma (SCC) treated with chemo-radiotherapy. If active malignancy is present in the context of an ADF, this represents locally advanced disease with poor outcome, rarely amenable to curative surgical intervention. In these patients, endocopic treatment should be considered to alleviate symptoms, coupled with chemo-radiotherapy if appropriate. The physiological state of the patient must also be thoroughly assessed, to ensure that the risks of major morbidity and mortality after surgery are minimised, and

that the patient would be able to recover from such intervention. Patients should be carefully optimised, and where indicated, the pre-operative placement of a feeding jejunostomy and a venting gastrostomy to improve the nutritional and metabolic state, and to minimise continued soiling of the airway, should be performed.

Once a patient is deemed to have an ADF curable by surgery, secondary factors relating to the ADF and surrounding tissue become important considerations. A larger defect, a history of previous local radiotherapy and endoscopic intervention are all factors which make surgery more challenging. Also, the location of the ADF is important, as more proximally sited fistulae are amenable to repair through a neck incision, yet for distal ADF a thoracotomy is mandated, carrying a greater risk of major morbidity and mortality. If there has been significant local contamination, then it may be prudent not perform a synchronous reconstruction, as the likelihood of an anastomotic dehiscence increases. In these patients, a delayed reconstruction confers improved chances of better recovery. However, given the heterogenous aetiology of ADF, each case should be considered with a view to an individualised treatment plan.

At induction, for tracheo-oesophageal fistulae (TOF), it is important that the endotracheal tube balloon is sited distal to the fistula. This will avoid inadvertent damage to the cuff whilst dissecting and exposing the fistula, and negate the possibility of ventilatory embarrassment intra-operatively. Furthermore, this manoeuvre minimises further contamination of the respiratory tract by manipulation of the affected structures during surgery.

ADF exploration and repair

This may involve either an incision in the neck for proximal fistulae, or a thoracotomy for more distal ADFs. In the neck, dissection must proceed to mobilise the thyroid with careful identification and preservation of the recurrent laryngeal nerves and parathyroid glands. The oesophagus should be circumferentially mobilised, as this manoeuvre will allow the pharyngo-laryngeal complex to be gently pulled superiorly and away from the thoracic inlet, to provide good access to the fistula. Once the fistula has been identified, it can be dissected free and a primary repair of the oesophagus and trachea with absorbable sutures can be performed. It is critical that the fistula is accessible from both sides of the neck to ensure complete control of the airway during the repair, whilst also facilitating a pedicled strap muscle interposition flap. This reinforces the repair by providing a physical barrier between the two suture lines.

In the thorax, a similar approach is used with an intercostal flap which is carefully prepared at the time of thoracotomy. Once the fistula has been identified, again, it is dissected free and a primary repair performed, with the intercostal flap placed between the suture lines.

Exclusion

Exclusion surgery involves isolating the oesophagus from alimentary tract continuity, both proximal and distal to the fistula. This involves an incision in the neck to access the proximal oesophagus, where, once circumferentially mobilised, it is transected above the fistula and brought to the skin as an oesophagostomy. If the fistula is very proximal, then the superior oesophagus may be left in situ, and a large T-tube placed in the lumen with the distal limb of the tube brought to the skin.

Next, a laparotomy is performed where the oesohagogastric junction (OGJ) is mobilised and the stomach transected below this, from the lesser curve through to the fundus. This manoeuvre excludes the oesophagus from the GI tract entirely, whilst preserving the majority of the stomach for future reconstruction. The small stomach remnant attached to the OGJ is brought to the abdominal wall, where a generous gastrostomy is fashioned. This allows retrograde access to the excluded oesophagus, for both endoscopic surveillance and therapy, and facilitates venting of oesophageal mucous.

Our unit policy is to defer reconstruction as a second, staged procedure. This allows the patient a period of recovery, whilst respiratory and nutritional optimisation continues. Furthermore, by fashioning an anastomosis at the index operation in a potentially contaminated surgical field, there is a higher chance of a leak. If this were to occur, there is substantial risk of fistula recurrence. Where possible, the stomach is used a conduit, and is brought to the neck through the retrosternal space, thus avoiding the need for a repeat thoracotomy. If there is insufficient proximal oesophagus, the stomach may be anastomosed directly to the inferior pharyngeal constrictors.

Resection

This is normally reserved for large or recurrent fistulae. For proximally sited ADF - those affecting the trachea, this will involve resection of the oesophagus, via a transthoracic approach. The fistula is identified, and the oesophagus dissected away around it. However, the oesophageal tissue intimately involved with the fistula is left in situ, thus avoiding direct dissection of the trachea and minimising the risk of an air leak. The tracheal defect with the overlying oesophageal tissue is then primarily closed, with the latter acting as a buttress reinforcing the tracheal repair. Typically, a gastric conduit is utilised for reconstruction, necessitating a laparotomy.

For more distal ADF, those affecting the bronchus intermedius and more distal, a thoracotomy is performed to identify the fistula. A segmentectomy or lobectomy of the lung can be performed, dependent on the size of the defect and the quality of the surrounding parenchyma. Thus, the affected distal airway and the fistula are excised *en*

bloc. The oesophageal defect can be repaired primarily, utilising an intercostal flap to reinforce the repair, or an oesophageal resection is performed if the defect is very large and unlikely to heal. In these instances, given the anastomosis will be at a distinct site from the ADF, a synchronous reconstruction can be performed safely.

In our experience, tracheal resection is a very challenging operation, with the risk of significant short and long-term complications [2, 3]. Owing to the limited vascularity of the trachea, healing, particularly in this cohort of patients, may be protracted, necessitating prolonged mechanical ventilation. Thus, we have preferred to avoid such an operative intervention. However, for very large TOFs, or those where a circumferential injury to the trachea is present (such as cuff related fistulae), or where other intervention has failed, tracheal resection and reconstruction may be indicated. Mathisen et al provide an operative description and experience of this technique [3].

Results

Preceding history and previous intervention

The median age at diagnosis of ADF was 56 years (range 29–73 years). Three patients had a previous diagnosis of oesophageal malignancy; all were treated with chemo- and/or radiotherapy, and one with surgical resection in addition. Two patients had a prior diagnosis of Tuberculosis (TB) and had received anti-microbial therapy in the past, and one patient previously had surgical intervention following a post-emetic oesophageal leak. In two patients, no obvious cause of ADF was identified, likely representing congenital fistulae that had persisted into adulthood. Of these cases, two patients (1 and 6) developed oesophageal strictures after their initial treatment. Patient 1 had undergone several balloon dilations and stent placements, with the stent subsequently eroding into the airway (Fig. 1). Similarly, patient 6 also received a stent which directly caused the fistula. Table 1 summarises key patient factors.

ADF characteristics

The two patients with an unknown cause of fistula had a very long history of symptoms, and had been managed in the community with a diagnosis of asthma (Table 2). The median time to ADF development for the three patients with a malignancy was 15 months (range 3–21), with the shortest time affecting a patient who had an oesophageal lymphoma (Patient 7). She had a complete response to chemotherapy, with a residual fistula persisting (Fig. 2). Both patients with TB had a long interval after curative medical therapy, although they had suggestive symptoms for some time prior to referral. Most patients presented with recurrent chest infections and symptoms suggestive of aspiration. Of these, one patient

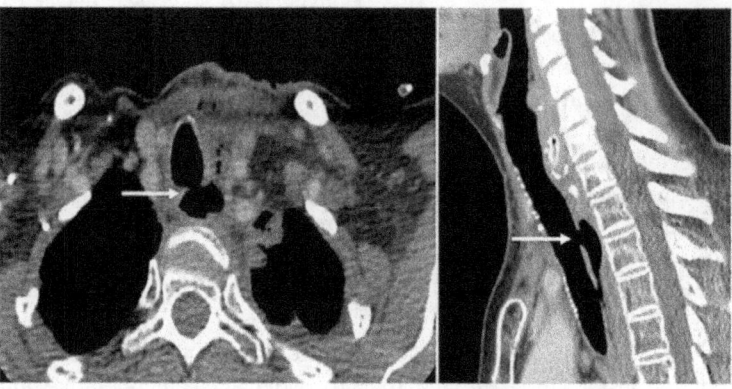

Fig. 1 CT scan of Patient 1 demonstrating the aerodigestive fistula (arrows)

(4) presented with acute respiratory failure owing to overwhelming infection caused by aspiration. Of interest, he had a fistula affecting the very proximal trachea (Fig. 3).

The size of the fistula ranged from 3 to 16 mm, with the larger defects affecting those who had a prior diagnosis of carcinoma or who underwent surgical treatment. The location of the fistula in relation to the airway too was variable, reflecting the site of underlying disease. Those thought to be congenital were very proximal. Those secondary to TB were both distal, involving the smaller bronchi and lung parenchyma at the original Ghon focus. Patient 6 presented with Boerhaave's Syndrome, and was initially managed with surgery to repair the oesophageal defect. However, he subsequently re-leaked, which again was managed surgically with a repair over a T-tube, but then developed a stricture at the site of injury, which was treated with an oesophageal stent. This eroded into the airway at its proximal extent, causing a fistula at 24 cm, with subsequent referral to our unit (Fig. 4).

After the diagnosis of ADF, three patients underwent further endotherapy in an attempt to manage the fistula prior to referral to our unit. Patient 1 had 3 oesophageal stents placed, but given the proximal location of the ADF, these all slipped distally. Patient 3, who had developed an ADF between the airway and a gastric conduit, most likely after a sub-clinical leak, had endoclips placed via flexible gastroscopy which failed to close the ADF. Patient 6 too had a stent[s] placed to treat the fistula without the desired effect.

Surgical intervention for ADF treatment

Three patients (3, 4, 8) underwent a primary repair of their ADF. Patient 3 required a thoracotomy given that the ADF was communicating with a gastric conduit and Patients 4 and 8 had proximally-sited fistulae approached through the neck. For the former case, an intercostal flap was interposed between the suture lines and for the latter two, the strap muscles were similarly utilised. These fistulae were small and the quality of tissue was sufficiently good to enable primary repair. Patient 4 presented as an acute emergency following aspiration -intubated- and a laparotomy was performed prior to repair, in order to place a feeding jejunostomy and venting gastrostomy (Table 3).

Table 1 Preceding history and intervention, prior to the diagnosis of ADF

Patient	Age at ADF Diagnosis (years)	Sex	Preceding Diagnosis	Preceding Intervention	Chemo-Radiotherapy	Preceding Treatment Related Complication	Previous Endotherapy
1	60	F	SSC[a] Proximal Oesophagus	Definitive chemo-radiotherapy	Chemo-radiotherapy	Radiotherapy related stricture	-×2 stents -×3 dilations
2	57	M	TB[b]	Medical therapy	–	–	–
3	59	M	Adenocarcinoma Distal Oesophagus	Ivor-Lewis Oesophagectomy	Neo-adjuvant chemotherapy	Anastomotic leak	–
4	73	M	Unknown	–	–	–	–
5	32	F	TB[b]	Medical Therapy	–	–	–
6	33	M	Boerhaave's Syndrome	Repair of leak	–	Re-leak; stricture	-× 1 stent
7	55	F	Oesophageal B Cell lymphoma	Chemotherapy	Chemotherapy	–	–
8	29	F	Unknown	–	–	–	–

[a]SCC- Squamous Cell Carcinoma; [b] TB- Tuberculosis

Table 2 Anatomical and Clinical Features of the ADFs

Patient	Time to ADF Development (months)	Fistula Site	Fistula Size (mm)	Main Symptoms	Endotherapy to Treat ADF
1	15	Proximal trachea 20 cm	12	Aspiration	×3 stents
2	> 30 years	Oesophagus-right bronchus intermedius 30 cm	12	Recurrent chest infections	–
3	21	Gastric conduit-lung 25 cm	16	Recurrent chest infections	Endoclip
4	> 30 years	Proximal trachea 17 cm	5	Aspiration; Respiratory embarrassment	–
5	144	Distal oesophagus-lung 38 cm	15	Haemoptysis	–
6	3	Oesophagus-carina 24 cm	15	Recurrent chest infections	×3 stents
7	3	Oesophagus- left main bronchus 26 cm	5	Recurrent chest infections	–
8	> 20 years	Proximal trachea 17 cm	3	Recurrent chest infections	–

Two patients (1 and 6) underwent an oesophageal exclusion operation. These were both performed as staged procedures with delayed reconstruction. The reason for performing this operation was that in both patients there was sufficient concern regarding the state of tissue. Patient 1 had previous radiotherapy for an oesophageal SCC, on a background of achalasia requiring a myotomy via thoracotomy several years previously. The degree of tissue inflammation, scarring and adhesions precluded a transthoracic resection. Thus, through a neck incision, the oesophagus was transected above the fistula and an oesophagostomy fashioned with a synchronous repair of the fistula. Distally, the oesophagus and OGJ was transected and a venting gastrostomy fashioned. After a period of optimisation and treatment of longstanding respiratory disease, the patient underwent reconstruction utilising a gastric conduit through the retrosternal space. Patient 6 too had severe inflammation and adhesions in

the chest following his surgical management of Boerhaave's syndrome. Exclusion and subsequent reconstruction with a colonic conduit (he had previously undergone a distal gastrectomy for benign ulcer disease) was performed. In both cases, the native tissues were poor enough to carry a high risk of leak with primary anastomosis at index surgery.

Patient 2 had a distal ADF, approached through a thoracotomy. The right bronchus intermedius was involved, and the ADF and affected parenchyma was excised as a segmentectomy, with oesophageal repair. Patient 5 underwent an exploration of the fistula through a thoractomy with a lobectomy. The fistula, along with associated necrotic parenchyma was excised *en bloc*, with a subsequent suture repair of the oesophagus. Patient 7, after chemotherapy for lymphoma, underwent an oesophageal resection. Again, severe residual inflammation was noted at the time of the surgery precluding repair of a small (5 mm) fistula. In addition, our oncology colleagues felt there was

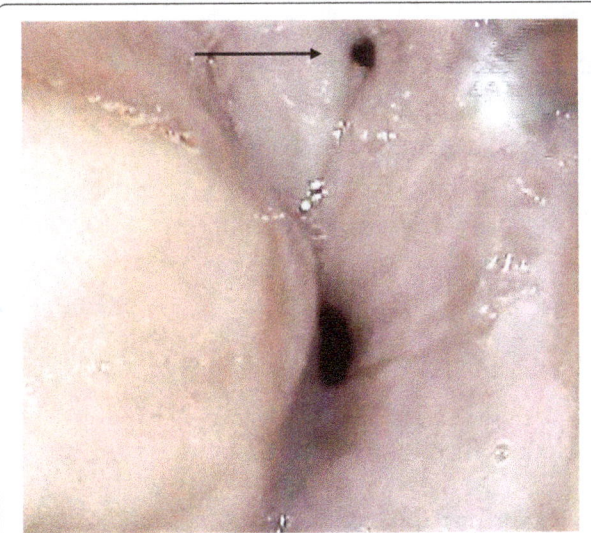

Fig. 2 Residual ADF (arrow) following treatment for oesophageal lymphoma

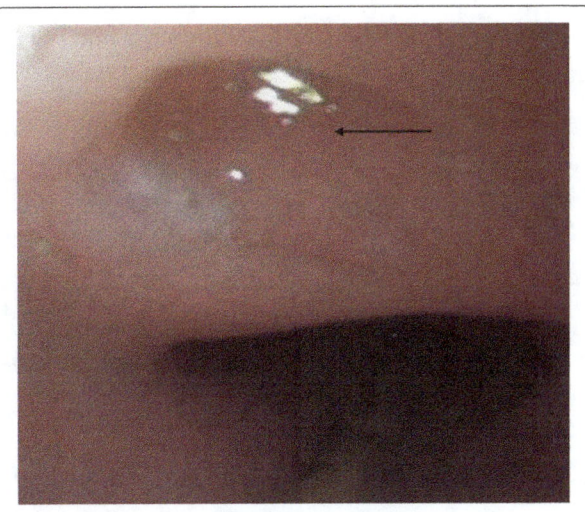

Fig. 3 ADF (arrow) in a proximal location, as seen by oesophagoscopy

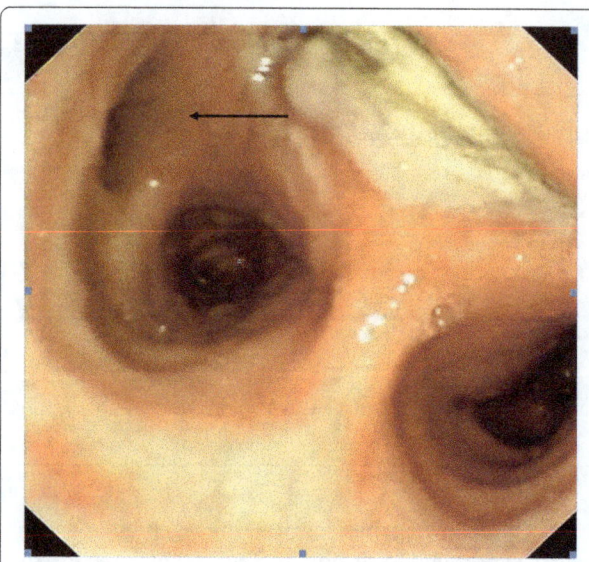

Fig. 4 A bronchoscopic image of the ADF (arrow) close to the carina

a reasonable risk of future recurrence of lymphoma, thus a resection was advocated. A primary repair of the left main bronchus was performed, utilising a flap muscle graft. A single-phase operation was performed as the anastomosis was at a distinct site to the fistula.

Morbidity and mortality

Three patients suffered from complications following surgery. Patient 2 developed a severe respiratory infection on Day 4 following surgery, requiring bronchoscopic washout. Patient 7 suffered a small anastomotic leak, necessitating prolonged nil oral alimentation. Her nutrition was maintained with jejunal feeding, and a contrast swallow at

7 weeks confirmed complete healing of the leak, after which gradual oral feeding was commenced.

Patient 4, who presented with respiratory failure, was affected by severe post-operative recurrent chest infections, and an inability to wean off mechanical ventilation. This had been anticipated, and hence a tracheostomy had been placed at the time of surgery. Despite 4 months of intensive management, he passed away with respiratory failure and multiple organ dysfunction. He represents the only mortality in this series.

Normal oral alimentation following surgery was achieved in all patients, bar patient 4. The time to attain this milestone ranged from 2 to 3 weeks in all cases, with the exception of patient 7 who had suffered a leak. She required supplemental enteral feeding at home for a short period. We reserve the use of contrast studies and formal swallow assessment for the very proximal fistulae, where the risk of leak and aspiration is highest. At the time of last follow-up, no patient demonstrated clinical evidence of recurrent ADF.

Hospital episodes statistics (HES)

We performed a search of the English national HES database to assess the reported incidence of ADFs in the UK between 2000 and 2012 (Table 4). Only 71 cases were found. However, we noted that the terms used in the HES system to record an episode or event related to an ADF were difficult to identify and, we suspect, many patients with an ADF were not coded correctly and thus not recorded. Of the 71 cases, 17 (23.9%) underwent documented treatment: 9 (12.7%) were treated surgically and 8 (11.3%) underwent oesophageal stent placement. Most patients (56.4%) presented with respiratory symptoms. The 30-day and 90-day mortality rates were 32.4 and 42.3% respectively, although for cases

Table 3 Surgical Intervention for the Correction of ADF, and Post-Operative Complications

Patient	Operation	Incision	Phases	Reconstruction	Complications
1	Oesophageal Exclusion and fistula repair with strap muscle	Left collar Right PL[a] thoracotomy Laparotomy	2 phase	Retrosternal Gastric conduit	–
2	Fistula Repair with intercostal muscle	Right PL[a] thoracotomy	1 phase	n/a	Respiratory infection
3	Fistula Repair with intercostal muscle	Right PL[a] thoracotomy	1 phase	n/a	–
4	Fistula Repair with strap muscle	Bilateral collar Laparotomy	1 phase	n/a	Respiratory failure RIP
5	Right lower lobe resection and fistula repair	Right PL[a] mini-thoracotomy	1 phase	n/a	–
6	Oesophageal Exclusion and fistula repair	Left collar Right PL[a] thoracotomy Laparotomy	2 phase	Retrosternal Colonic conduit	–
7	Oesophagectomy and fistula repair with intercostal muscle	Left collar Right PL[a] thoracotomy Laparotomy	1 phase	Retrosternal Gastric conduit	Anastomotic leak
8	Fistula Repair with strap muscle	Bilateral collar	1 phase	n/a	–

[a]PL- Postero-lateral

Table 4 HES data search for ADFs between 2000 and 2012 ([a] denotes hospitals that perform ≥20 oesophageal cancer resections per year)

HES data (2000–2012)	n	%	p
Age ≥ 70 years	35	49.3	
Sex			
Female	35	49.3	
Male	36	50.7	
Treatment	17	24	
Surgery	9	12.7	
Stenting of oesophagus	8	11.3	
Unknown	54	76	
Presenting Clinical Feature			
Pneumonia	18	25.4	
Pleural effusion	22	31	
Pulmonary embolus	1	1.4	
Ischaemic cardiac event	1	1.4	
Unknown	29	40.8	
All Hospitals			
30-day mortality	23	32.4	
90-day mortality	30	42.3	
Specialist Centres[a]	16	22.5	
30-day mortality	4	25	0.473
90-day mortality	5	31.3	0.311

managed in high-volumes centres this fell to 25 and 31.3% respectively.

Discussion

This series demonstrates the techniques, challenges and strategies utilised in the surgical management of ADFs. The key aspect in the approach to such intervention is the multi-disciplinary nature of care, utilising the experience of several distinct surgical specialities. Pre-operative respiratory optimisation should be aggressive, and ideally patients should be weaned off artificial ventilation prior to surgery [2, 3]. As the HES data demonstrates, apart from being rare, there is a deficiency in accurate diagnosis, coding and documentation of this condition.

The range of operations that can be utilised reflect the nature of underlying disease [1–4]. The determinants of which operation will be performed are mainly the site and size of the ADF, and the state of the affected tissue-itself a reflection of the preceding disease and treatment. For the most proximal ADFs, an approach through a neck incision is the most desirable. A pivotal stratagem here involves mobilising the oesophagus circumferentially. This manoeuvre allows the more distal structures to be brought superiorly into the wound, making further

surgery easier and away from the rigid confines of the thoracic inlet. If necessary, the medial clavicle and sternoclavicular joint can be excised, a procedure which does not cause future disability [7]. Distal ADFs necessitate a thoracotomy. These ADFs can cause significant damage to the lung parenchyma, affecting the compliance by causing fibrosis [8]. Thus, where necessary, we advocate a lobar or segmental resection, with closure of the associated distal bronchi. Where an oesophagectomy is indicated, we favour leaving a cuff of oesophageal tissue around the trachea. This enables a dissection plane away from the airway, and the remnant tissue can be incorporated into the repair. This manoeuvre also lessens the future risk of tracheal stenosis [3].

Although not universally favoured, we have found the oesophageal exclusion operation a beneficial option in specific patients. Gross contamination of the airway, or in patients who have had a previous leak or radiotherapy, results in significant inflammation and adhesions in the thorax. Attempting a resection in this circumstance is hazardous, and if there is no definite indication to resect, the oesophagus can be safely left in situ. It is important that a generous venting gastrostomy is sited, from where the oesophagus can be accessed. We have successfully performed a retrograde endoscopy through this, and administered therapeutic agents required for treatment of disuse oesophagitis. Most importantly, it enables venting of oesophageal mucous. Some authors favour a single operation rather than a staged approach for resection or repair and reconstruction [3, 7]. In our experience, fashioning an anastomosis in a contaminated field increases the chance of a leak. In such an event, the fistula has a high chance of recurrence. Most importantly, however, a significant leak may necessitate a far more morbid operative intervention. Indeed, any resultant fistula is likely to be more difficult to treat, if this remains at all possible.

Several other series also demonstrate the complexity of surgical intervention [1–4, 9]. A feature of these reports is that experience is limited to a few specialist units where an expertise in ADF management is present. This results in better outcomes, and facilitates an environment where management is continually improved. In our series, there was one post-operative death. The remaining patients all achieved normal alimentation soon after surgery, with no evidence of ADF recurrence at a median of 32 months. These results are comparable to other dedicated units. Mathisen et al demonstrated a mortality rate of 10.5% in a series of 38 patients, many of whom underwent tracheal reconstruction, with excellent long-term outcomes [3]. In a subsequent report, highlighting 35 years' experience in the management of ADFs, the operative mortality rate fell to 2.8%, reflecting the effect of concentrating cases in specialist units [1].

Shen et al similarly report a low mortality rate of 5.7%, with a post-operative complication rate of 54.3%, and an oesophageal leak rate of 11.4% [9]. Baisi et al reported on 31 patients, of whom 26 underwent simple closure of the oesophageal and tracheal defects. Operative mortality was 3.2%, with a recurrence rate of 6.4% [10].

Non-operative techniques can be used to manage ADFs. Oesophageal stenting is the most common intervention, and although it plays a key role in some patients, they can themselves *cause* fistulae and may affect future surgical intervention [11, 12]. Newer endoscopic techniques utilising endoscopic suturing, clip placement or tissue glue, may have an increasing role in the management of ADFs in the future. Thus, early referral to a dedicated unit is advocated, as the *whole* management of the patient can be pursued where the complete skill-set, including access to novel treatments, is present. By focusing care in specific units, the expertise in all facets of management and outcomes can continually improve.

Conclusion

In summary, for a select group of patients an operative approach can be a truly life-saving intervention. Although surgery is not without risk, it offers the best chance of cure of ADF with a very low risk of recurrence and a return to normal oral alimentation.

Abbreviations
ADF: Aerodigestive Fistula; HES: Hospital Episodes Statistics; MDT: Multidisciplinary Team; OGJ: Oesophago-Gastric Junction; TB: Tuberculosis; TOF: Tracheo-Oesophageal Fistula

Acknowledgements
N/A

Funding
No funding to declare

Authors' contributions
Each author has participated sufficiently in the work to take public responsibility for this manuscript as per the guidelines of the International Committee of Medical Journal Editors (ICMJE) criteria. YQ and MM designed the study, acquired and analysed the data and drafted the manuscript; SM collected HES data and assisted in writing the manuscript; BM, JG, MH and DL assisted in interpretation of the data and critically revising the intellectual content. All authors approved the final version of the manuscript and are accountable for all aspects of accuracy and integrity related to this work.

Competing interests
The authors declare that they have no competing interests.

Author details
[1]Department of Oesophago-Gastric Surgery, University College London Hospital, 250 Euston Road, London NW1 2BU, UK. [2]Department of Surgery and Cancer, Imperial College London, London, UK. [3]Department of Thoracic Medicine, University College London Hospital, London, UK. [4]Department of Thoracic Surgery, University College London Hospital, London, UK.

References
1. Muniappan A, Wain JC, Cameron D, et al. Surgical treatment of nonmalignant tracheoesophageal fistula: a thirty-five year experience. Ann Thorac Surg. 2013;95:1141–6.
2. Macchiarini P, Verhoye J-P, Chapelier A, et al. Evaluation and outcome of different surgical techniques for postintubation tracheoesophageal fistulas. J Thorac Cardio Vasc Surg. 2000;119(2):268–76.
3. Mathisen DJ, Grillo HC, Wain JC, et al. Management of Acquired Nonmalignant Tracheoesophageal Fistula. Ann Thorac Surg. 1991;52:759–65.
4. Meunier B, Stasik C, Raoul JL, et al. Gastric bypass for malignant esophagotracheal fistula: a series of 21 cases. Eur J Card Thorac Surg. 1998; 13:184–98.
5. Grillo HC. Acquired tracheoesophageal fistula and bronchoesophageal. In: Frillo HC, ed. Surgery of the Trachea and Bronchi. New York: BC Dekker Inc., 2003, 341–356.
6. Bartels HE, Stein HJ, Siewert JR. Tracheobronchial lesions following oesophagectomy: prevalence, predisposing factors and outcome. Br J Surg. 1998;85:403–6.
7. Barkley C, Orringer MB, Iannettoni MD, Yee J. Challenges in reversing esophageal discontinuity operations. Ann Thorac Surg. 2003;76:989–95.
8. Diddee R, Shaw IH. Acquired trachea-oesophageal fistula in adults. BJA: CEACCP. 2006;6(3):105–8.
9. Shen KR, Allen MS, Cassivi SD, et al. Surgical management of acquired nonmalignant tracheoesophageal and Bronchoesophgageal fistulae. Ann Thorac Surg. 2010;90:914–9.
10. Baisi A, Bonavina L, Narne S, et al. Benign trachea-esophageal fistula: results of surgical therapy. Dis Esoph. 1999;12:209–11.
11. Desiree van den Bongard HJ, Boot H, Baas P, Taal BG. The role of parallel stent insertion in patients with esophagorespiratory fistulas. Gastointest Endosc. 2002;55:110–5.
12. Ellul JP, Morgan R, Gold D, et al. Parallel self-expanding covered metal stents in the trachea and oesophagus for the palliation of complex high tracheo-oesophageal fistula. Br J Surg. 1996;83:1767–8.

19

Diastolic dysfunction is common and predicts outcome after cardiac surgery

Thomas S. Metkus[1]*(iD), Alejandro Suarez-Pierre[2], Todd C. Crawford[2], Jennifer S. Lawton[2], Lee Goeddel[3], Jeffrey Dodd-o[3], Monica Mukherjee[1], Theodore P. Abraham[4] and Glenn J. Whitman[2]

Abstract

Background: Diastolic dysfunction (DD) identified on echocardiography predicts mortality after cardiac surgery, however the most useful diastolic parameters for assessment and the association of DD with prolonged mechanical ventilation, ICU re-admission, and hospital length of stay are not established.

Methods: We included patients that underwent coronary artery bypass grafting (CABG), aortic valve replacement (AVR) or a combined procedure (CAB-AVR) from 2010 to 2016, and who had preoperative transthoracic echocardiography (TTE) at our institution within 6 months of the operation. Diastolic function was graded using the transmitral E and A waves and the septal tissue Doppler velocity. We performed logistic regression to assess the association of grade of DD with a composite endpoint of death, prolonged mechanical ventilation, ICU readmission during hospitalization, and hospital length of stay longer than 14 days.

Results: Between 2010 and 2016, 577 patients were eligible for inclusion. DD was common, with 42% of the cohort manifesting grade II or grade III DD. Rates of death and prolonged ventilation increased across grades of DD and across quartiles of increasing LV filling pressure, assessed by the E/e' ratio. Adjusting for age, sex, procedure, systolic and diastolic function, both systolic (odds ratio 0.68 95% CI 0.55–0.85 per inter-quartile increase in LVEF) and diastolic function (odds ratio 1.31 95% CI 1.04–1.66 per increasing DD grade) both independently predicted outcome.

Conclusion: Diastolic dysfunction is common among patients undergoing cardiac surgery and is associated with death, prolonged mechanical ventilation, and prolonged hospital and ICU length of stay independent of systolic dysfunction.

Keywords: CABG, AVR, Echocardiography, Diastolic dysfunction, Mechanical ventilation

Background

Diastolic dysfunction (DD) consists of abnormalities in myocardial relaxation and increased left ventricular stiffness leading to elevated cardiac filling pressures and, in the extreme form, decreased stroke volume [1, 2]. DD is a cardinal manifestation of heart failure with preserved ejection fraction (HFpEF) [3] and is impacted by volume status [4], positive pressure ventilation [5–7], and revascularization [8]. Diastolic function assessed by echocardiography has been shown to be associated with atrial fibrillation after cardiac surgery in some [9] but not all [10] studies, and various echocardiographic markers of diastolic function may predict outcomes including death,

major morbidity, and difficulty separating from cardiopulmonary bypass [11–17]. The specific diastolic parameters most useful for predicting outcomes after cardiac surgery are not clear, and the association of DD with important outcomes including prolonged need for mechanical ventilation, intensive care unit re-admission and prolonged length of stay have not been established.

The purpose of this study was to assess the association of pre-operative diastolic function assessed by echocardiography with post-operative outcomes following coronary artery bypass grafting (CABG), aortic valve replacement (AVR) or combined CABG and AVR. We hypothesized that a higher grade of DD would be associated with an increased risk of postoperative mortality, prolonged hospital length of stay, and need for prolonged mechanical ventilation after surgery.

* Correspondence: tmetkus1@jhmi.edu
[1]Division of Cardiology, Johns Hopkins University School of Medicine, 600 N. Wolfe Street, Blalock 524 D2, Baltimore, MD 21287, USA
Full list of author information is available at the end of the article

Methods

We performed a retrospective study to determine the association of echocardiographic DD with outcomes after CAB, AVR, or CAB-AVR. We hypothesized that higher grade of DD assessed using the transmitral E and A waves and the septal tissue Doppler velocity (e') and higher cardiac filling pressures estimated by the ratio of E to e' velocity would both be associated with higher risk of postoperative mortality, prolonged hospital length of stay, and need for prolonged mechanical ventilation after surgery. The study was approved by the Johns Hopkins Hospital institutional review board.

Patient population

Between 2010 and 2016, 2596 patients underwent CAB, 809 patients underwent AVR, and 386 underwent CAB-AVR. The present study included patients undergoing isolated CAB, isolated AVR and combined CAB-AVR between July 2010 and July 2016 who had a full transthoracic echocardiogram at our institution within the 6 months prior to surgery, who were in sinus rhythm pre-operatively, and had measurable mitral inflow pattern, systolic function, and tissue Doppler as described below. Using these criteria, 577 patients were included in the current study.

Echocardiography

We extracted data from echocardiography reports for eligible patients. Studies were performed by certified sonographers and interpreting physicians were expert practicing echocardiographers at the Johns Hopkins Hospital. Diastolic function was assessed using transmitral diastolic flow profile including peak early diastolic velocity (E wave velocity) and peak late diastolic filling velocity (A wave velocity) [1, 2]. We assessed septal annular velocity (e') using Tissue Doppler Imaging (TDI) consistent with recommended guidelines [1, 2]. The ratio of E to e' velocity was assessed [1, 2] as a surrogate for LV filling pressure [18]. The choice of parameters used to assess diastolic function was made on the basis of guideline-recommended approaches and anticipated feasibility of obtaining measurements on both transthoracic and intra-operative trans-esophageal echocardiography. Using the mitral inflow patterns from the 2016 guidelines on echocardiographic assessment of diastolic function [2], we graded diastolic function as follows:

Grade 0: normal left ventricular ejection fraction, e' > 7 cm/s and E/e' < 14

Grade I: E/A < 0.9 and E < 50 cm/s

Grade I: E/A < 0.8 with E > 50 cm/s or 0.8 < E/A < 2 AND E/e' < 14

Grade II: E/A < 0.8 with E > 50 cm/s or 0.8 < E/A < 2 AND E/e' > 14

Grade III: E/A > 2

Statistics

Demographic and clinical characteristics were compared across grades of diastolic function using the Kruskal-Wallis test for continuous variables and Pearson's chi-squared test for categorical variables. We report the percentage of patients suffering death, prolonged mechanical ventilation or both across grades of diastolic function and across quartiles of E/e' ratio. We performed logistic regression to assess the association of grade of DD with a composite endpoint of events of a priori clinical interest: death within 30 days, prolonged mechanical ventilation, ICU readmission during hospitalization, and hospital length of stay longer than 14 days. Univariate models and models which adjusted for clinical factors of a priori clinical interest were performed. Covariates included age, sex, procedure (CABG v. AVR v. CAB-AVR), and systolic function. A two-tailed P value less than 0.05 was considered statistically significant. All analyses were performed using StataSE version 14.0 (StataCorp Inc., College Station, TX).

Results

Between 2010 and 2016, 577 patients were eligible for inclusion. The specific procedures included CABG alone in 77%, AVR alone in 16% and a combined procedure in 6%. A median of 4 (interquartile range (IQR) 1.5–10) days passed between the transthoracic echocardiogram used to grade diastolic function and the operation. DD was common, with 42% of the cohort manifesting grade II or grade III DD compared to 58% of the group with grade 0 or grade I. Most patients had preserved systolic function, with median LVEF 55% (IQR 45–60%).

Demographic and clinical characteristics are shown in the Table 1 for the entire cohort and across grades of diastolic function. Patients with more advanced DD were older, had higher body-mass index, more concomitant systolic dysfunction, had a higher prevalence of known heart failure, diabetes, and elevated creatinine.

Outcomes across grades of diastolic function are shown in the Table 1. Patients with more advanced DD had higher post-operative creatinine levels, longer hospital length of stay, higher rates of prolonged mechanical ventilation post-operatively, and higher rates of in hospital mortality. The patients who had AVR had higher rate of grade 2 or 3 diastolic dysfunction compared to those who underwent CABG alone (67.2% v. 34.8%, $p < 0.001$).

Figure 1 displays increasing rates of mortality, prolonged ventilation, and a composite of mortality and prolonged ventilation across increasing grade of DD. Rates of death and prolonged ventilation also increased across quartiles of increasing LV filling pressure, assessed by the E/e' ratio, as shown in Fig. 2. The median E/e' in quartile 1 was 8.2 (interquartile range (IQR) 7.1–8.9), quartile 2 was 11.1 (IQR 10.4–11.6), quartile 3 was 14.7 (IQR 13.7–15.9) and quartile 4 was 22.7 (IQR 19.5–27.6). There were

Table 1 Demographic and clinical characteristics and outcomes of the cohort and across grades of diastolic function

Diastolic grade (N)	Total (577)	Grade 0 (155)	Grade 1 (179)	Grade 2 (203)	Grade 3 (40)	P
Age (years)	66 (58–74)	62 (53–69)	66 (58–75)	70 (60–78)	69.5 (61–78.5)	0.0001
Timing of echo pre-op (days)	4 (1.5–10)	2.5 (1–8)	3 (1.4–6.3)	5 (2–26)	7.1 (2.3–13.2)	0.0001
Female sex	160 (27.7%)	25 (16%)	46 (26%)	80 (39%)	9 (23%)	0.0001
Height (cm)	172.7 (165–179)	175.3 (167.6–180.3)	172.7 (165–180.3)	170.2 (162.6–177.8)	172.7 (162.6–179.1)	0.0003
Weight (kg)	84.8 (74.5–98.1)	85.3 (74–96)	83.9 (74.5–94.4)	86 (75.2–103.3)	84.3 (72.5–102)	0.4
Body-mass index (kg/m2)	28.6 (25.5–32.6)	27.7 (25.3–31.2)	28.3 (25.2–31.9)	29.9 (26.5–35.0)	29.4 (25.4–32.8)	0.001
E (cm/s)	80.5 (64.2–98.7)	76.9 (66–90.8)	62.8 (51.4–72)	96.7 (82.2–112)	115.5 (96.4–134)	0.0001
A (cm/s)	79.5 (64.4–97.2)	71.4 (61.2–87.1)	78.5 (65.8–89.3)	95.4 (75.5–116)	39.9 (32.2–54.6)	0.0001
Decel time (ms)	222 (188–269)	220 (187–259)	235 (202–288)	226 (191–272)	156 (130–191.5)	0.0001
LVEF (%)	55 (45–60)	60 (55–65)	55 (45–60)	55 (40–60)	30 (22.5–50)	0.0001
e' (cm/s)	6.1 (4.9–7.3)	8.1 (7.4–9.4)	5.9 (5–6.7)	5.0 (4.0–6.0)	5.1 (4.4–6.2)	0.0001
E/e' ratio	12.6 (9.6–17.1)	9.1 (7.7–11.1)	11 (9.3–12.1)	17.9 (15.8–22.8)	23.1 (18.0–27.6)	0.0001
Septal thickness (cm)	1.2 (1.0–1.4)	1.1 (1.0–1.3)	1.2 (1.0–1.4)	1.2 (1.1–1.4)	1.1 (1.0–1.3)	0.0003
Posterior wall thickness (cm)	1.0 (0.9–1.2)	1.0 (0.8–1.1)	1.0 (0.9–1.2)	1.1 (0.9–1.2)	1.1 (1.0–1.3)	0.0001
End-diastolic diameter (cm)	4.6 (4.2–5.1)	4.6 (4.2–4.9)	4.6 (4.1–5.0)	4.7 (4.2–5.2)	5.4 (5.0–5.9)	0.0001
Prior MI	223 (38.7%)	44 (28%)	71 (40%)	92 (45%)	16 (40%)	0.01
Prior heart failure	228 (39.5%)	40 (26%)	57 (32%)	100 (49%)	31 (78%)	0.0001
Prior arrhythmia	24 (4.2%)	3 (2%)	8 (4%)	10 (5%)	3 (8%)	0.3
Diabetes	244 (42.3%)	47 (30%)	59 (33%)	116 (57%)	22 (55%)	0.0001
Hypertension	324 (56.1%)	77 (50%)	98 (55%)	126 (62%)	23 (58%)	0.1
Moderate or worse chronic lung disease	28 (4.9%)	5 (3%)	11 (6%)	10 (5%)	2 (5)	0.7
Peripheral vascular disease	67 (11.6%)	12 (8%)	14 (8%)	33 (16%)	8 (20%)	0.008
Creatinine	1.0 (0.9–1.3)	1.0 (0.9–1.2)	1.0 (0.9–1.2)	1.1 (0.9–1.3)	1.3 (1.0–2.3)	0.0001
Procedure						0.0001
CAB alone	446 (77.3%)	10 (6%)	19 (11%)	52 (26%)	13 (33%)	
AVR alone	94 (16.3%)	138 (89%)	153 (85%)	132 (65%)	23 (57%)	
CAB-AVR	37 (6.4%)	7 (5%)	7 (4%)	19 (9%)	4 (10%)	
Post-op creatinine	1.2 (1.0–1.6)	1.1 (1.0–1.4)	1.1 (1.0–1.4)	1.3 (1.0–1.9)	1.7 (1.2–2.9)	0.0001
Acute kidney injury (> 2× increase in creatinine)	35 (6%)	8 (5%)	7 (4%)	19 (9%)	1 (3%)	0.09
Length of hospital stay (days)	10 (8–15)	9 (7–13)	10 (8–14)	11 (7–17)	20.5 (12.5–24)	0.0001
Reintubation	16 (2.8%)	4 (3%)	5 (3%)	7 (3%)	0	0.7
ICU readmission	24 (4.2%)	7 (5%)	4 (2%)	10 (5%)	3 (8%)	0.4
Prolonged ventilation > 24 h	46 (8%)	6 (4%)	11 (6%)	22 (11%)	7 (18%)	0.009
AF	103 (17.9%)	29 (19%)	25 (14%)	39 (19%)	10 (25%)	0.3
In-hospital mortality	17 (3%)	3 (2%)	0	11 (5%)	3 (8%)	0.004

Data is displaced as median (interquartile range) for continuous variables and N(%) for categorical variables

increasing adverse events with increasing E/e' ratio, with highest event rates in the highest quartile of E/e', corresponding to an E/e' ratio of 15 or higher. Diastolic dysfunction grade 2 or 3 remained associated with the composite of death or prolonged mechanical ventilation when the cohort was stratified by CABG alone versus AVR. In the CABG alone group, 5.8% of the group with diastolic function grade 0 or 1 suffered the composite endpoint compared to 11.6% of those with Diastolic dysfunction grade 2 or 3 ($p = 0.031$). In the AVR group, 4.7% of the group with diastolic function grade 0 or 1 suffered the composite endpoint compared to 18.2% of those with Diastolic dysfunction grade 2 or 3 ($p = 0.035$).

Univariate logistic regression models for associations with the composite endpoint of death, prolonged mechanical

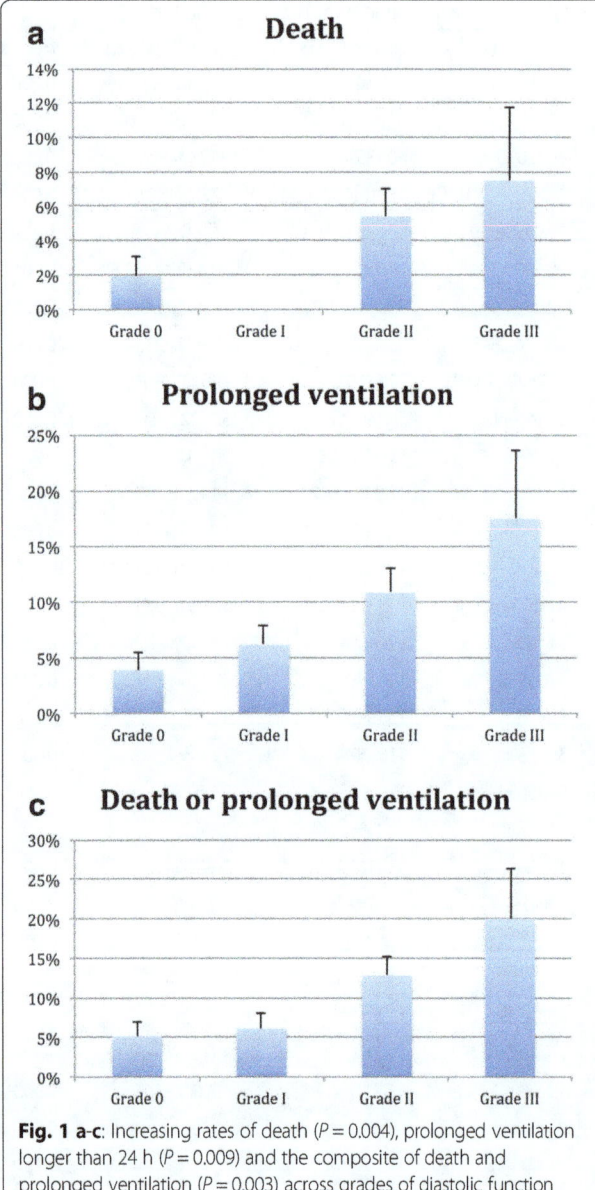

Fig. 1 a-c: Increasing rates of death (*P* = 0.004), prolonged ventilation longer than 24 h (*P* = 0.009) and the composite of death and prolonged ventilation (*P* = 0.003) across grades of diastolic function

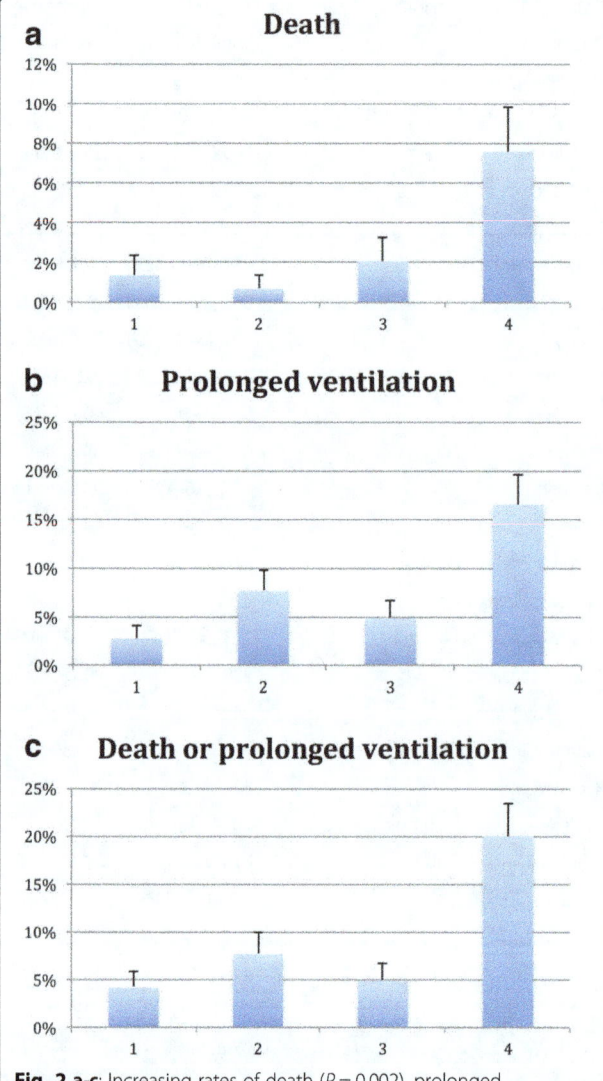

Fig. 2 a-c: Increasing rates of death (*P* = 0.002), prolonged ventilation longer than 24 h (*P* = 0.001) and the composite of death and prolonged ventilation (*P* = 0.0001) across quartiles of increasing LV filling pressure, estimated by the E/e' ratio

ventilation, ICU readmission, and hospital length of stay longer than 14 days are shown in Fig. 3, panel A. Both systolic function (odds ratio 0.63 95% CI 0.52–0.76 per inter-quartile increase in LVEF) and diastolic function (odds ratio 1.62 95% CI 1.34–1.96 per increasing DD grade) were associated with outcome in univariate models. A multivariable model is shown in Fig. 3, B. In the model including age, sex, procedure, systolic and diastolic function, both systolic (odds ratio 0.68 95% CI 0.55–0.85 per inter-quartile increase in LVEF) and diastolic function (odds ratio 1.31 95% CI 1.04–1.66 per increasing DD grade) independently predicted outcome. Similar findings were obtained in considering quartile of E/e' ratio: increasing quartile of E/e' ratio was associated with the composite outcome in a univariate model (odds ratio 1.61 95% CI 1.34–1.92 per

inter-quartile increased in E/e' ratio) and the model adjusted for age, sex, procedure, and systolic function (odds ratio 1.40 95% CI 1.14–1.72 per inter-quartile increase in E/e' ratio).

Discussion

In a cohort of 577 patients undergoing cardiac surgery, we report the association of echocardiographic diastolic function with outcome. Our major findings include 1) DD is common among patients undergoing CAB, AVR or both, 2) higher grade of DD and higher LV filling pressure assessed by echocardiography is associated with higher risk of mortality and need for prolonged ventilation and 3) both systolic and diastolic function independently predict outcome after cardiac surgery.

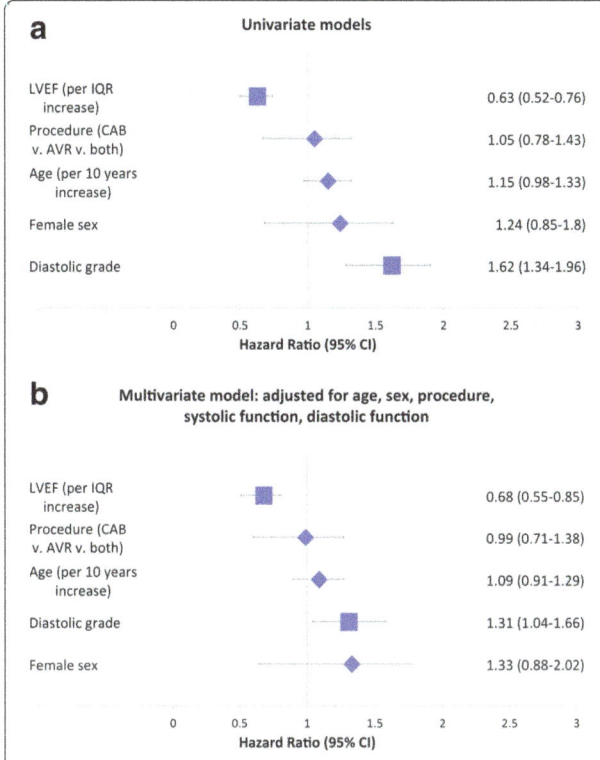

Fig. 3 Univariate (Panel **a**) and multivariate (Panel **b**) logistic regression models for associations with the composite endpoint of death, prolonged mechanical ventilation, ICU readmission, and hospital length of stay longer than 14 days

We report that DD is common among patients undergoing cardiac surgery, with 42% of patients manifesting grade II or higher DD. These findings are consistent with community based cohorts, demonstrating abnormal diastolic function in between 27 and 56% of a community based sample [19, 20] and more common still among patients with underlying conditions also associated with cardiac surgical disease such as age, diabetes, renal insufficiency, coronary disease hypertension, and obesity [19, 21, 22]. Conditions that cause left ventricular hypertrophy, such as aortic stenosis and systemic hypertension, contribute uniquely to DD. Increased LV wall thickness and LV mass contribute to diastolic dysfunction by decreasing ventricular compliance and increasing left ventricular stiffness. These alterations contribute to changes in both the passive and active filling properties of the ventricle [1]. Furthermore, as the LV wall becomes thicker, there is regional dyssynchrony in contraction that can be observed which further contributes to diastolic dysfunction [23]. Given that DD is common in cardiac surgical patients, has prognostic value, and can be impacted by specific treatments as discussed below, consideration should be given to screening for DD prior to cardiac surgery.

We demonstrate that DD is associated with prolonged ventilation, death, and longer ICU and hospital length of stay. Other studies have also correlated diastolic grade with mortality [11, 13] and adverse events [15] after cardiac surgery, and the ratio of E to e' which is a surrogate for LV filling pressure has also been shown to predict postoperative morbidity [12]. The unifying feature responsible for this adverse prognosis may be elevated left heart filling pressure which has itself been associated with mortality [24] and length of stay after surgery [25]. Other putative mechanisms of adverse prognosis include DD predisposing to atrial fibrillation, which has been suggested in some [9] but not all [10] studies. DD has been shown to correlate with difficulty separating from cardiopulmonary bypass [14] and to be associated with postoperative pulmonary edema which could explain need for prolonged ventilation [17].

We report that echocardiographic systolic and DD both predict outcome independently. While systolic function is commonly utilized as a risk marker prior to cardiac surgery [13, 26, 27], less attention has been paid to DD. DD has been shown to independently improve prognostic ability when considered with systolic dysfunction, improving model performance by 5.9% above that provided by the Society of Thoracic Surgeons' risk score alone [13]. If future studies confirm our findings, an assessment of diastolic function or left heart filling pressure could be used to further refine prognosis prior to surgery or to delay surgery until diastolic indices improve after change in loading conditions or volume status [4, 18] or revascularization after myocardial infarction [8].

Although there are no treatments targeted specifically at the cellular perturbations underlying DD [3], several clinical parameters can be modified to improve diastolic function. Intra-aortic balloon pumping can improve diastolic function [28] and high levels of positive end-expiratory pressure on the ventilator can influence diastolic function by changing preload sensitivity [6, 7] and exacerbating defects in myocardial relaxation [5]. The calcium sensitizing agent levosimendan improves diastolic function at time of CABG by decreasing relaxation time and deceleration time, suggesting improved myocardial relaxation, and nitrate infusions have similar albeit less pronounced effects [29]. Control of heart rate is also important in patients with DD. Those patients with restrictive myocardial filling complete LV filling in early diastole and are thus "heart rate dependent," as stroke volume is fixed and longer diastole will not improve filling [1, 2]. Such patients would benefit from permissively higher heart rates [30]. In contrast, those patients with an impaired relaxation filling pattern- grade I DD- benefit from longer filling periods and slower heart rates due to the prolonged myocardial relaxation time. Thus, once DD is identified prior to cardiac surgery, there are several therapeutic implications. Whether treating DD in this manner or via techniques or agents to be developed improves surgical outcomes should be a major focus of future research.

Limitations of our study include its retrospective, observational nature. Thus, we can assess for associations but cannot infer causality of DD and post-surgical outcomes. Our study focuses only on those patients in sinus rhythm in whom diastolic function can be graded, however patients with paced rhythms, mitral valve disease, and mitral annular calcification, and arrhythmia such as atrial fibrillation are major subsets of the cardiac surgical population; thus, although diastolic function cannot always be graded in these populations, markers of left ventricular filling pressure such as E/e' ratio should be used. Our data set did not include details on completeness of revascularization and detailed conduct of cardiopulmonary bypass, and the association of diastolic function with these parameters needs to be more fully characterized in future studies. Finally, not all patients in practice will have adequate transthoracic echocardiographic windows and image quality for assessment of diastolic function, and correlation of our findings with those on intra-operative trans-esophageal echocardiography would be useful.

Conclusions

In conclusion, DD is common among patients undergoing CAB, AVR and CAB-AVR and is associated with death, prolonged mechanical ventilation, and prolonged hospital and ICU length of stay independent of systolic dysfunction. Future studies should assess treatments targeted at improving diastolic function in cardiac surgical patients and the impact of therapy on post-operative outcomes.

Abbreviations

AVR: Aortic valve replacement; CABG: Coronary artery bypass grafting; CI: Confidence interval; DD: Diastolic dysfunction; HFPEF: Heart failure with preserved ejection fraction; IQR: Interquartile range; LVEF: Left ventricular ejection fraction; TDI: Tissue Doppler imaging; TTE: Transthoracic echocardiography

Authors' contributions

All authors participated in conception and design of the study. TM obtained organized and cleaned the dataset. TM, AS, TC, and LG performed data analyses. All authors provided data interpretation and results interpretation. TM drafted the article and all authors provided critical revisions of the article. All authors provided final approval of the article.

Competing interests

The authors declare they have no competing interests.

Author details

[1]Division of Cardiology, Johns Hopkins University School of Medicine, 600 N. Wolfe Street, Blalock 524 D2, Baltimore, MD 21287, USA. [2]Division of Cardiac Surgery, Johns Hopkins University School of Medicine, Baltimore, MD, USA. [3]Department of Anesthesia and Critical Care Medicine, Johns Hopkins University School of Medicine, Baltimore, MD, USA. [4]Division of Cardiology, Department of Medicine, University of California, San Francisco, 505 Parnassus Ave., Suite M344 San Francisco, San Francisco, CA, USA.

References

1. Nagueh SF, Appleton CP, Gillebert TC, Marino PN, Oh JK, Smiseth OA, Waggoner AD, Flachskampf FA, Pellikka PA, Evangelisa A. Recommendations for the evaluation of left ventricular diastolic function by echocardiography. Eur J Echocardiogr. 2009;10(2):165–93.
2. Nagueh SF, Smiseth OA, Appleton CP, Byrd BF 3rd, Dokainish H, Edvardsen T, Flachskampf FA, Gillebert TC, Klein AL, Lancellotti P, et al. Recommendations for the evaluation of left ventricular diastolic function by echocardiography: an update from the American Society of Echocardiography and the European Association of Cardiovascular Imaging. Eur Heart J Cardiovasc Imaging. 2016;17(12):1321–60.
3. Sharma K, Kass DA. Heart failure with preserved ejection fraction: mechanisms, clinical features, and therapies. Circ Res. 2014;115(1):79–96.
4. Hurrell DG, Nishimura RA, Ilstrup DM, Appleton CP. Utility of preload alteration in assessment of left ventricular filling pressure by Doppler echocardiography: a simultaneous catheterization and Doppler echocardiographic study. J Am Coll Cardiol. 1997;30(2):459–67.
5. Chin JH, Lee EH, Kim WJ, Choi DK, Hahm KD, Sim JY, Choi IC. Positive end-expiratory pressure aggravates left ventricular diastolic relaxation further in patients with pre-existing relaxation abnormality. Br J Anaesth. 2013;111(3):368–73.
6. Juhl-Olsen P, Frederiksen CA, Hermansen JF, Jakobsen CJ, Sloth E. Echocardiographic measures of diastolic function are preload dependent during triggered positive pressure ventilation: a controlled crossover study in healthy subjects. Crit Care Res Pract. 2012;2012:703196.
7. Juhl-Olsen P, Hermansen JF, Frederiksen CA, Rasmussen LA, Jakobsen CJ, Sloth E. Positive end-expiratory pressure influences echocardiographic measures of diastolic function: a randomized, crossover study in cardiac surgery patients. Anesthesiology. 2013;119(5):1078–86.
8. Hedman A, Samad BA, Larsson T, Zuber E, Nordlander R, Alam M. Improvement in diastolic left ventricular function after coronary artery bypass grafting as assessed by recordings of mitral annular velocity using Doppler tissue imaging. Eur J Echocardiogr. 2005;6(3):202–9.
9. Melduni RM, Suri RM, Seward JB, Bailey KR, Ammash NM, Oh JK, Schaff HV, Gersh BJ. Diastolic dysfunction in patients undergoing cardiac surgery: a pathophysiological mechanism underlying the initiation of new-onset post-operative atrial fibrillation. J Am Coll Cardiol. 2011;58(9):953–61.
10. Barbara DW, Rehfeldt KH, Pulido JN, Li Z, White RD, Schaff HV, Mauermann WJ. Diastolic function and new-onset atrial fibrillation following cardiac surgery. Ann Card Anaesth. 2015;18(1):8–14.
11. Vaskelyte J, Stoskute N, Kinduris S, Ereminiene E. Coronary artery bypass grafting in patients with severe left ventricular dysfunction: predictive significance of left ventricular diastolic filling pattern. Eur J Echocardiogr. 2001;2(1):62–7.
12. Jun NH, Shim JK, Kim JC, Kwak YL. Prognostic value of a tissue Doppler-derived index of left ventricular filling pressure on composite morbidity after off-pump coronary artery bypass surgery. Br J Anaesth. 2011;107(4):519–24.
13. Afilalo J, Flynn AW, Shimony A, Rudski LG, Agnihotri AK, Morin JF, Castrillo C, Shahian DM, Picard MH. Incremental value of the preoperative echocardiogram to predict mortality and major morbidity in coronary artery bypass surgery. Circulation. 2013;127(3):356–64.
14. Denault AY, Couture P, Buithieu J, Haddad F, Carrier M, Babin D, Levesque S, Tardif JC. Left and right ventricular diastolic dysfunction as predictors of difficult separation from cardiopulmonary bypass. Can J Anaesth. 2006;53(10):1020–9.
15. Swaminathan M, Nicoara A, Phillips-Bute BG, Aeschlimann N, Milano CA, Mackensen GB, Podgoreanu MV, Velazquez EJ, Stafford-Smith M, Mathew JP, et al. Utility of a simple algorithm to grade diastolic dysfunction and predict outcome after coronary artery bypass graft surgery. Ann Thorac Surg. 2011;91(6):1844–50.

16. Zaid RR, Barker CM, Little SH, Nagueh SF. Pre- and post-operative diastolic dysfunction in patients with valvular heart disease: diagnosis and therapeutic implications. J Am Coll Cardiol. 2013;62(21):1922–30.

17. Cho DH, Park SM, Kim MN, Kim SA, Lim H, Shim WJ. Presence of preoperative diastolic dysfunction predicts postoperative pulmonary edema and cardiovascular complications in patients undergoing noncardiac surgery. Echocardiography. 2014;31(1):42–9.

18. Ommen SR, Nishimura RA, Appleton CP, Miller FA, Oh JK, Redfield MM, Tajik AJ. Clinical utility of Doppler echocardiography and tissue Doppler imaging in the estimation of left ventricular filling pressures: a comparative simultaneous Doppler-catheterization study. Circulation. 2000;102(15):1788–94.

19. Kuznetsova T, Herbots L, Lopez B, Jin Y, Richart T, Thijs L, Gonzalez A, Herregods MC, Fagard RH, Diez J, et al. Prevalence of left ventricular diastolic dysfunction in a general population. Circ Heart Fail. 2009;2(2):105–12.

20. Yamada H, Goh PP, Sun JP, Odabashian J, Garcia MJ, Thomas JD, Klein AL. Prevalence of left ventricular diastolic dysfunction by Doppler echocardiography: clinical application of the Canadian consensus guidelines. J Am Soc Echocardiogr. 2002;15(10 Pt 2):1238–44.

21. Boyer JK, Thanigaraj S, Schechtman KB, Perez JE. Prevalence of ventricular diastolic dysfunction in asymptomatic, normotensive patients with diabetes mellitus. Am J Cardiol. 2004;93(7):870–5.

22. Fischer M, Baessler A, Hense HW, Hengstenberg C, Muscholl M, Holmer S, Doring A, Broeckel U, Riegger G, Schunkert H. Prevalence of left ventricular diastolic dysfunction in the community. Results from a Doppler echocardiographic-based survey of a population sample. Eur Heart J. 2003;24(4):320–8.

23. Stork T, Mockel M, Danne O, Voller H, Eichstadt H, Frei U. Left ventricular hypertrophy and diastolic dysfunction: their relation to coronary heart disease. Cardiovasc Drugs Ther. 1995;9(Suppl 3):533–7.

24. Salem R, Denault AY, Couture P, Belisle S, Fortier A, Guertin MC, Carrier M, Martineau R. Left ventricular end-diastolic pressure is a predictor of mortality in cardiac surgery independently of left ventricular ejection fraction. Br J Anaesth. 2006;97(3):292–7.

25. Mounsey JP, Griffith MJ, Heaviside DW, Brown AH, Reid DS. Determinants of the length of stay in intensive care and in hospital after coronary artery surgery. Br Heart J. 1995;73(1):92–8.

26. Fukui T, Shibata T, Sasaki Y, Hirai H, Motoki M, Takahashi Y, Nakahira A, Suehiro S. Long-term survival and functional recovery after isolated coronary artery bypass grafting in patients with severe left ventricular dysfunction. Gen Thorac Cardiovasc Surg. 2007;55(10):403–8.

27. Velazquez EJ, Lee KL, Jones RH, Al-Khalidi HR, Hill JA, Panza JA, Michler RE, Bonow RO, Doenst T, Petrie MC, et al. Coronary-artery bypass surgery in patients with ischemic cardiomyopathy. N Engl J Med. 2016;374(16):1511–20.

28. Khir AW, Price S, Henein MY, Parker KH, Pepper JR. Intra-aortic balloon pumping: effects on left ventricular diastolic function. Eur J Cardiothorac Surg. 2003;24(2):277–82.

29. Malik V, Subramanian A, Hote M, Kiran U. Effect of Levosimendan on diastolic function in patients undergoing coronary artery bypass grafting: a comparative study. J Cardiovasc Pharmacol. 2015;66(2):141–7.

30. Kushwaha SS, Fallon JT, Fuster V. Restrictive cardiomyopathy. N Engl J Med. 1997;336(4):267–76.

20

Is isolated aortic valve replacement sufficient to treat concomitant moderate functional mitral regurgitation? A propensity-matched analysis

Robert A. Sorabella, Anna Olds, Halit Yerebakan, Dua Hassan, Michael A. Borger, Michael Argenziano, Craig R. Smith and Isaac George[*] ⓘ

Abstract

Background: A significant proportion of patients presenting for isolated aortic valve replacement (AVR) demonstrate some degree of functional mitral regurgitation (fMR). Guidelines addressing concomitant mitral valve intervention in those patients with moderate fMR lack strong evidence-based support. Our aim is to determine the effect of untreated moderate fMR at the time of AVR on long-term survival.

Methods: All patients undergoing isolated AVR from 2000 to 2013 at our institution were retrospectively reviewed. Patients were stratified according to severity of preoperative fMR; 0–1+ MR (Group NoMR, $n = 1826$) and 2–3+ MR (Group MR, $n = 330$). All patients in Group MR were propensity-matched with patients in Group NoMR to control for differences in baseline characteristics. The primary outcome of interest was overall survival.

Results: Propensity analysis matched 330 patients from each group. Mean age was 77.9 ± 10.0 years and 50.6% were male. There were no differences in baseline demographics, echocardiographic parameters, or co-morbidities between groups. Kaplan-Meier analysis showed significantly worse medium and long-term survival in Group MR compared to Group NoMR (log-rank $p = 0.02$). Follow-up echocardiography showed slightly more severe MR in Group MR (1.1 ± 0.7 MR vs. 0.8 ± 0.7 NoMR, $p = 0.03$) at 1 year.

Conclusions: Patients undergoing isolated AVR with concomitant 2–3+ fMR experience poorer long-term survival than those patients with no or mild fMR. This suggests that mitral valve intervention may be necessary in patients undergoing AVR with clinically significant fMR.

Keywords: Aortic valve replacement, Mitral valve disease, Mitral regurgitation

Background

Surgical aortic valve replacement (AVR) remains the most common valvular operation with over 50,000 procedures performed in the United States in 2013 alone [1]. In addition to correction of primary aortic valve pathology, current American Heart Association guidelines recommend mitral valve intervention for patients presenting with concomitant severe functional mitral regurgitation (fMR) as a result of their aortic valve disease [2–4]. However, according to published literature, up to two-thirds of patients with aortic stenosis or insufficiency (AS, AI, respectively) can present with moderate or less fMR, and significant debate persists on whether these patients warrant mitral valve repair at the time of AVR [5–12].

The traditional, conservative perspective assumes that non-severe fMR regresses following isolated AVR due to left ventricular reverse remodeling and removal of afterload obstruction, which subsequently leads to improved mitral leaflet coaptation. Although this phenomenon occurs to some extent following AVR, some reports suggest that patients may still be left with clinically

* Correspondence: isaacgeorge@hotmail.com
Division of Cardiothoracic Surgery, New York Presbyterian Hospital - Columbia University College of Physicians and Surgeons, 177 Fort Washington Ave, MHB 7GN-435, New York, NY 10032, USA

significant fMR even at late follow-up, which may lead to worsened long-term survival [13–15]. However, these studies are limited by small sample sizes and lack of extended follow-up, and fail to yield definitive conclusions. Therefore, the aim of this study is to determine the impact of uncorrected moderate fMR at the time of AVR on late survival in comparison to patients with no or mild fMR in a large patient population. These results may have important clinical implications in defining the appropriate treatment strategy for patients with combined aortic and moderate functional mitral valve disease, particularly in the modern era of transcatheter valve therapy.

Methods
Patient selection

All patients undergoing isolated AVR at NY Presbyterian-Columbia University Medical Center between January 2000 and December 2013 were retrospectively reviewed for inclusion into the study. Patients with severe fMR (4+), primary mitral valve disease, prior mitral surgery, or cardiogenic shock at the time of surgery were excluded from the analysis. A total of 2156 patients met inclusion and exclusion criteria, and patients were stratified according to degree of preoperative fMR: 0–1+ MR (Group NoMR, $n = 1826$) and 2–3+ MR (MR, $n = 330$). Functional MR was defined as MR with normal mitral valve morphology regardless of severity of left ventricular dysfunction as evaluated by preoperative transthoracic or transesophageal echocardiography. Degree of MR was assessed using a 0–4+ scale, as graded by a blinded echocardiographer (0 = no MR, 1 + =mild MR, 2 + =moderate MR, 3 + =moderate-severe MR, 4 + =severe MR). Given the significant underlying differences in demographics and co-morbid conditions between groups, a propensity-matched analysis was performed using a subset of the overall cohort. The study was approved by the Columbia University Institutional Review Board and need for individual patient consent was waived.

Clinical and follow-up data were collected from the electronic medical record and mortality data for patients lost to follow up were collected from United States Social Security Death Index. Baseline demographics, co-morbidities [congestive heart failure, prior myocardial infarct, severe chronic kidney disease (eGFR < 30 mL/min), diabetes mellitus, end-stage renal disease needing dialysis, cerebrovascular disease, peripheral vascular disease, and chronic obstructive pulmonary disease], preoperative echocardiographic measurements, operative details, postoperative complications and length of stay, follow-up echocardiographic data, and survival data were collected for analysis.

Statistical analysis

All analyses were conducted using SPSS version 22 (IBM corporation, Armonk, NY). Continuous variables are presented as mean ± standard deviation and compared using independent samples t-tests, or median and interquartile range and compared using Mann-Whitney U test where appropriate. Categorical variables are presented as total count and percentage of the group, and compared using Pearson's chi-square test or Fisher's exact test where applicable. Kaplan-Meier analysis was used for comparison of survival, and survival curves were compared using the log-rank test. In order to control for differences in preoperative variables between groups, a propensity-matched analysis was performed. Patients were assigned a propensity score and matched using the nearest neighbor Greedy 5 to 1 digit matching algorithm (MatchIt package in R 3.0.2, R foundation for Statistical Computing, Vienna, Austria). Covariates included in calculation of the propensity score included age at surgery, gender, body mass index, preoperative ejection fraction, preoperative tricuspid regurgitation, preoperative hemoglobin, indication for surgery, and history of severe chronic kidney disease, cerebrovascular disease, myocardial infarction, peripheral vascular disease, chronic obstructive pulmonary disease, diabetes mellitus, need for hemodialysis, congestive heart failure, or prior cardiac surgery. Matching was done in a 1:1 fashion and matched 330 patients from each group for comparison. All p-values≤0.05 were considered statistically significant.

Results
Overall cohort analysis

Baseline characteristics, operative details, and outcomes of the overall cohort analysis are presented in Table 1. Patients in Group MR were significantly older, had lower BMIs, and generally had more preoperative co-morbidities than those in Group NoMR. Preoperative echocardiograms revealed significantly lower left ventricular ejection fractions and higher rates of severe aortic stenosis (AS) and severe tricuspid regurgitation (TR) in Group MR. Analysis of postoperative complications showed that patients in Group MR had a significantly higher 30-day mortality rate (3.6% MR vs. 1.5% NoMR, $p = 0.007$) and experienced significantly longer postoperative lengths of stay and higher rates of postoperative respiratory failure.

Kaplan-Meier analysis of survival in the overall cohort (Fig. 1A) showed significantly worse medium- and long-term survival for patients in Group MR (log rank $p < 0.001$). In addition, follow-up echocardiograms showed more severe MR at 1 year in Group MR (1.1 ± 0.7 MR vs. 0.6 ± 0.7 NoMR, $p < 0.001$) compared to Group NoMR, although the mean severity of MR in both groups fell in the trace-to-mild range.

Table 1 Overall Cohort Analysis

	NoMR	MR	p-value
Demographics			
Total, n	1826	330	–
Age, years (mean ± SD)	69.3 ± 14.5	78.1 ± 10.1	< 0.001
Male, n (%)	1061 (58.1)	174 (52.7)	0.07
BMI, kg/m² (mean ± SD)	28.0 ± 5.8	27.2 ± 5.6	0.03
Co-morbidities, n (%)			
Myocardial infarction	156 (8.5)	66 (20.0)	< 0.001
Congestive heart failure	329 (18.0)	111 (33.6)	< 0.001
Severe CKD	81 (4.4)	39 (11.8)	< 0.001
Diabetes	361 (19.8)	84 (25.5)	0.02
Dialysis	26 (1.4)	9 (2.7)	0.09
Baseline echocardiography			
LVEF, % (mean ± SD)	52.1 ± 12.0	46.1 ± 14.2	< 0.001
3–4+ AI, n (%)	424 (23.2)	65 (19.7)	0.16
Severe AS, n (%)	1472 (80.6)	287 (87.0)	0.006
3–4+ TR, n (%)	16 (0.9)	11 (3.3)	< 0.001
Operative details			
Re-operations, n (%)	324 (17.7)	96 (29.1)	< 0.001
CPB time, minutes (mean ± SD)	88.9 ± 32.0	92.5 ± 33.2	0.06
XCL time, minutes (mean ± SD)	62.3 ± 19.8	63.3 ± 18.8	0.39
Outcomes			
30-day mortality, n (%)	27 (1.5)	12 (3.6)	0.007
Post-op LOS, days (median, IQR)	7, 5–9	8, 6–11	< 0.001
Re-op for bleeding	60 (3.3)	12 (3.6)	0.74
Respiratory failure, n (%)	91 (5.0)	26 (7.9)	0.03
New need for dialysis, n (%)	18 (1.0)	3 (0.9)	0.90
Echocardiographic follow-up			
1-year MR grade (mean ± SD)	0.6 ± 0.7	1.1 ± 0.7	< 0.001

Abbreviations: AI = aortic insufficiency, AS = aortic stenosis, BMI = body mass index, CKD = chronic kidney disease, CPB = cardiopulmonary bypass, IQR = interquartile range, LOS = length of stay, LVEF = left ventricular ejection fraction, MR = mitral regurgitation, TR = tricuspid regurgitation, XCL = aortic cross-clamp

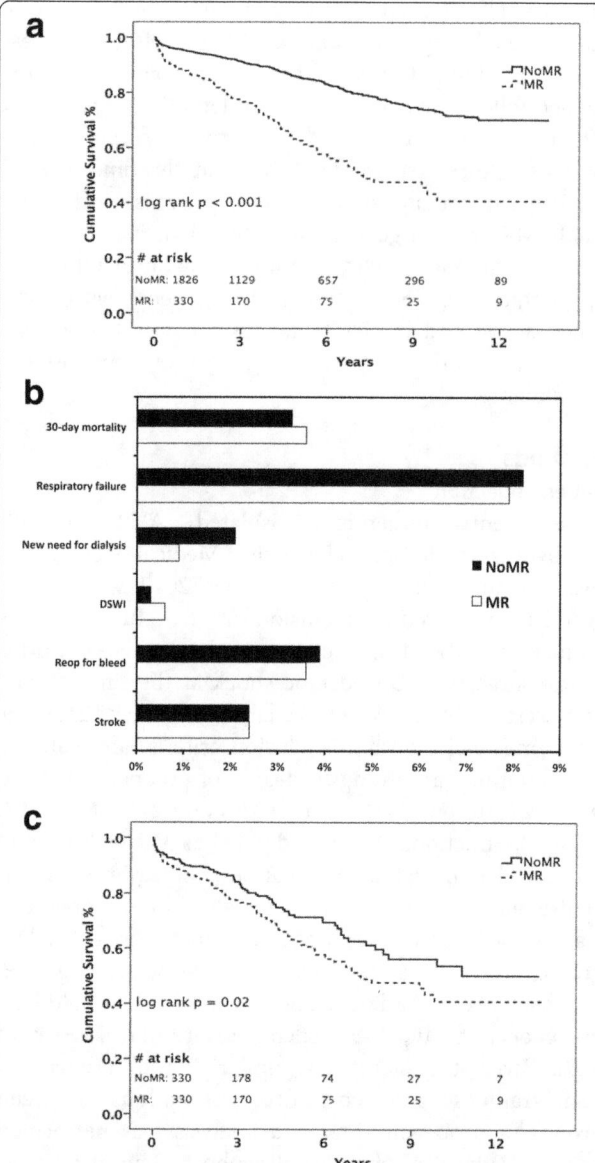

Fig. 1 a Kaplan-Meier analysis of long-term survival in overall cohort stratified by treatment group, (**b**) Postoperative complications of propensity-matched cohort by treatment group, (**c**) Kaplan-Meier analysis of long-term survival in propensity-matched cohort by treatment group. (Abbreviations: DSWI = deep sternal wound infection)

Propensity-matched analysis

In view of the significant baseline differences between the groups MR and NoMR, a propensity-matched analysis was performed. A total of 330 patients were identified in each group following propensity matching. Baseline characteristics are shown in Table 2. Mean age was 77.9 ± 10.0 years and 50.6% of patients were male. There were no significant differences in co-morbidities. Propensity-matched preoperative echocardiographic data is presented in Table 3. There was no difference in preoperative ejection fraction or prevalence of severe AI, severe AS, or severe TR. Propensity-matched operative details are presented in Table 4. There was no difference in patients undergoing re-operative sternotomy or a

minimally invasive approach. The vast majority of patients (n = 298 (90.3%) in MR vs. n = 299 (90.6%) in NoMR, p = 0.9) underwent bioprosthetic AVR with no differences between groups.

Propensity-matched postoperative complications and perioperative mortality are shown in Fig. 1B. There was no difference in 30-day mortality between groups (3.6% MR vs. 3.3% NoMR, p = 0.83). Additionally, there were no differences in postoperative complication rates or post-operative length of stay [8 (IQR 6–11) days MR vs. 8 (IQR 6–12) days NoMR, p = 0.47). Kaplan-Meier

Table 2 Propensity-Matched Baseline Characteristics

	NoMR	MR	p-value
Demographics			
Total, n	330	330	–
Age, years (mean ± SD)	77.7 ± 10.0	78.1 ± 10.1	0.66
Male, n (%)	160 (48.5)	174 (52.7)	0.28
BMI, kg/m^2 (mean ± SD)	27.2 ± 5.8	27.2 ± 5.7	0.99
Co-morbidities, n (%)			
Myocardial infarction	64 (19.4)	66 (20.2)	0.85
Congestive heart failure	111 (33.6)	111 (33.6)	1.00
Cerebrovascular disease	33 (10.0)	43 (13.0)	0.22
Severe CKD	33 (10.0)	39 (11.8)	0.45
Peripheral vascular disease	31 (9.4)	31 (9.4)	1.00
COPD	46 (13.9)	45 (13.6)	0.91
Diabetes	84 (25.5)	66 (25.5)	1.00
Dialysis	9 (2.7)	9 (2.7)	1.00

Abbreviations: BMI = body mass index, CKD = chronic kidney disease, COPD = chronic obstructive pulmonary disease

Table 3 Propensity-Matched Baseline Echocardiographic Data

	NoMR	MR	p-value
Ejection fraction			
LVEF, % (mean ± SD)	46.7 ± 14.7	46.1 ± 14.2	0.61
LVEF > 50%, n (%)	162 (50.9)	158 (47.9)	0.76
LVEF 30–50%, n (%)	124 (37.6)	128 (38.8)	0.75
LVEF < 30%, n (%)	44 (13.3)	44 (13.3)	1.00
Aortic insufficiency, n (%)			
None/Trace (0)	136 (41.2)	128 (38.8)	0.52
Mild (1+)	92 (27.9)	76 (23.0)	0.15
Moderate (2+)	47 (14.2)	61 (18.5)	0.14
Moderately-Severe/Severe (3–4+)	55 (16.7)	65 (19.7)	0.31
Aortic stenosis, n (%)			
None	33 (10.0)	34 (10.3)	0.90
Mild	1 (0.3)	2 (0.6)	0.56
Moderate	3 (0.9)	7 (2.1)	0.20
Severe	293 (88.8)	287 (87.0)	0.47
Mitral regurgitation, n (%)			
None/Trace	172 (52.1)	0 (0)	< 0.001
Mild	158 (47.9)	0 (0)	< 0.001
Moderate/Moderately-Severe	0 (0)	330 (100)	< 0.001
Tricuspid regurgitation			
None	217 (65.8)	216 (65.5)	0.94
Mild	69 (20.9)	66 (20.0)	0.77
Moderate	34 (10.3)	37 (11.2)	0.71
Severe	10 (3.0)	11 (3.3)	0.82

Abbreviations: LVEF = left ventricular ejection fraction

Table 4 Propensity-Matched Operative Characteristics

	NoMR	MR	p-value
Re-operation, n (%)	105 (31.8)	96 (29.1)	0.45
Minimally invasive approach, n (%)	17 (5.2)	15 (4.5)	0.72
CPB time, minutes (mean ± SD)	89.5 ± 26.6	92.5 ± 33.2	0.19
XCL time, minutes (mean ± SD)	61.9 ± 18.2	63.3 ± 18.8	0.36
Prosthesis type, n (%)			
Biological	299 (90.6)	298 (90.3)	0.90
Mechanical	26 (7.9)	26 (7.9)	1.00
Homograft	5 (1.5)	6 (1.8)	0.76

Abbreviations: CPB = cardiopulmonary bypass, XCL = aortic cross-clamp

survival analysis of the propensity-matched cohort (Fig. 1C) showed significantly worse medium and long-term survival in Group MR (log rank $p = 0.02$). At 1-year follow-up, mean MR severity was significantly worse in Group MR, although both groups fell in the trace-to-mild range (1.1 ± 0.7 MR vs. 0.8 ± 0.7 NoMR, $p = 0.03$).

Discussion

Concomitant fMR in patients presenting for surgical AVR remains a challenging clinical problem. Although the predominant opinion is that fMR should improve following correction of aortic valve pathology, it is not clear that postoperative relief of left ventricular pressure-volume overload is sufficient to cause significant regression of moderate fMR, which may subsequently limit functional status and postoperative survival. While it seems that mild preoperative fMR will regress following isolated AVR, studies have shown that many patients with moderate preoperative fMR still demonstrate a clinically significant level of postoperative regurgitation on follow-up [6–23]. Given the lack of well-defined treatment guidelines for these patients and small sample sizes used in prior studies, further investigation of the late effects of isolated AVR on moderate fMR is required.

The current study is, to the best of our knowledge, the largest single-center experience and the only propensity-matched analysis in this patient population. We have demonstrated that unaddressed moderate to moderate-severe (2–3+) fMR at the time of isolated AVR leads to equivalent perioperative survival but worsened medium- and long-term survival compared to patients with no or mild preoperative fMR. We did not detect a difference in postoperative complication rates or postoperative length of stay between groups. One-year echocardiographic follow-up revealed that patients with 2–3+ preoperative fMR had slightly but significantly worse residual MR compared to patients with mild or no preoperative fMR. While the post-AVR left ventricular reverse remodeling may improve fMR severity to some degree, our findings show that preoperative 2–3+ fMR in isolated AVR patients presages poorer late survival.

Review of our overall cohort analysis showed that patients with 2–3+ fMR are sicker than patients with no or mild fMR. Patients in Group MR were significantly older with worse renal and cardiac function, as evidenced by higher rates of congestive heart failure and lower ejection fractions. Group MR patients also had more severe TR, suggesting higher degrees of pulmonary hypertension and right ventricular dysfunction. Several prior studies addressing this population demonstrated similar findings [9, 11, 14]. Although it is possible that the worse prognosis of Group MR patients in the overall analysis is a direct effect of a greater degree of fMR, it is more likely that these patients simply have more advanced cardiovascular disease resulting in worsened overall survival. While our propensity-matched analysis allowed us to control for some of these baseline differences to more specifically evaluate the effect of preoperative fMR, it is worth noting that patients presenting with 2–3+ fMR in the setting of aortic valve disease generally have more advanced cardiac disease than their counterparts with no or mild fMR, and should be treated accordingly.

While many studies have demonstrated that severe MR should be repaired during concomitant AVR, controversy remains concerning the correct management of moderate and moderate-severe MR [2–4, 19–24]. Late survival in prior studies comparing patients with 2–3+ preoperative MR to patients with no or mild MR has varied. Given that the question at hand is whether or not isolated AVR is sufficient treatment for these patients, those studies that found a survival difference generally concluded that mitral intervention should be considered in patients with moderate or greater preoperative MR [6, 7, 13, 19–23]. However, several other studies, including the largest single-center study from the Mayo Clinic ($n = 190$), found no difference in survival between the two groups, suggesting that mitral intervention may be unnecessary [8, 11]. Nonetheless, large baseline demographic differences among groups are present in these studies, fundamentally confounding interpretation of the data. Given the clinical equipoise in the conclusions of prior studies and the potential that moderate fMR may simply be an indicator of more advanced disease rather than a causative entity leading to poorer late survival, a propensity-matched analysis was essential to control for key baseline differences and remove confounding comorbidities. After propensity-matching, our data suggest that a lower bar for mitral intervention in these patients may be warranted. Further study into specific patient subgroups may be necessary to clarify the tradeoff between additional perioperative risk and late mortality with combined aortic and mitral surgery.

Our data suggest that patients with moderate, concomitant fMR undergoing AVR would benefit from mitral intervention, although the logical follow-up question to that observation is to ask whether mitral valve repair or replacement would confer the lowest perioperative mortality and the highest late survival in this population. A Cardiothoracic Surgery Trials Network study from Acker and colleagues evaluated the performance of mitral valve repair vs. replacement for patients with ischemic MR not undergoing AVR and found no difference in perioperative or 1-year survival, but the recurrence rate of moderate or severe MR was higher in the repair group [25]. Although not directly applicable to patients with combined aortic and mitral valve disease, follow-up of this randomized trial could help to predict which mitral intervention confers a greater survival benefit to patients.

Few studies exist that directly address AVR/mitral repair vs. AVR/mitral replacement in the fMR subgroup. In 2003, the Cleveland Clinic group published a study addressing all patients who underwent combined AVR with either mitral valve repair or replacement for any reason, not solely for fMR [26]. While there was no difference in perioperative survival between mitral repair and replacement, they found that concomitant mitral repair with AVR resulted in significantly improved survival at 5, 10, and 15-year follow-up compared to mitral valve replacement with AVR [26]. However, only 7% of the total population had fMR in the Cleveland Clinic series, which again highlights the need for a large randomized trial evaluating the appropriate therapy for patients with aortic valve disease and significant concomitant fMR [26].

There are several limitations to our study. It is a retrospective, single-center study that reflects the treatment biases of our clinical team. We have attempted to limit preoperative baseline differences by propensity matching, but it is possible that our propensity-matched groups do not accurately reflect the true population based on unmeasured covariates. Follow-up survival information did not include the cause of late death, so all comparisons of mortality reflect all-cause mortality and not death from cardiovascular causes. Finally, formal quantification of MR using more advanced echocardiographic parameters, such PISA derived metrics, will be necessary in future studies; these measurements are now a standard part of our echocardiographic analysis, but were not available for the majority of this patient dataset during our study period.

Conclusions

In conclusion, patients undergoing isolated AVR with concomitant moderate and moderate-severe preoperative fMR have worse medium- and long-term survival, and continue to have elevated MR severity at 1 year, compared to patients with no or mild preoperative fMR. These results indicate the need for mitral valve intervention at the time of AVR in patients with moderate or greater fMR. Given our results and those from prior studies, a randomized trial is needed to definitively clarify the optimal treatment strategy for this population, and to determine whether mitral valve repair or replacement at the time of AVR for moderate or greater preoperative fMR is superior.

Abbreviations

AI: aortic insufficiency; AS: aortic stenosis; AVR: aortic valve replacement; fMR: functional mitral regurgitation; TR: tricuspid regurgitation

Authors' contributions

RS, AO, HY, DH, MAA, MA, CRS, IG all contributed to data collection, study idea, and writing and revisions of the manuscript. All authors read and approved the final manuscript.

Competing interests

Isaac George is a consultant for Medtronic and for Edwards Lifesciences Inc. Craig Smith is the Surgical Principal Investigator of the PARTNER and PARTNER II Trials, for which travel and customary expenses associated with Trial management are reimbursed by the sponsor, Edwards LifeSciences.

References

1. Society for Thoracic Surgery Adult Cardiac Surgery Database, 2014 Harvest 1-Exectuive summary, 2014.
2. Nishimura RA, Otto CM, Bonow RO, Carabello BA, Erwin JP, Guyton RA, et al. 2014 AHA/ACC guideline for the Management of Patients with Valvular Heart Disease: a report of the American College of Cardiology/American Heart Association task force on practice guidelines. Circulation. 2014;129(23):2440–92.
3. Nishimura RA, Otto CM, Bonow RO, Carabello BA, Erwin JP, Fleisher LA, et al. 2017 AHA/ACC focused update of the 2014 AHA/ACC guideline for the management of patients with valvular heart disease: a report of the American College of Cardiology/American Heart Association task force on clinical practice guidelines. Circulation. 2017;135(25):e1159–95.
4. Bonow RO, Brown AS, Gillam LD, Kapadia SR, Kavinsky CJ, Lindman BR, et al. ACC/AATS/AHA/ASE/EACTS/HVS/SCA/SCAI/SCCT/SCMR/STS 2017 appropriate use criteria for the treatment of patients with severe aortic stenosis: a report of the American College of Cardiology Appropriate use Criteria Task Force, American Association for Thoracic Surgery, American Heart Association, American Society of Echocardiography, European Association for Cardio-Thoracic Surgery, heart valve society, Society of Cardiovascular Anesthesiologists, Society for Cardiovascular Angiography and Interventions. J Am Soc Echocardiogr. 2018;31(2):117–47.
5. Come P, Riley M, Ferguson JF, Morgan JP, McKay RG. Prediction of severity of aortic stenosis: accuracy of multiple noninvasive parameters. Am J Med. 1988;85:29–37.
6. Barreiro CJ, Patel ND, Fitton TP, Williams JA, Bonde PN, Chan V et al. Aortic Valve Replacement and Concomitant Mitral Valve Regurgitation in the Elderly: Impact on Survival and Functional Outcome. Circulation 2005; 112(s1):I-443-I-447.
7. Harling L, Saso S, Jarral OA, Kourliouros A, Kidher E, Athanasiou T. Aortic

valve replacement for aortic stenosis in patients with concomitant mitral regurgitation: should the mitral valve be dealt with? Eur J Cardiothorac Surg. 2011;40:1087–96.
8. Absil B, Dagenais F, Mathieu P, Metras J, Perron J, Baillot R, et al. Does moderate mitral regurgitation impact early or mid-term clinical outcome in patients undergoing isolated aortic valve replacement for aortic stenosis? Eur J Cardiothorac Surg. 2003;24:217–22.
9. Takeda K, Matsumiya G, Sakaguchi T, Miyagawa S, Yamauchi T, Shudo Y, et al. Impact of untreated mild-to-moderate mitral regurgitation at the time of isolated aortic valve replacement on late adverse outcomes. Eur J Cardiothorac Surg. 2010;37:1033–8.
10. Lim JY, Jung SH, Kim JB, Chung CH, Lee JW, Song H. Management of concomitant mild to moderate functional mitral regurgitation during aortic valve surgery for severe aortic insufficiency. J Thorac Cardiovasc Surg. 2014; 148(2):441–6.
11. Wan CKN, Suri RM, Li Z, Orszulak TA, Daly RC, Schaff HV, et al. Management of moderate functional mitral regurgitation at the time of aortic valve replacement: is concomitant mitral valve repair necessary? J Thorac Cardiovasc Surg. 2009;137(3):635–40.
12. Ruel M, Kapila V, Price J, Kulik A, Burwash IG, Mesana TG. Natural history and predictors of outcome in patients with concomitant functional mitral regurgitation at the time of aortic valve replacement. Circulation. 2006; 114(s1):I-541–6.
13. Moazami N, Diodato MD, Moon MR, Lawton JS, Pasque MK, Herren RL, et al. Does functional mitral regurgitation improve with isolated aortic valve replacement? J Card Surg. 2004;19:444–8.
14. Caballero-Borrego J, Gomez-Doblas JJ, Cabrera-Bueno F, García-Pinilla JM, Melero JM, Porras C, et al. Incidence, associated factors and evolution of non-severe functional mitral regurgitation in patients with severe aortic stenosis undergoing aortic valve replacement. Eur J Cardiothorac Surg. 2008;34:62–6.
15. Brasch AV, Khan SS, DeRobertis MA, Kong JH, Chiu J, Siegal RJ. Change in mitral regurgitation severity after aortic valve replacement for aortic stenosis. Am J Cardiol. 2000;85:1271–4.
16. Alghamdi AA, Elmistekawy EM, Singh SK, Latter DA. Is concomitant surgery for moderate functional mitral regurgitation indicated during aortic valve replacement for aortic stenosis? A systematic review and evidence-based recommendations. J Card Surg. 2010;25(2):182–7.
17. Waisbren EC, Stevens LM, Avery EG, Picard MH, Vlahakes GJ, Agnihotri AK. Changes in mitral regurgitation after replacement of the stenotic aortic valve. Ann Thorac Surg. 2008;86(1):56–62.
18. Kowalówka AR, Onyszczuk M, Wańha W, Deja MA. Do we have to operate on moderate functional mitral regurgitation during aortic valve replacement for aortic stenosis? Interact Cardiovasc Thorac Surg. 2016;23(5):806–9.
19. Jeong DS, Park PW, Sung K, Kim WS, Yang JH, Jun TG, et al. Long-term clinical impact of functional mitral regurgitation after aortic valve replacement. Ann Thorac Surg. 2011;92(4):1339–45.
20. Joo HC, Chang BC, Cho SH, Youn YN, Yoo KJ, Lee S. Fate of functional mitral regurgitation and predictors of persistent mitral regurgitation after isolated aortic valve replacement. Ann Thorac Surg. 2011;92(1):82–7.
21. Matsumura Y, Gillinov AM, Toyono M, Oe H, Yamano T, Takasaki K, et al. Echocardiographic predictors for persistent functional mitral regurgitation after aortic valve replacement in patients with aortic valve stenosis. Am J Cardiol. 2010;106(5):701–6.
22. Unger P, Dedobbeleer C, Van Camp G, Plein D, Cosyns B, Lancellotti P. Mitral regurgitation in patients with aortic stenosis undergoing valve replacement. Heart. 2010;96(1):9–14.
23. Schubert SA, Yarboro LT, Madala S, Ayunipudi K, Kron IL, Kern JA, et al. Natural history of coexistent mitral regurgitation after aortic valve replacement. J Thorac Cardiovasc Surg. 2016;151(4):1032–42.
24. Eynden FV, Bouchard D, El-Hamamsy I, Butnaru A, Demers P, Carrier M, et al. Effect of aortic valve replacement for aortic stenosis on severity of mitral regurgitation. Ann Thorac Surg. 2007;83(4):1279–84.
25. Acker MA, Parides MK, Perrault LP, Moskowitz AJ, Gelijns AC, Voisine P, et al. Mitral-valve repair versus replacement for severe ischemic mitral regurgitation. New Engl J Med. 2014;370:23–32.
26. Gillinov AM, Blackstone EH, Cosgrove DM, White J, Kerr P, Marullo A, et al. Mitral valve repair with aortic valve replacement is superior to double valve replacement. J Thorac Cardiovasc Surg. 2003;125:1372–87.

21

Aortic arch cannulation with the guidance of transesophageal echocardiography for Stanford type A aortic dissection

Hao Ma[†], Zhenghua Xiao[†], Jun Shi, Lulu Liu, Chaoyi Qin and Yingqiang Guo[*]

Abstract

Background: Aortic arch cannulation for an antegrade central perfusion during the surgery for Stanford type A aortic dissection can be performed within median sternotomy. We summarize the safety and convenient profile of the central cannulation strategy using the guidance of transesophageal echocardiography (TEE) in comparison to traditional femoral cannulation strategy.

Methods: Sixty-two patients with acute Stanford type A aortic dissection underwent aortic arch surgery in our hospital. All the patients were operated by the same surgeon. Cannulation was performed in 33 patients through the aortic arch under the guidance of TEE (Group A) and in 29 patients through the femoral artery (Group F). Under moderate hypothermic circulatory arrest, the brain is continuously perfused in an anterograde manner through the brachiocephalic and left common carotid arteries. Preoperative characeristics and surgical information were collected for each patient. Additionally, 30-day mortality rate and the incidence of the temporary neurological dysfunction were recorded as the outcomes. To compare the categorical variables, we used the chi-squared test. Continuous variables were compared using the t-test.

Results: Preoperative characteristics were almost similar between the two groups. The mean operation time (7.33 ± 1.14 h vs. 8.93 ± 2.59 h, $P = 0.002$) and the mean cardiopulmonary bypass (CPB) time (260.97 ± 45.14 min vs. 298.28 ± 95.89 min, $P = 0.024$) were significantly shorter in Group A than those in Group F. The 30-day mortality rates were 9.09 and 27.59% in Groups A and F, respectively ($P = 0.057$). And the incidences of temporary neurological dysfunction were 39.39 and 65.52% in Group A and F, respectively ($P = 0.040$).

Conclusions: Aortic arch cannulation with the guidance of TEE during the aortic arch surgery is a simple, fast, safe, and less invasive technique for establishing cardiopulmonary bypass for Stanford type A aortic dissection.

Keywords: Cannulation site, Aortic arch cannulation, Transesophageal echocardiography, Femoral cannulation, Stanford type a aortic dissection

Background

Stanford type A aortic dissection is a devastating event associated with major morbidity and mortality and requires immediate surgical repair. During surgery for type A aortic dissection, the choice of cannulation site is of great importance to improve the outcomes of the operation [1]. For the past decades, various cannulation sites have been used. Femoral arterial cannulation (FC) has been used for cardiopulmonary bypass since the 1950s [2] and it has been reported to be the standard cannulation site, but it can bring a risk of distal re-entry, perfusion of the false lumen, malperfusion syndrome and cerebral embolization because of retrograde perfusion in the dissected aorta [3, 4]. Axillary arterial cannulation was firstly described by Villard et al. in 1976, but it was infrequently used for arterial inflow until 1995 when the Cleveland Clinic published positive results in 35 patients after axillary arterial cannulation [5]. It provides antegrade cerebral perfusion to reduce the risk of stroke and retrograde embolization. However, it also involves some local

* Correspondence: drguoyq@hotmail.com
[†]Hao Ma and Zhenghua Xiao contributed equally to this work.
Department of Cardiovascular Surgery, West China Hospital, Sichuan University, Chengdu 610041, China

complications such as injury of the artery or the brachial plexus which can lead to arm ischemia, insufficient CPB flow, atherosclerosis of the artery, and often requires side graft sewn to the vessel [1, 6]. Subclavian artery cannulation is a more time consuming procedure and provides a cumbersome antegrade cerebral perfusion (ACP) because of selective ACP through only the right carotid artery during periods of systemic circulatory arrest [7]. What's more, if the type A aortic dissection extends beyond the brachiocephalic artery, or if the patient has an incomplete circle of Willis, the surgeons would choose not to cannulate via sites like subclavian artery, innominate artery or axillary artery [4, 8]. Transapical aortic cannulation is an old technique that was initially described in the early 1970s [9], but it is limited to those patients with severely calcified ascending aortas and easy to bleed at the access site [10]. Recently, direct cannulation into the dissected ascending aorta has been reported by several surgeons [11–13] and that it can be performed rapidly without an additional incision. During the early 20th century, several surgeons tried to combine transesophageal echocardiography (TEE) with arterial cannulation to reduce the risk of cannulating into the false lumen [14, 15]. These techniques have been described in numerous studies and have been widely used. However, the question on which cannulation site is the optimal site remains controversial.

The present study was undertaken to compare the experience and results in patients undergoing surgery for Stanford type A aortic dissection using two different cannulation sites: the aortic arch under the guidance of TEE and the femoral artery. We compare the two methods and try to provide helpful information regarding the selection of the cannulation method for aortic arch surgery.

Patient selection for surgery

This retrospective study was approved by the Institutional Review Board. Individual patient consent was not required. All patients with Stanford type A aortic dissection irrespective of the dissection flap in our hospital underwent computed tomography angiography (CTA) and transthoracic echocardiography (TTE) for diagnosis and operative planning. Cannulation sites were decided individually upon patient status and surgeon preference. From December 2015 to April 2017, 62 patients with acute Stanford type A aortic dissection underwent aortic arch surgery in our hospital. All the patients were operated by the same surgeon. Cannulation was performed in 33 patients through the aortic arch with the guidance of TEE (Group A) and in 29 patients through the femoral artery (Group F). Almost all of the 33 patients in Group A were complicated cases, wherein other conventional cannulation methods were precluded because of the involvement of the axillary and femoral arteries by the dissection flap. Clinical backgrounds and preoperative clinical condition of the patients are presented in Table 1.

Surgical technique

After general anesthesia and intubation, standard median sternotomy was performed, and cardiopulmonary bypass (CPB) was instituted by cannulating either the aortic arch with the guidance of TEE (Group A) or the femoral artery (Group F).

Aortic arch cannulation technique

Group A received aortic arch cannulation with the guidance of TEE, where in a TEE probe was inserted through the esophagus. Following the median sternotomy and

Table 1 Preoperative patient characteristics

Variable	Group A($n = 33$)	Group F($n = 29$)	Total($n = 62$)	P value
Age(means±S.D.)	46.48 ± 10.32	47.90 ± 9.93	47.15 ± 10.08	0.756
Male	29(87.88%)	21(72.41%)	50(83.33%)	0.124
BMI	26.05 ± 4.25	23.32 ± 3.11	24.77 ± 3.97	0.060
Smoke	23(69.70%)	11(37.93%)	54.84(%)	0.012
Drink	18(54.55%)	6(20.69%)	38.71(%)	0.006
Marfan's syndrome	2(6.06%)	3(10.34%)	5(8.06%)	0.658
Hypertension	19(57.58%)	11(37.93%)	30(48.39%)	0.122
Coronary heart disease	2(6.06%)	1(3.45%)	3(4.84%)	1.000
Respiratory disease	2(6.06%)	2(6.90%)	4(6.45%)	1.000
Liver dysfunction	6(18.18%)	4(13.79%)	10(16.13%)	0.902
Renal dysfunction	4(12.12%)	3(10.34%)	7(4.84%)	1.000
Chronic aortic dissection	5(15.15%)	5(17.24%)	10(16.13%)	1.000
History of aortic dissection	2(6.06%)	0	2(3.23%)	0.494
Cardiac reoperation	2(6.06%)	0	2(3.23%)	0.494

systemic heparinization, the pericardium was opened slowly. A concentric pledget reinforced purse-string suture was placed through the adventitial layer on the lesser curvature of the aortic arch. A modified Potts Courmand style 18 gauge needle was used to puncture the aorta inside the purse-string suture. Once pulsatile bleeding was confirmed, a 0.035-in. flexible guide wire was introduced through the needle. After TEE confirmed the presence of the guide wire in the true lumen of the descending aorta, the needle was taken out, and the cannula was advanced over the guide wire. TEE confirmed the accurate positioning of the cannulation into the true lumen. After double-stage cannulas were inserted into the superior and inferior venae cavae, a CPB was established, and the patient started to cool down. The TEE was performed by cardiologists (Fig. 1)

Femoral cannulation technique

Group F received femoral cannulation. Cannulation of the right or the left femoral artery was surgically exposed prior to sternotomy. The venous cannulation was performed with a double-stage cannula via the right atrium. Then, a CPB was established, the patient started to cool down, and a standard median sternotomy was performed.

We used selective antegrade cerebral perfusion whenever total arch replacement was required, and the brain was selectively antegrade perfused with a rate of 5 ml/kg/min and a temperature of 25 °C to 27 °C. An ice pack was applied on the head to maintain cerebral hypothermia until CPB was restarted. Myocardial protection was obtained by means of an antegrade infusion of cold blood cardioplegia. The patients underwent David and Bentall operations, ascending aortic replacements, total aortic arch replacements, hemi-arch replacements, descending aortic stented elephant trunk implantation, or other operations (Table 2).

CPB time was defined as the cumulative time on full-body CPB, including moderate hypothermic circulatory arrest (MHCA). MHCA time was defined as the cumulative time of full-body circulatory arrest, which is equivalent to the brain perfusion time. Operation time was defined as the time from incision to closure. Cross time was defined as the time from clamping the aorta to opening the aorta. Stroke was defined as

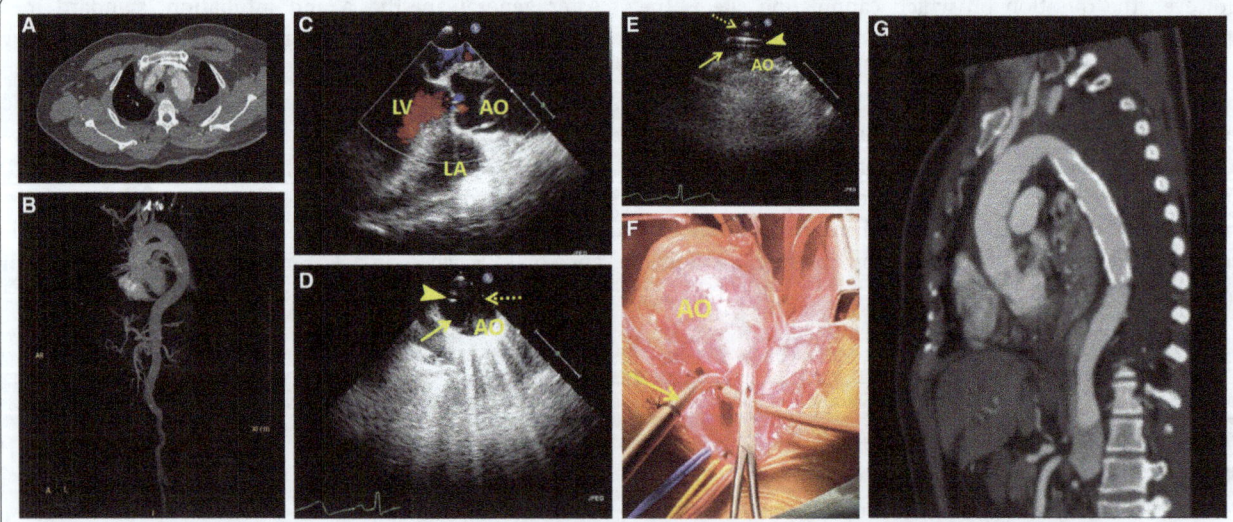

Fig. 1 Perioperative images. **a-b** Computed tomography angiography (CTA) before the operation revealing a Stanford type A aortic dissection extending from the aortic root to the bilateral iliac artery. **c** Transesophageal echocardiography (TEE) showing a mild aortic regurgitation, an enlarged root (47) and ascending aorta (48–52), and an ejection fraction of 69%. **d** Transesophageal echocardiography (TEE) image. TEE showing the guide wire (arrow-head) present in the true lumen (arrow) of the descending aorta. The false lumen is depicted by a dotted-arrow. **e** Transesophageal echocardiography (TEE) image. TEE confirming the accurate positioning of the cannulation into the true lumen (arrow). Arrow-head is the false lumen. **f** The 20 Fr cannulation (Medtronic, arrow) advanced over the guide wire and cannulated into the true lumen of the aortic arch. **g** Postoperative CTA image revealing the patency of the three-branched vessels and the optimal position of the graft. Perioperative image. Computed tomography (CTA) before the operation revealing a Stanford type A aortic dissection extending from the aortic root to the bilateral iliac artery. Transthoracic echocardiography (TEE) image. Transthoracic echocardiography (TEE) showing a mild aortic regurgitation, an enlarged root (47) and ascending aorta (48–52), and an ejection fraction of 69%. Transesophageal echocardiography (TEE) image. TEE showing the guide wire (arrow-head) present in the true lumen(arrow) of the descending aorta. The false lumen is depicted by a dotted-arrow. Transthoracic echocardiography (TEE). TEE confirming the accurate positioning of the cannulation into the true lumen (arrow). Arrow-head is the false lumen. Transthoracic echocardiography (TEE). The 20 Fr cannulation (Medtronic, arrow) advanced over the guide wire and cannulated into the true lumen of the aortic arch. Postoperative CTA image. Postoperative CTA image revealing the patency of the three-branched vessels and the optimal position of the graft

Table 2 Techniques used

Technique	Group A(n = 33)	Group F(n = 29)	Total(n = 62)	P value
Total arch replacement	31(93.94%)	20(68.97%)	51(82.26%	0.010
Hemiarch repair	0	6(20.69%)	6(9.68%)	0.008
Aortic debranching	2(6.06%)	1(3.45%)	3(4.83%)	1.000
Ascending aorta replacement	33(100%)	29(100%)	62(100%)	–
Elephant trunk	33(100%)	19(65.52%)	52(83.87%)	0.001
Aortic valve replacement	15(45.45%)	13(44.83%)	28(45.16%)	0.961
Aortic valve plastic	15(45.45%)	7(24.14%)	22(35.48%)	0.080
Coronary artery bypass	2(6.06%)	1(3.45%)	3(4.83%)	1.000
Mitral valve plastic	3(9.09%)	1(3.45%)	4(6.45%)	0.616
Tricuspid valve plastic	2(6.06%)	3(10.34%)	5(8.06%)	0.658
Repair of ruptured sinus of Valsalva aneurysm	0	1(3.45%)	1(1.61%)	0.468
Left vertebral artery reconstruction	0	1(3.45%)	1(1.61%)	0.468
Repair of auricular septal defect	1(3.03%)	0	1(1.61%)	1.000

a new postoperative focal neurologic deficit or cerebral hemorrhage that persisted for more than 72 h, or a new focal lesion of the brain detected by a computed tomography scan. Temporary neurologic dysfunction was defined as a focal neurologic deficit lasting for less than 72 h, or postoperative delirium, agitation, confusion, or decreased level of consciousness without any new structural abnormality observed on imaging [16, 17].

Statistical analysis

Patient data were analyzed using SPSS 22.0 for Windows. Categorical variables are presented as numbers and percentages, and continuous variables are presented as mean and standard deviation values. To compare the categorical variables, we used the chi-squared test. Continuous variables were compared using the t-test.

Methods

Sixty-two patients with acute Stanford type A aortic dissection underwent aortic arch surgery in our hospital. All the patients were operated by the same surgeon. Cannulation was performed in 33 patients through the aortic arch under the guidance of TEE (Group A) and in 29 patients through the femoral artery (Group F). Under moderate hypothermic circulatory arrest, the brain is continuously perfused in an anterograde manner through the brachiocephalic and left common carotid arteries. Preoperative characeristics and surgical information were collected for each patient. Additionally, 30-day mortality rate and the incidence of the temporary neurological dysfunction were recorded as the outcomes. To compare the categorical variables, we used the chi-squared test. Continuous variables were compared using the t-test The Methods include the sentences

mentioned above and the part of the surgery process in the text.

Results
Patient characteristics

A total of 62 patients were diagnosed with acute Stanford type A aortic dissection by contrast-enhanced computer tomography and echocardiography, and they underwent elective ascending aortic surgery from December 2015 to April 2017. Patient characteristics are presented in Table 1. No significant differences in age, gender, body mass index (BMI), Marfan's syndrome, hypertension, coronary heart disease, respiratory disease, liver dysfunction, renal dysfunction and cardiac reoperation were found. However, the rates of patients who smoke (69.70% vs. 37.94%, $P = 0.012$) and drink (54.55% vs. 20.69%, $P = 0.006$) were higher in Group A than in Group F. Liver dysfunction was defined as the assay index of laboratory examination that was used to evaluate the liver function were unusual. Renal dysfunction was defined as the value of creatinine > 120 mmol/L.

Intraoperative parameters

We determined that the puncture and cannulation of the aortic arch were possible in 33 of the 62 patients, and none of them experienced intraoperative difficulties. Additionally, femoral cannulation was performed in the remaining 29 patients, except that two patients required another cannulation through the innominate artery because of the presence of malperfusion in their right arms when the ascending aortas were cross-clamped. The techniques used are shown in Table 2. All the patients underwent ascending aorta replacement. Hemiarch repair was performed in 6

Table 3 Intraoperative variables

Variables	Group A(n = 33)	Group F(n = 29)	Total(n = 62)	P value
Operation time(h)	7.33 ± 1.14	8.93 ± 2.59	8.08 ± 2.10	0.002
CPB time(min)	260.97 ± 45.14	298.28 ± 95.89	278.42 ± 75.11	0.024
Cross time(min)	170.67 ± 41.72	193.55 ± 57.97	181.37 ± 50.87	0.089
The lowest temperature during CPB(°C)				
Nasopharyngeal temperature	25.49 ± 2.07	26.05 ± 2.78	25.75 ± 2.42	0.259
Anal temperature	27.14 ± 1.73	27.36 ± 2.64	27.24 ± 2.18	0.114
MHCA time(min)	40.97 ± 7.98	37.00 ± 9.39	39.28 ± 8.75	0.287
Absence of circulatory arrest	2(6.06%)	6(20.69%)	8(12.90%)	0.131
Hct after CPB (%)	27.92 ± 4.14	26.62 ± 4.95	27.31 ± 4.55	0.463
Maximum internal time of twice myocardial perfusion during CPB(min)	71.70 ± 14.80	69.71 ± 24.69	70.77 ± 19.90	0.001
Minimun hemoglobin concentration during operation(g/L)	77.23 ± 15.48	74.35 ± 10.18	75.88 ± 13.24	0.849
Maximum serum lactic acid concentration during operation(mol/L)	9.06 ± 4.70	10.34 ± 6.27	9.66 ± 5.48	0.192

CPB cardiopulmonary bypass, *MHCA* moderate hypothermic circulatory arrest

patients (0% vs. 20.69%, $P = 0.008$), whereas total arch replacement was performed in 51 patients (93.04% vs. 28.97%, $P = 0.010$). Aortic debranching was performed in 3 patients (6.06% vs. 3.45%, $P = 1.000$). A total of 52 patients underwent elephant trunk procedure (100% vs. 5.52%, $P = 0.001$); 28 patients needed aortic valve replacement because of severe aortic valve regurgitation (45.45% vs. 44.83%, $P = 0.961$); and 22 patients needed aortic valve plastic surgery (45.45% vs. 24.14%, $P = 0.080$). Concomitant cardiac procedures included coronary artery bypass in 4.84% ($n = 3$) of the patients because the coronary arteries were affected by the dissection, mitral valve plastic surgery in 6.45% ($n = 4$), tricuspid valve plastic surgery in 8.06% ($n = 5$), repair of ruptured sinus of Valsalva aneurysm in 1.61% ($n = 1$), left vertebral artery reconstruction in 1.61% ($n = 1$), and repair of atrial septal defect in 1.61% ($n = 1$). In general, we concluded that the surgeries were more complicated in Group A.

Surgical duration and intraoperative data summary are shown in Table 3. After starting the extracorporeal circulation, the body temperature was cooled to 25 °C to 27 °C in all patients (nasopharyngeal temperature of 25.49 °C ± 2.07 °C vs. 26.05 °C ± 2.78 °C, $P = 0.259$; anal temperature of 27.14 °C ± 1.73 °C vs. 27.36 °C ± 2.64 °C, $P = 0.144$). No significant differences in MHCA time, absence of circulatory arrest, Hct after CPB, minimum hemoglobin concentration, and maximum serum lactic acid concentration during operations were found. However, the mean operation time (7.33 ± 1.14 h vs. 8.93 ± 2.59 h, $P = 0.002$) and the mean CPB time (260.97 ± 45.14 min vs. 298.28 ± 95.89 min, $P = 0.024$) were significantly shorter in Group A than in Group F. One patient required a second run of extracorporeal circulation to stop the hemorrhage after the termination of extracorporeal circulation.

Postoperative parameters

Table 4 shows the postoperative parameters. The length of intensive care unit (ICU) stay (5.50 ± 3.35 vs. 4.62 ± 1.75, $P = 0.200$) and intubation time (43.54 ± 36.38 vs. 36.52 ± 27.54, $P = 0.393$) were similar in both groups as the same with the need for tracheostomy (9.09% vs. 6.90%, $p = 1.000$), thoracentesis (30.30% vs. 44.83%, $p = 0.237$), and thoracic cavity closed-chest drainage (6.06% vs. 3.45%, $p = 1.000$). No significant intergroup differences existed in the frequency of hemorrhage requiring rethoracotomy, which occurred in only one patient in Group A; sepsis, which occurred in one patient (3.03%) in Group A and in one patient (3.45%) in Group F; renal failure, which occurred in two patients (6.06%) in Group A and in three patients (10.34%) in Group F; multiple organ failure, which occurred in two patients (6.06%) in Group A and in two patients (6.90%) in Group F; circulatory failure, which occurred in one patient (3.03%) in Group A and in four patients (13.79%) in Group F; intestinal ischemia, which occurred in one patient (3.45%) in Group F; limb ischemia, which occurred in one patient (3.45%) in Group F; or rehospitalization, which occurred in one patient (3.45%) in Group F only. The rate of temporary neurological dysfunction (TND) was significantly lower in Group A than in Group F (39.39% vs. 65.52%, $p = 0.040$) and the wake time was significantly shorter in Group A than in Group F (7.22 ± 3.78 vs. 12.35 ± 12.64, $p = 0.046$). No statistical difference in in-hospital mortality was found between the two groups; however, a trend toward a lower 30 day mortality (9.09% vs. 27.59%, $p = 0.057$) was observed in Group A.

Discussion

The optimal cannulation site for the repair of acute Stanford type A aortic dissection remain unknown. The

Table 4 Postoperative variables

Variables	Group A(n = 33)	Group F(n = 29)	Total(n = 62)	P value
Length of ICU stay(days)	5.50 ± 3.35	4.62 ± 1.75	5.12 ± 2.79	0.200
Fail to come out of ICU	5(15.15%)	8(27.59%)	13(20.97%)	0.230
Re-enter ICU	3(9.09%)	1(3.45%)	4(6.54%)	0.616
Wake time(h)	7.22 ± 3.78	12.35 ± 12.64	9.59 ± 9.29	0.046
Fail to wake	5(15.15%)	5(17.24%)	10(16.13%)	1.000
Intubation time(hours)	43.54 ± 36.38	36.52 ± 27.54	40.37 ± 32.57	0.393
Fail to remove the intubation	5(15.15%)	6(20.69%)	11(17.74%)	0.569
Tracheostomy	3(9.09%)	2(6.90%)	5(8.06%)	1.000
Length of remove chest tube(days)	11.48 ± 3.90	9.30 ± 3.70	10.52 ± 3.93	0.913
Chest tube drainage(ml/24 h)	688.63 ± 363.03	715.31 ± 435.82	701.31 ± 396.12	0.385
Fail to remove chest tube	4(12.12%)	6(20.69%)	10(16.13%)	0.569
Thoracentesis	10(30.30%)	13(44.83%)	23(37.10%)	0.237
Thoracic cavity closed drainage	2(6.06%)	1(3.45%)	3(4.84%)	1.000
Hemorrhage requiring rethoracotomy	1(3.03%)	0	1(1.61%)	1.000
Sepsis	1(3.03%)	1(3.45%)	2(3.23%)	1.000
Temporary neurological dysfunction	13(39.39%)	19(65.52%)	32(51.61%)	0.040
Stroke	3(9.09%)	1(3.45%)	4(6.54%)	0.616
Renal failure	2(6.06%)	3(10.34%)	5(8.06%)	0.658
Circulatory failure	1(3.03%)	4(13.79%)	5(8.06%)	0.176
Multiple organ failure	2(6.06%)	2(6.90%)	4(6.54%)	1.000
Intestinal ischemic	0	1(3.45%)	1(1.61%)	0.468
Limb ischemic	0	1(3.45%)	1(1.61%)	0.468
30-day-mortality	3(9.09%)	8(27.59%)	11(17.74%)	0.057
Rehospitalization	0	1(3.45%)	1(1.61%)	0.468

most common site for cannulation in this setting was the femoral artery until the late 1990s [18]. However, femoral artery cannulation has a risk of distal re-entry, false lumen perfusion, organ malperfusion, and cerebral embolization because of retrograde perfusion in the dissected aorta [3, 4]. As an alternative cannulation technique, direct ascending cannulation has been advocated by the Hannover group [19] and has been developed through the guidance of TEE by some surgeons [20, 21]. Our center considered FC as the normal cannulation technique in the repair of the Stanford type A aortic dissection and has begun to use aortic arch cannulation with the guidance of TEE since 2015.

Aortic arch cannulation with the guidance of TEE is easy, fast, and straightforward, and ensures antegrade flow in the aorta and could be advantageous compared with the axillary and femoral cannulations. If the three branches of the aortic arch and bilateral femoral arteries are all affected by the aortic dissection, this proves to be the best procedure to cannulate through the aortic arch. Opening another surgical area is not required, thus establishing CPB becomes faster, which is highly beneficial to a patient experiencing hemodynamic instability.

Moreover, no additional incisions are required and surgeons do not need to repair the cannulation site, thereby avoiding injuries in other peripheral arteries. With the guidance of TEE, we did not introduce perfusion of the false lumen because the cannulation was directly inserted into the false lumen. Surgoens can use a large-diameter cannulation to provide sufficient perfusion during CPB and shorten the time of cooling the body temperature, cutting down the time of surgery as a whole. What's more, this cannulation technique tends to provide selective antegrade cerebral perfusion to protect the brain from edema, stroke and other neurological complications and retrograde cerebral embolization. However, this technique has one negative outcome, which is the risk of aortic rupture at the cannulation site. Khaladj et al. [19] reported that only 1 of 122 patients (0.8%) had an aortic rupture caused by aortic cannulation in patients with Stanford type A aortic dissection. Hiroyuki et al. [18] did not report aortic ruptures after aortic cannulation of 82 patients for 20 years. Moreover, we did not cause any aortic rupture at the cannulation site in the 33 patients in the study. Therefore, the danger of aortic rupture at the cannulation site is extremely low.

In Group A, the aortic arch cannulation with the guidance of TEE was technically feasible and safe in all 33 patients. Using careful and safe cannulation techniques, we encountered no difficulties related to the cannulation procedure and did not transfer to a different cannulation site. We did not observe any malperfusion phenomenon or problems directly related to aortic arch cannulation. However, in Group F, we found intraoperative malperfusion of the right upper limb, as evidenced by the decreased blood pressure of the right radial artery; and of the left brain hemisphere, as evidenced by the decreased cerebral oxygen saturation. This phenomenon may be caused by the malperfusion of the innominate artery. We suspected that this phenomenon may have been caused by the following: (1) the diameter of the cannula, which was limited by the diameter of the femoral artery, was too small to provide enough blood for the upper limbs and the brain; and (2) some blood may have flowed into the false lumen after the CPB was started; thus, the perfusion flow was lower than the value that detected by the instrument. This phenomenon required no treatment other than the additional cannulation inserted into the innominate artery. Moreover, intestinal ischemia was detected through the abdominal computed tomography (CT) scan of one of the two patients. The patients were fasted for more than 1 week and were given parenteral nutrition. Furthermore, no femoral arterial rupture was present in these patients. A patient's left dorsalis pedis artery pulsation was non-palpable during the first week post-operation and muscle force was weaker in the left lower limb than in the right lower limb. The temperature was lower in the left lower limb than in the other parts of the body. These results may have been caused by malperfusion because the cannulation was inserted into the left femoral artery of this patient.

Mortality with acute Stanford type A aortic dissection remains high with an average 30 day mortality rate of approximately 17%, which progressively increases to 25% in octogenarians [22]. In our single-center study, we reported a 30 day mortality rate of 17.74% in 62 patients. Our study shows that aortic arch cannulation with the guidance of TEE has a positive effect on 30 day mortality. Stefan and colleagues [23] found that the cannulation strategy used for the initial bypass has no impact on mortality, even though the femoral cannulation is performed more often in a sick patient group, as categorized by ASA classification. In another study, the risk for early mortality was driven by the preoperative clinical and hemodynamic status before the operation rather than by the cannulation technique [24]. In the retrospective study of Masahiro and colleagues [1], the mean operative time, mean CPB time, and interval time between the start of operation and start of CPB was significantly shorter in the central group, and central cannulation had a positive effect on mortality (6.8% vs. 17.3%, $p < 0.001$). In conclusion, their study showed that a direct central cannulation through the ascending aorta is successful in repairing type A dissection and produced surgical results that are superior to those of femoral cannulation. Hiroyuki and colleagues [18] found a trend toward a reduced mortality rate in patients with aortic cannulation, although no statistical differences in postoperative mortalities and morbidities between the aortic and femoral cannulation groups were present. The large German Registry for acute aortic dissection (GERAADA) [25] with 2137 patients does not show significant influence of the cannulation site on any outcome parameter.

Preoperative and postoperative neurologic symptoms were present in approximately 7 and 20%, respectively, of the patients [22]. In our study, preoperative neurologic symptoms did not differ between the two groups, but a significantly lower rate of TND was present in Group A than in Group F. Moreover, the patients who received aortic arch cannulation with the guidance of TEE tended to recover quicker than those who received the femoral cannulation. This effect will prevent cerebral embolization because of retrograde perfusion in the dissected aorta caused by the femoral cannulation. The risk of stroke between the two groups did not differ. With adequate cerebral perfusion and cerebral monitoring using the bilateral cerebral oxygen, a moderate hypothermic arrest with temperatures between 25 °C and 27 °C is acceptable in both groups. In the study by Stefan and colleagues [23], no differences in neurologic symptoms regarding the perfusion strategy were found. In another singer-center study by Stefan and colleagues [24], their data showed a new neurologic event in 11% of all patients, which did not differ between femoral and central cannulation. In other studies [1, 18, 24], the rate of short-term and postoperative neurology in patients receiving different cannulation techniques did not differ.

Moreover, the mean operation time and mean CPB time were significantly shorter in Group A than in Group F. This result may be attributed to the aortic arch cannulation with the guidance of TEE, which does not require another incision; and to the flow of the cannulation, which is larger than that of the femoral cannulation. Moreover, LV asynergy or pseudoaneurysm on the apex and aortic valve regurgitation in the early postoperative period by TTE were absent.

Conclusion

Direct aortic arch cannulation using the Seldinger technique with the guidance of TEE may be a simple, accurate, fast, and safe cannulation technique to establish CPB during the surgery to treat type A aortic dissection. This technique is an appropriate approach for patients with peripheral arteries affected by the aortic dissection or those with hemodynamic instability.

Limitation

Limitations of the present study are the relatively small number of patients from a single institution and the non-randomized and retrospective study design. Moreover, the cannulation site was not randomly chosen but individually decided depending on patient status. Therefore, further studies with large patient populations are necessary.

Abbreviations

ACP: Antegrade cerebral perfusion; BMI: Body mass index; CPB: Cardiopulmonary bypass; CT: Computed tomography; CTA: Computed tomography angiography; FC: Femoral arterial cannulation; GERAADA: German Registry for acute aortic dissection; ICU: Intensive care unit; MHCA: Moderate hypothermic circulatory arrest; TEE: Transesophageal echocardiography; TND: Temporary neurological dysfunction; TTE: Transthoracic echocardiography

Authors' contributions

HM and ZX and YG carried out the conception and drafted the manuscript; ZX, JS and YG give the administrative support; JS, CQ and LL provided the materials or patients of the study; HM collected and assembled the data; Data was analyzed and interpreted by HM; All authors read and approved the final manuscript.

Competing interests

The authors declare that they have no competing interests.

References

1. Osumi M, Wada H, Morita Y, et al. Safety and efficacy of ascending aorta cannulation during repair of acute type a aortic dissection (PA29-04): "presented at the 65th annual scientific meeting of the Japanese Association for Thoracic Surgery". Gen Thorac Cardiovasc Surg. 2014;62(5): 296–300.
2. Lillehei CW, Cardozo RH. Use of median sternotomy with femoral artery cannulation in open cardiac surgery. Surg Gynecol Obstet. 1959;108(6): 706–14.
3. Benedetto U, Mohamed H, Vitulli P, et al. Axillary versus femoral arterial cannulation in type a acute aortic dissection: evidence from a meta-analysis of comparative studies and adjusted risk estimates. Eur J Cardiothorac Surg. 2015;48(6):953–9.
4. Attaran S, Safar M, Saleh HZ, et al. Cannulating a dissecting aorta using ultrasound-epiaortic and transesophageal guidance. Heart Surg Forum. 2011;14(6):E373–5.
5. Sabik JF, Lytle BW, McCarthy PM, et al. Axillary artery: an alternative site of arterial cannulation for patients with extensive aortic and peripheral vascular disease. J Thorac Cardiovasc Surg. 1995;109(5):885–90. discussion 890-1
6. Wada S, Yamamoto S, Honda J, et al. Transapical aortic cannulation for cardiopulmonary bypass in type a aortic dissection operations. J Thorac Cardiovasc Surg. 2006;132(2):369–72.
7. Schurr UP, Emmert MY, Berdajs D, et al. Subclavian artery cannulation provides superior outcomes in patients with acute type-a dissection: long-term results of 290 consecutive patients. Swiss Med Wkly. 2013;143:w13858.
8. Nouraei SM, Nouraei SA, Sadashiva AK, et al. Subclavian cannulation improves outcome of surgery for type a aortic dissection. Asian Cardiovasc Thorac Ann. 2007;15(2):118–22.
9. Zwart HH, Krallos A, Kwan-Gett CS, et al. First clinical application of transarterial closed-chest left ventricular (TaCLV) bypass. Trans Am Soc Artif Intern Organs. 1970;16:386–91.
10. Golding LA. New cannulation technique for the severely calcified ascending aorta. J Thorac Cardiovasc Surg. 1985;90(4):626–7.
11. Reece TB, Tribble CG, Smith RL, et al. Central cannulation is safe in acute aortic dissection repair. J Thorac Cardiovasc Surg. 2007;133(2):428–34.
12. Minatoya K, Karck M, Szpakowski E, et al. Ascending aortic cannulation for Stanford type a acute aortic dissection: another option. J Thorac Cardiovasc Surg. 2003;125(4):952–3.
13. Imanaka K, Kyo S, Tanabe H, et al. Fatal intraoperative dissection of the innominate artery due to perfusion through the right axillary artery. J Thorac Cardiovasc Surg. 2000;120(2):405–6.
14. Gobolos L, Philipp A, Foltan M, et al. Surgical management for Stanford type a aortic dissection: direct cannulation of real lumen at the level of the Botallo's ligament by Seldinger technique. Interact Cardiovasc Thorac Surg. 2008;7(6):1107–9.
15. Di Eusanio M, Ciano M, Labriola G, et al. Cannulation of the innominate artery during surgery of the thoracic aorta: our experience in 55 patients. Eur J Cardiothorac Surg. 2007;32(2):270–3.
16. Hagl C, Ergin MA, Galla JD, et al. Neurologic outcome after ascending aorta-aortic arch operations: effect of brain protection technique in high-risk patients. J Thorac Cardiovasc Surg. 2001;121(6):1107–21.
17. Ergin MA, Galla JD, Lansman SL, et al. Hypothermic circulatory arrest in operations on the thoracic aorta. Determinants of operative mortality and neurologic outcome. J Thorac Cardiovasc Surg. 1994;107(3):788–97. discussion 797-9
18. Kamiya H, Kallenbach K, Halmer D, et al. Comparison of ascending aorta versus femoral artery cannulation for acute aortic dissection type a. Circulation. 2009;120(11 Suppl):S282–6.
19. Khaladj N, Shrestha M, Peterss S, et al. Ascending aortic cannulation in acute aortic dissection type A: the Hannover experience. Eur J Cardiothorac Surg. 2008;34(4):792–6. disussion 796
20. Inoue Y, Takahashi R, Ueda T, et al. Synchronized epiaortic two-dimensional and color Doppler echocardiographic guidance enables routine ascending aortic cannulation in type a acute aortic dissection. J Thorac Cardiovasc Surg. 2011;141(2):354–60.
21. Brinster DR, Parrish DW, Meyers KS, et al. Central aortic cannulation for Stanford type a aortic dissection with the use of three-dimensional and two-dimensional transesophageal echocardiography. J Card Surg. 2014; 29(5):729–32.
22. Rylski B, Hoffmann I, Beyersdorf F, et al. Acute aortic dissection type a: age-related management and outcomes reported in the German registry for acute aortic dissection type a (GERAADA) of over 2000 patients. Ann Surg. 2014;259(3):598–604.
23. Klotz S, Bucsky BS, Richardt D, et al. Is the outcome in acute aortic dissection type a influenced by of femoral versus central cannulation? Ann Cardiothorac Surg. 2016;5(4):310–6.
24. Klotz S, Heuermann K, Hanke T, et al. Outcome with peripheral versus central cannulation in acute type a dissection dagger. Interact Cardiovasc Thorac Surg. 2015;20(6):749–53. discussion 754
25. Conzelmann LO, Weigang E, Mehlhorn U, et al. Mortality in patients with acute aortic dissection type a: analysis of pre- and intraoperative risk factors from the German registry for acute aortic dissection type a (GERAADA). Eur J Cardiothorac Surg. 2016;49(2):e44–52.

22

The impact of pericardial approach and myocardial protection onto postoperative right ventricle function reduction

Marco Zanobini[1], Claudia Loardi[1], Paolo Poggio[1], Gloria Tamborini[1], Fabrizio Veglia[1], Alessandro Di Minno[1], Veronika Myasoedova[1], Liborio Francesco Mammana[1], Raoul Biondi[1], Mauro Pepi[1], Francesco Alamanni[1] and Matteo Saccocci[1,2]* (iD)

Abstract

Background: The reduction of RV function after cardiac surgery is a well-known phenomenon. It could persist up-to one year after the operation and often leads to an incomplete recovery at follow-up echocardiographic control. The aim of the present study is to analyze the impact of different modalities of pericardial incision (lateral versus anterior) and of myocardial protection protocols (Buckberg versus Custodiol) onto postoperative RV dynamic by relating two- and three-dimensional echocardiographic parameters in patients undergoing mitral valve repair through minimally invasive or traditional surgery approach.

Methods: We have analyzed 44 consecutive patients with severe degenerative mitral regurgitation who underwent mitral reparation with different surgical approach and cardioplegia type: Group 1 (17 pts): sternotomy with Buckberg cardioplegia protocol; Group 2 (10 pts): sternotomy with Custodiol cardioplegia; Group 3 (17 pts): mini-invasive surgery with Custodiol cardioplegia. Two-dimensional transthoracic echocardiography was performed pre- and 6 months post-surgery to evaluate RV function by tricuspid annular plane systolic excursion (TAPSE).

Results: All patients underwent successful and uneventful. A postoperative TAPSE reduction was found in all groups. However, mini-invasive patients experienced a significant reduced variation versus traditional surgery.

Conclusions: Mini-invasive mitral repair, with lateral incision of pericardium, reduces postoperative TAPSE fall, while cardioplegia protocol fails to have an impact onto longitudinal RV function. In our study, the RV seems to experience a clinically irrelevant geometrical modification too, whose entity appears to be less evident in case of lateral pericardial approach. These results could strengthen the use of minimally invasive approach also to preserve RV function.

Keywords: Mitral valve, Valve repair, Minimally invasive surgery, Right ventricle, Cardioplegia, Echocardiography

Background

Right ventricular function is widely known as a determinant of exercise capacity and as significant prognostic value in the evaluation of surgical outcome [1, 2]. During and immediately after cardiac surgery, it is known that there is a decrease of two-dimensional indexes of right ventricle systolic performance [3–5]. Recovery to basal values is often incomplete and an echocardiographic dysfunction can persist even at one year after surgery [6].

Physiopathology of right ventricle behavior following cardiac surgery is a largely debated issue and several hypotheses have been suggested: 1) myocardial hypothermia [7]; 2) cardiopulmonary bypass use [8]; 3) pericardial adhesions [9]. Pericardial opening need [10] and modality of cardioplegia delivery, retrograde cardiac protection seems to be less effective in preserving right ventricle function, [11] appear to be mainly involved.

Two-dimensional echocardiography represents the reference method for cardiac surgery patients' follow up;

---

* Correspondence: matteo.saccocci@unimi.it
[1]Department of Cardiac Surgery, Centro Cardiologico Monzino IRCCS, University of Milan, Via Parea, 4, 20138 Milan, Italy
[2]Heart Center, University Hospital of Zürich, University of Zürich, Zürich, CH, Switzerland

however, regarding the evaluation of right ventricle performance, it has important limitations due to its particular anatomy. The recent introduction of 3-dimensional echocardiographic images allows a more complete evaluation of right ventricle contraction, showing that two-dimensional indexes decrease failed to be accompanied by concomitant parallel right ventricle three-dimensional functional changes [3].

Unfortunately, 3D echocardiograms can be performed only by highly specialized experienced operators. Indeed, 2D measurements like tricuspid annular plane systolic excursion (TAPSE) is still largely used in right ventricular evaluation.

The aim of the present study is to evaluate the impact of the type of pericardial incision (lateral versus anterior) in combination of different myocardial protection protocols onto postoperative right ventricular systolic function in order to further investigate the superiority of minimally invasive approach in mitral valve surgery.

Methods

Population and study protocol

All patients were enrolled in our Center and operated by the same surgeon. Written informed consent to participate in this observational study, which was approved by Centro Cardiologico Monzino Institutional Review Board, was obtained from all patients. The study protocol conforms to the ethical guidelines of the Declaration of Helsinki as reflected in a priori approval by the institution's human research committee.

To achieve the aim of this study, we compared 2- and 3-dimensional echocardiographic parameters in patients undergoing minimally invasive or traditional (full sternotomy) mitral valve repair (MVR) focusing onto the impact of pericardial incision and cardioplegia protocol.

We retrospectively analyze data of 44 consecutive patients (mean age 54 ± 12 years; 34 males/10 females) with severe mitral regurgitation related to degenerative dysfunction due to mitral valve prolapse who underwent mitral valve reparation at our Center by the same Surgeon. We subdivided them in 3 groups according to surgical approach and cardioplegia type (Fig. 1):

1. Group 1: traditional sternotomy operation with Buckberg cardioplegia protocol (blood mixed antegrade-retrograde solution) – 17 patients
2. Group 2: traditional sternotomy operation with Custodiol cardioplegia (crystalloid antegrade administration) – 10 patients
3. Group 3: mini-invasive surgery (4 cm right antero-lateral thoracotomy) with Custodiol cardioplegia (crystalloid antegrade administration) – 17 patients

Mini-invasive mitral surgery tends to be performed with single shot cardioplegia protocol, like Custodiol, while Buckberg protocol seems to be more protective and versatile for traditional surgery. The design of the study permits to investigate independently surgical approach and cardioplegia making a comparison between groups with same pericardial access (group 1 and 2) but different myocardial protection and between groups with same cardioplegia protocol but different incision of the pericardium (group 2 and 3).

Clinical and echocardiographic baseline patients' characteristics are shown in Table 1. Composition of cardioplegic solutions is reported in Table 2.

Exclusion criteria were persistent or paroxysmal atrial fibrillation, urgent intervention with hemodynamic instability, poor echocardiographic acoustic apical window, tricuspid regurgitation major than 1 degree (scale 1 to 4),

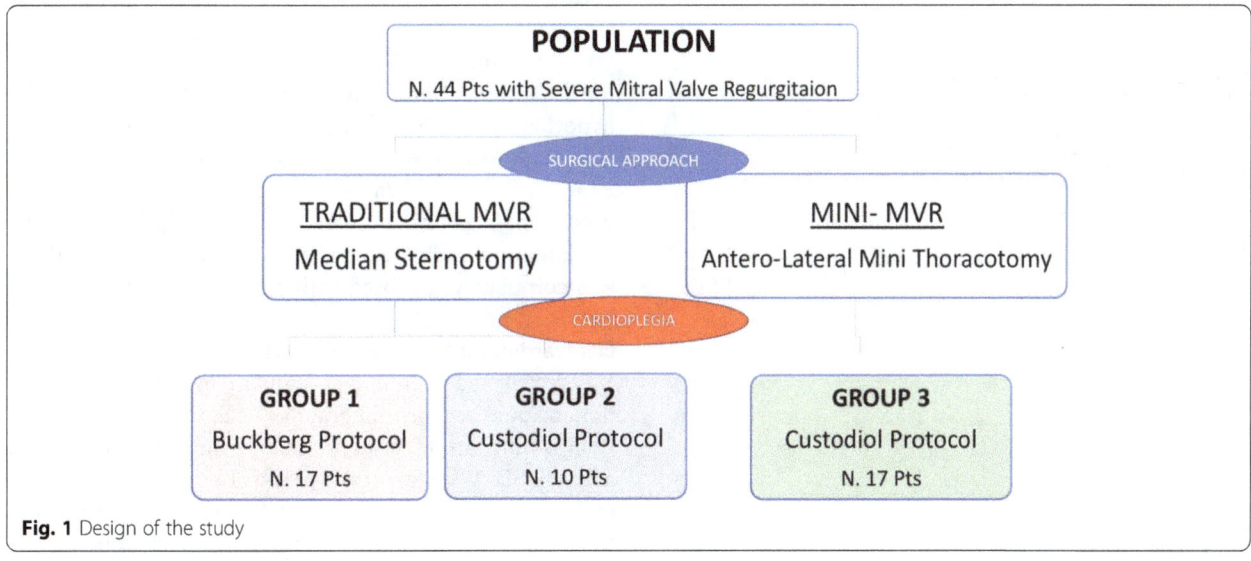

Fig. 1 Design of the study

Table 1 Clinical and echocardiographic groups' baseline characteristics

	Group 1 (n = 17)	Group 2 (n = 10)	Group 3 (n = 17)	P value
Age, y	54.8 ± 11.9	59.2 ± 10.2	50.9 ± 12.2	0.14
Male, n (%)	13 (76%)	7 (70%)	14 (82%)	0.18
BSA (m²)	1.9 ± 0.2	1.8 ± 0.2	1.8 ± 0.1	0.32
EuroSCORE 2*	0.98%	0.96%	0.95%	0.45
LVEF	60.4 ± 6.4	58.2 ± 4.1	64.5 ± 4.7	0.32
TAPSE (mm)	24.5 ± 4.8	27.4 ± 5.3	23.5 ± 4	0.17
SPAP (mmHg)	33.9 ± 4.8	32.3 ± 5.1	34.9 ± 2.7	0.83
RVEF (3D)	62.2 ± 8.9	60.5 ± 8.2	58.5 ± 6.1	0.56
RVSV (3D)	68.3 ± 23.9	54.1 ± 18.8	68 ± 13.1	0.21
RVESV (3D)	43.4 ± 22.5	34.7 ± 11.7	48.5 ± 11.6	0.34†
RVEDV (3D)	111.7 ± 42.8	88.8 ± 26.1	116.5 ± 19.8	0.18φ
MVP Type				
Posterior leaflet prolapse	17	9	17	
Anterior leaflet prolapse	2	1	1	

*EuroSCORE 2 denotes the European System for Cardiac Operative Risk Evaluation (2nd version)
†p = 0.04 Group 2 versus 3
φp = 0.03 Group 2 versus 3
BSA Indicates body surface area, *LVEF* Left ventricular ejection fraction, *TAPSE* Tricuspid annular plane systolic excursion, *SPAP* Systolic pulmonary arterial pressure, *RVEF* Right ventricular ejection fraction, *RVSV* Right ventricular stroke volume, *RVESV* Right ventricular end-systolic volume, *RVEDV* Right ventricular end-diastolic volume, *MVP* Mitral valve prolapse

concomitant surgery procedures or mitral valve replacement, major pulmonary diseases justifying a right ventricular dysfunction or pulmonary hypertension, previous cardiac surgery and preoperative reduced LV function (Ejection fraction < 40%). Two-dimensional (2D-) and three-dimensional (3D-) transthoracic echocardiography (TTE) was performed preoperative (24–48 h before surgery) and 6 months after surgical operation.

Table 2 Composition of cardioplegic solutions used in the study

Ingredient	Buckberg cold induction 4.1	Buckberg cold maintenance 4.1	Buckberg "hot shot"	Custodiol
Na⁺	140	140	140	15
K⁺	20	10	8	9
Mg⁺⁺	13	9	6	4
Ca⁺⁺	–	–	–	0.015
Hystidine	–	–	–	198
Tryptophan	–	–	–	2
Ketoglutarate	–	–	–	1
Mannitol	–	–	–	30
Glucose	6	6	8	–
pH	7.2	7.4	7.5	7.02–7.2

All ingredients are expressed in mmol/L

Surgical procedures

Traditional MVR patients (group 1 and 2) underwent complete median sternotomy and anterior opening of the pericardium with a reversed T incision. Standard cardiopulmonary bypass (CBP) was implanted with ascending aortic cannulation and bicaval venous cannulation.

In Group 1 Buckberg cardioplegia was adopted, consisting in a three-phases myocardial protection protocol:

1. Cold induction: delivery of cold cardioplegic solution (8–12 °C) antegrade and retrograde for 2 min each until complete cardioplegic arrest was achieved (flow 200 ml/min, in hypertrophied hearts increase to 300 ml/min)
2. Reinfusions with cold blood cardioplegia: during aortic cross-clamping, multidose cold blood cardioplegia was applied at intervals of 20 min to maintain cardioplegic arrest and myocardial hypothermia. Infusions were delivered retrograde for 1 min (flow 200 ml/min)
3. Warm terminal reperfusion ("hot shot"): normothermic substrate-enriched blood cardioplegia was applied before aortic unclamping. The warm reperfusate was delivered via coronary sinus for 1 min and followed by a brief (20–30 s) retrograde administration of normothermic blood [12].

In Group 2 Custodiol protocol protection (single antegrade injection of crystalloid intracellular cold cardioplegia in 6–8 min) was employed.

Minimally invasive mitral valve repair (Group 3) was performed through a small (5 cm) right antero-lateral thoracotomy and with a lateral supra-phrenic pericardial incision. Peripheral CBP was implanted using femoral vessels for arterial and venous cannulation. Similarly to Group 2, a single antegrade dose of Custodiol cardioplegia was administered.

All interventions were performed in moderate hypothermia (32 °C) with a direct left atriotomy through Waterstone's groove. Depending on patient's mitral alteration we used different surgical repairing techniques always supported by annuloplasty with a prosthetic ring implantation (Table 3). In each group the pericardium was completely re-closed with a continuous suture.

Echocardiographic measurements

We performed a complete standard M-mode and two-dimensional echocardiographic examinations using a Philips ultrasound system (iE33, Andover, MA, USA) and an S5–1 sector array probe. LV end-diastolic and end-systolic volumes, as well as biplane ejection fraction were measured in apical four- and two chamber views

Table 3 Intraoperative groups' characteristics

	Group 1 (n = 17)	Group 2 (n = 10)	Group 3 (n = 17)	P value
CPB time (min)	113 ± 17	105 ± 18	131 ± 23	0.21
Cross-clamp time (min)	95 ± 13	93 ± 12	112 ± 12	0.24
Complete prosthetic semi-rigid ring	3	2	2	0.32
Incomplete band	14	8	15	0.25
Annular plication	1	0	0	0.43
Quadrangular resection	6	4	7	0.44
Triangular resection	9	5	9	0.28
Sliding-plasty	5	4	6	0.12
Artificial chordae positioning	2	1	1	0.23
Papillary muscle plication	1	0	0	0.34

CPB Indicates cardio-pulmonary bypass

with the area–length method. Systolic pulmonary arterial pressure was non-invasively acquired using Doppler echo method from the systolic right ventricle–right atrial gradient, calculated from the systolic trans-tricuspid regurgitant flow peak velocity by the modified Bernoulli equation. Right atrial (RA) pressure was derived by means of the inferior vena cava (IVC) collapsibility index measured from the subcostal view [13]. To estimate tricuspid annular plane systolic excursion (TAPSE), defined as the difference in the displacement of the right ventricle base from end-diastole to end-systole, from the apical four-chamber view, the M-mode cursor was positioned at the junction of the tricuspid valvular plane with the right ventricle free [14, 15].

3D- Real-time TTE was performed during same echocardiographic session utilizing an X3–1 matrix array probe. The 3D-measurement were acquired using 'full volume' mode from the apical view, adapted to improve the visualization of the right ventricular chamber. We registered Two datasets for each patient. To perform off-line post-processing and three-dimensional reconstruction we used a commercially available dedicated system (Echo View, Tom Tec Imaging Inc., Munich, Germany) equipped with a four-dimensional right ventricle analysis software [16].

Statistical analysis

Data were managed in Microsoft Excel 2016 and analyzed with SPSS 22.0 software (SPSS, Inc., Chicago, IL) and SAS system (SAS Institute Inc., Cary, NC). Each echocardiographic parameter was evaluated pre- and 6 months post-surgery. Continuous variables were presented as mean ± SD and compared with an unpaired t-test, while categorical data were expressed as percentages or numbers and compared with χ^2 test.

A between-groups comparison examining the impact of pericardial approach and type of cardioplegia on right ventricular function over time was made with an analysis of variance and co-variance (ANOVA test) adjusted for patients' age, sex, body surface area and right ventricular features basal values.

A p value < 0.05 was considered as statistically significant.

Results

All enrolled patients underwent mitral valve repair surgery without significant complications. After six month after surgery (185 ± 23 days), all cases had residual mitral regurgitation inferior to 1 degree (scale 1 to 4). At least one good quality, three-dimensional right ventricle dataset was acquired in all patients before surgery and six months after the surgery. Tables 4 and 5 and Panel A (Fig. 2) shows the mean values of the two-dimensional and three-dimensional parameters for each step of the study in both groups.

Table 4 Two-dimensional and three-dimensional echocardiographic parameters measured at pre- and 6 months post-surgery

Variable	Pre-surgery	Sixth month	P Within Group
TAPSE (mm)			
Group 1	24.5 ± 4.8	14.9 ± 3	< 0.0001
Group 2	27.4 ± 5.3	19.3 ± 4.2	0.0003
Group 3	23.5 ± 4	21.5 ± 4.1	0.013
SPAP (mmHg)			
Group 1	33.9 ± 4.8	25.7 ± 2.9	< 0.0001
Group 2	32.3 ± 5.1	28.3 ± 6.5	0.054
Group 3	34.9 ± 8.1	25.2 ± 3.1	0.049
RVEDV (ml)			
Group 1	111.7 ± 42.8	93.1 ± 26.2	0.016
Group 2	88.8 ± 26.1	72.2 ± 21.3	0.002
Group 3	116.5 ± 19.8	105.2 ± 20.6	0.039
RVESV (ml)			
Group 1	43.4 ± 22.5	39.2 ± 13.6	0.244
Group 2	34.7 ± 11.7	29.2 ± 9.2	0.048
Group 3	48.5 ± 11.6	41 ± 9	0.005
3D RVEF (%)			
Group 1	62.2 ± 8.9	58.2 ± 5.4	0.021
Group 2	60.5 ± 8.2	59.5 ± 6.9	0.579
Group 3	58.5 ± 6.1	60.7 ± 6.8	0.207
3D RVSV (ml)			
Group 1	68.3 ± 23.9	53.9 ± 13.9	0.004
Group 2	54.1 ± 18.8	43 ± 14.1	0.0039
Group 3	68 ± 13.1	64.1 ± 15.9	0.349

TAPSE Indicates tricuspid annular plane systolic excursion, *SPAP* Systolic pulmonary arterial pressure, *RVEDV* Right ventricular end-diastolic volume, *RVESV* Right ventricular end-systolic volume, *RVEF* Right ventricular ejection fraction, *RVSV* Right ventricular stroke volume

Table 5 Inter-group comparison of two-dimensional and three-dimensional echocardiographic parameters variations (6 months post-surgery versus pre-operative values)

Delta variable	Group 1	Group 2	Group 3	P Group 1 vs 3	P Group 1 vs 2	P Group 3 vs 2
TAPSE(mm)	−9.5	−8.1	−2	< 0.0001	0.12	0.008
SPAP(mmHg)	−8.1	−4	−9.7	0.66	0.86	0.65
RVEDV (ml)	−18.6	−16.5	−11.3	0.54	0.93	0.51
RVESV (ml)	−4.2	−5.5	−7.4	0.49	0.69	0.91
3D RVEF (%)	−3.9	−0.9	2.2	0.04	0.22	0.74
3D RVSV(ml)	−14.4	−11.1	−3.9	0.18	0.66	0.45
2D LVEF (%)	−7.6	−8.1	−3.8	0.08	0.84	0.19

TAPSE indicates tricuspid annular plane systolic excursion, SPAP systolic pulmonary arterial pressure, RVEDV right ventricular end-diastolic volume, RVESV right ventricular end-systolic volume, RVEF right ventricular ejection fraction, RVSV right ventricular stroke volume, LVEF left ventricular ejection fraction

Preoperative left and right ventricular function were in normal range for all patients. Basal TAPSE was slightly greater, but did not reach statistical significance, in traditional surgery (Group 1 and 2, respectively 24.5 and 27.4 versus 23.5 for mini-invasive patients; $p = 0.17$). All the three groups had similar preoperative 3D right ventricular function and cross-clamping/extracorporeal circulation time.

Two-dimensional measurements

Postoperative TAPSE fall was found in each group (Table 4), but mini-invasive patients experienced a less marked variation (group 3: 21.5 ± 4.1 post- versus 23.5 ± 4 pre-; $p = 0.01$) compared to traditional surgery (Group 1 14.9 ± 3 post versus 24.5 ± 4.8 pre; $p < 0.0001$; Group 2 19.3 ± 4.2 post versus 27.4 ± 5.3 pre; $p = 0.0003$). The difference remained statistically significant after adjustment for patients' age, sex, body surface area and basal TAPSE (Group 3 versus 1 $p < 0.0001$ and Group 3 versus 2 $p = 0.008$).

Systolic pulmonary arterial pressure showed a similar postoperative fall in each group.

Left ventricular volumes and ejection fraction decreased after surgery in a similar manner in all patients.

Three-dimensional measurements

In Sterno-Buckberg patients (Group 1) end-systolic size-decreasing trend failed to reach statistical significance. However, in the other two groups (groups 2 and 3, Custodiol), both end-diastolic and end-systolic right ventricular volumes significantly diminished after surgery. Any inter-group size changes comparison showed a significant difference (Table 4).

In mini-invasive patients (group 3), right ventricular ejection fraction slightly augmented after surgery (60.7 ± 6.8 post versus 58.5 ± 6.1 pre; $p = 0.2$), while, in Group 1 decreased (58.2 ± 5.4 post versus 62.2 ± 8.9 pre; $p = 0.02$). In contrast, no significance difference was found in Group 2 (59.5 ± 6.9 post versus 60.5 ± 8.2 pre; $p = 0.58$). In addition, this variation was significantly different

between mini-invasive versus sternotomy-Buckberg patients ($p = 0.04$). Similarly, right ventricular stroke volume diminished after surgery in all patients without significant inter-group differences.

Discussion

The importance of RV function as an important physiopathology element in many different cardiovascular disease is a well-known phenomenon and it is an already validated prognostic index after cardiac surgery. In the past, obtaining an accurate postoperative evaluation of RV function has been made difficult by its complex anatomy and morphology. This problem was solved by the assessment of tricuspid annulus movement with 2D-Echocardiographic analysis that has been proved to be accurate, feasible, simple and reproducible in both normal and pathological patients [17]. The introduction of 3D-Echocardiography has permitted a big step forward in the evaluation of RV volume and function throughout the cardiac cycle [18, 19] permitting to calculate the right ventricular ejection fraction (RV-EF) that represents the global performance of the ventricle. The main limitation 3D-echocardiography is that is a technology usually available only in high-experienced center with skilled operators while 2D- TAPSE evaluation is an easy measurement for every echocardiographist.

Several studies report a reduction of TAPSE after cardiac surgery for congenital and acquired diseases [6, 20] without univocal explanation. Observing a postoperative TAPSE decrease, without variation in left ventricle function, has driven to interpret it as a simple modification with modest clinical impact. Many hypothesis have been presented in order to clarify this loss in RV performance measured at 2D-TTE, including cardiopulmonary bypass use [8, 21], geometrical changes of the right ventricular chamber (in association with interventricular septal paradoxical motion [22], intraoperative ischemia, right atrial injury due to cannulation procedure [23], poor myocardial protection [24], and

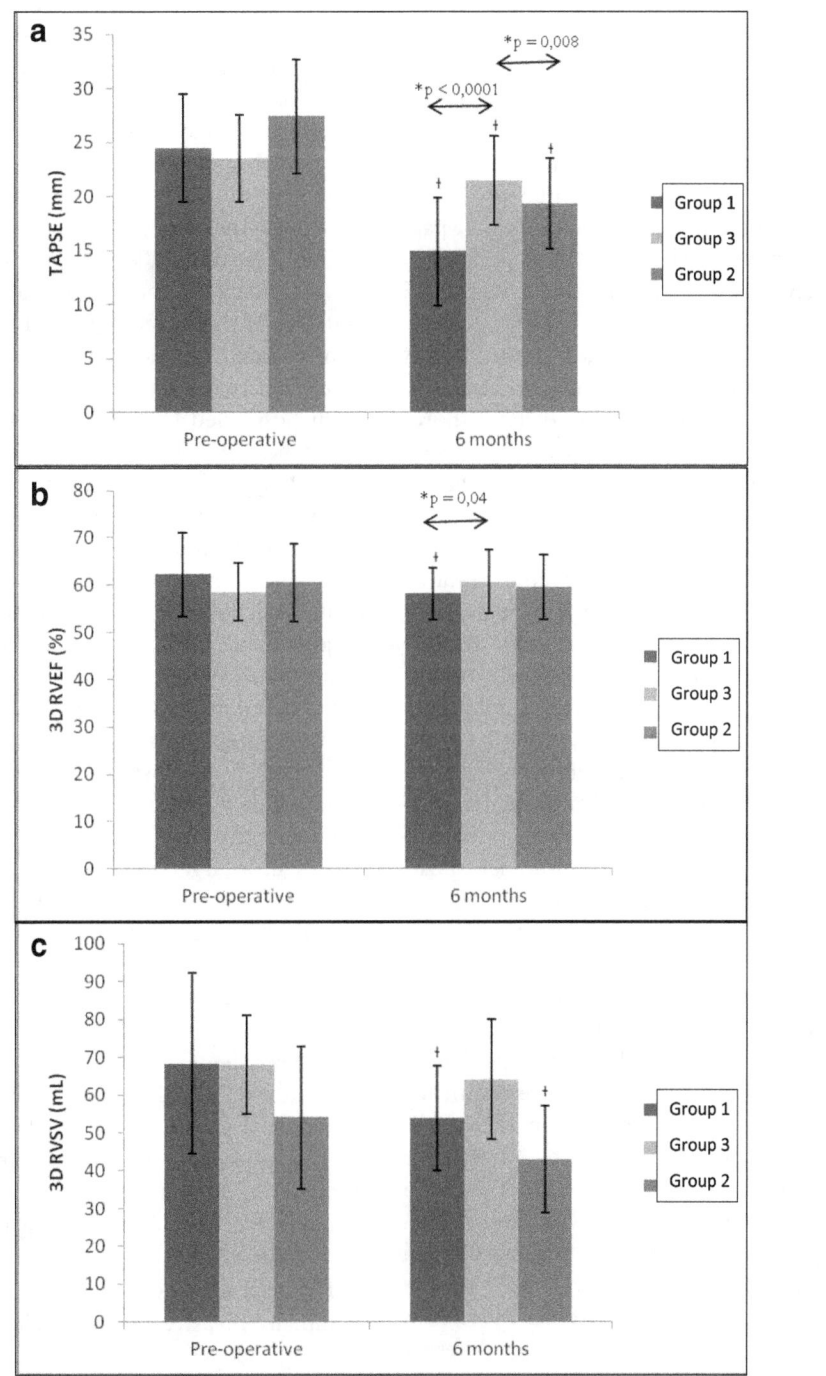

Fig. 2 PANEL **a** - Mean tricuspid annular plane systolic excursion (TAPSE) and 95% confidence intervals (CIs) measured preoperatively and at 6 months postoperatively. * Between-groups comparison. † $p < 0.05$ vs preoperative; PANEL **b** - Mean three-dimensional right ventricular ejection fraction (3D RVEF) and 95% confidence intervals (CIs) measured preoperatively and at 6 months postoperatively. * Between-groups comparison † $p < 0.05$ vs preoperative; Panel **c** - Mean three-dimensional right ventricular stroke volume (3D RVSV) and 95% confidence intervals (CIs) measured preoperatively and at 6 months postoperatively. † $p < 0.05$ vs preoperative

extra myocardial causes (pericardial disruption, changes in Fossa Ovalis and post-operative adherence of the right ventricle to the thoracic wall, 9). The role of pericardial injury has also been highlighted in our precedent study [25]. One of the major confounding factors comparing traditional and mini-invasive surgery is represented by the use of single shot cardioplegia protocol in mini-MVR. To eliminate this bias and to evaluate myocardial protection impact on TAPSE we designed this three groups study.

To minimize all other possible confounding factors and to eliminate inter-operators difference, we acquired data only from patient underwent MVR by the same surgeon and who had pre- and postoperative TTE by one dedicated echocardiographist. Surgical valve repair technique doesn't significantly differ within the 3 groups (Table 3) as well as the type of implanted prosthetic rings. Cross-clamping time and cardiopulmonary bypass time resulted comparable in all groups. The pericardial opening was entirely closed with a running suture in all patients.

TAPSE reduction was observed in all groups, but it has been significantly less marked in mini-invasive surgery group who underwent mini-anterolateral thoracotomy with supraphrenic lateral pericardial incision and Custodiol cardioplegia. Evaluating different cardioplegia protocol with same surgical approach (group 1 vs. 2) we did not find any significant differences. 3D-echocardiographic RV postoperative volume resulted comparable within the 3 groups. A slightly augmented RV ejection fraction was observed after mini-invasive surgery (group 3) while it decreased in patients underwent traditional median sternotomy despite the different cardioplegia protocol (group 1 Buckberg, group 2 Custodiol). According to these results, only different surgical approach impact RV function, in particular, lateral pericardial incision used in mini-invasive surgery is able to significantly limit right-ventricle longitudinal postoperative function decrease while the different type of cardioplegia protocol has no relevant effect on TAPSE.

To explain these findings more than a hypothesis can be provided. The first one could be that anterior pericardial incision modifies a portion of pericardium directly connected with the RV free wall while lateral opening, in the face of interatrial groove, does not interfere with RV motility. As we previously proposed [25], another explication could be linked to the shape itself of anterior pericardial incision. It consisted in a reversed T incision with a double opening line along the diaphragm that could modify the relationship between this muscle and the inferior RV wall leading to possible variations in longitudinal right ventricular contractile pattern and consequently to postoperative TAPSE fall. The different surgical repair techniques and prosthetic rings used to restore mitral valve competency and to assure long-term durability should not influence inter-group differences due to the homogenous distribution of them in the 3 groups. Different kind of resection or ring did not reach significant statistic difference within the study population (Table 3).

An additional important observation from this study is that, in parallel to the attended impairment of right ventricle long-axis function, also three-dimensional global systolic indexes showed a postoperative slight decreasing trend, which was less accentuated (or even inversed when talking about right ventricular ejection fraction) in mini-invasive group. In other words, it seems that, in our study, the right ventricle undergoes a kind of geometrical modifications too, which appear to be less affected by a lateral pericardial approach. Nevertheless, in our opinion, such tendency (which could be interpreted as clinically negligible since included in the normal range of measure variability) is partially different from what previously reported [3]. A prudent interpretation is justified by various considerations: 1) the increasing trend of right ventricular ejection fraction in mini-invasive group is not confirmed by a parallel stroke volume time-course; 2) the inter-group evaluation failed to show a statistically significant difference when comparing Group 3 vs Group 2 (thus perhaps suggesting a role played by cardioplegia too); 3) the intra-group three-dimensional variables variations were not significant in all groups.

Basing on these reasons, we believe that deeper investigations involving a greater patients' population and a longer follow up time (which could elucidate that such trend was only a temporary phenomenon, as also pointed out by postoperative right ventricular ejection fraction fluctuations described by Tamborini et al.,3) are required before drawing definitive conclusions.

We studied a relative small number of cases. Despite this limitation and even though our data should be confirmed in a larger population, statistical analysis clearly defined significant changes and differences in the three groups, being able to highlight how different surgical protocols resulted in diverse right ventricular function postoperative trends.

Study limitations

Main study limitation is represented by limited number of patients of the cohort analyzed and as well as the needed of longer echocardiographic follow-up. Larger population, different type of cardioplegia (Del Nido, St. Thomas, etc..) should be investigated.

Conclusions

Minimally invasive mitral repair with lateral pericardial opening reduces postoperative TAPSE fall while cardioplegia protocol fails to have an impact onto longitudinal RV function. In our study, the right ventricle seems to show a clinically irrelevant geometrical modification too, whose entity appears to be less evident in case of lateral pericardial approach. These results could strengthen the use of minimally invasive approach also to preserve right ventricle function.

Abbreviations

CBP: Cardiopulmonary bypass; IVC: Inferior vena cava; MVR: Mitral valve repair; TAPSE: Tricuspid annular plane systolic excursion; TTE: Transthoracic echocardiography

Authors' contribution

MS, MZ have contribute equally to this work. MS,CL,MZ,GT, MP data collection, study design. FV,MS, MZ statistical analysis. MS,MZ,CL,PP,ADM,VM,RB writing. MS,MZ,FA,MP,GT manuscript revision. All authors read and approved the final manuscript.

Competing interests

None of the authors have competing interest within this paper.

References

1. De Groote P, Millaire A, Foucher-Hossein C, et al. Right ventricular ejection fraction is an independent predictor of survival in patients with moderate heart failure. J Am Coll Cardiol. 1998;32:948–54.
2. Davila-Roman VG, Waggoner AD, Hopkins WE, Barzilai B. Right ventricular dysfunction in low output syndrome after cardiac operations: assessment by transesophageal echocardiography. Ann Thorac Surg. 1995;60:1081–6.
3. Tamborini G, Muratori M, Brusoni D, et al. Is right ventricular systolic function reduced after cardiac surgery? A two- and three- dimensional echocardiographic study. Eur J Echocardiogr. 2009;10:630–4.
4. Unsworth B, Casula R, Kyriacou A, et al. The right ventricular annular velocity reduction caused by coronary artery bypass graft surgery occurs at the moment of pericardial incision. Am Heart J. 2010;159:314–22.
5. Wranne B, Pinto FJ, Hammarström E, St Goar FG, Puryear J, Popp RL. Abnormal right heart filling after cardiac surgery: time course and mechanisms. Br Heart J. 1991;66:435–42.
6. Alam M, Hedman A, Nordlander R, Samad B. Right ventricular function before and after an uncomplicated coronary artery bypass graft as assessed by pulsed wave Doppler tissue imaging of the tricuspid annulus. Am Heart J. 2003;146:520–6.
7. Boldt J, Kling D, Dapper F, Hempelmann G. Myocardial temperature during cardiac operations: influence on right ventricular function. J Thorac Cardiovasc Surg. 1990;100:562–8.
8. Pegg T, Selvanayagam J, Karamitsos T, et al. Effects of off-pump versus on-pump coronary artery bypass grafting on early and late right ventricular function. Circulation. 2008;117:2202–10.
9. Joshi S, Salah A, Mendoza D, Goldstein SA, Fuisz AR, Lindsay J. Mechanism of paradoxical ventricular septal motion after coronary bypass grafting. Am J Cardiol. 2009;103:212–5.
10. Unsworth B, Casula R, Yadav H, et al. Contrasting effect of different operations on echocardiographic right ventricular long axis velocities, and implications for interpretation of post-operative values. Int J Cardiol. 2013;165:151–60.
11. Rangaraj A, Ghanta R, Umakanthan R, et al. Real-time visualization and quantification of retrograde cardioplegia delivery using near infrared fluorescent imaging. J Card Surg. 2008;23:701–8.
12. Rosenkranz ER, Okamoto F, Buckberg GD, et al. Safety of prolonged aortic clamping with blood cardioplegia. III. Aspartate enrichment of glutamate-blood cardioplegia in energy-depleted hearts after ischemic and reperfusion injury. J Thorac Cardiovasc Surg. 1986;91:428–35.
13. Pepi M, Tamborini G, Galli C, et al. A new formula for echo-Doppler estimation of right ventricular systolic pressure. J Am Soc Echocardiogr. 1994;7:20–6.
14. Hammarstrom E, Wranne B, Pinto FJ, Puryear J, Popp RL. Tricuspid annular motion. J Am Soc Echocardiogr. 1991;4:131–9.
15. Miller D, Farah MG, Keith F, Fox K, Schluchter M, Hoit BD. The relation between quantitative right ventricular ejection fraction andindices of tricuspidal annular motion and myocardial performance. J Am Soc Echocardiogr. 2004;17:443–7.
16. Niemann PS, Pinho L, Balbach T, et al. Anatomically oriented right ventricular volume measurements with dynamic three-dimensional echocardiography validated by 3-tesla magnetic resonance imaging. J Am Coll Cardiol. 2007;50:1668–76.
17. Tamborini G, Pepi M, Galli C, et al. Feasibility and accuracy of a routine echocardiographic assessment of right ventricular function. Int J Cardiol. 2007;115:86–9.
18. Tamborini G, Brusoni D, Torres Molinab JE, et al. Feasibility of a new generation three-dimensional echocardiography for right ventricular volumetric and functional measurements. Am J Cardiol. 2008;102:499–505.
19. Maffessanti F, Muraru D, Esposito R, et al. Age-, body size-, and sex-specific reference values for right ventricular volumes and ejection fraction by three-dimensional echocardiography: a multicenter echocardiographic study in 507 healthy volunteers. Circ Cardiovasc Imaging. 2013;6:700–10.
20. Hanseus KC, Bjorkhem GE, Brodin LA, Pesonen E. Analysis of atrioventricular plane movements by Doppler tissue imaging and M-mode in children with atrial septal defects before and after surgical and device closure. Pediatr Cardiol. 2002;23:152–9.
21. Forsberg L, Tamas E, Vanky F, Nielsen NE, Enqvall J, Nylander E. Left and right ventricular function in aortic stenosis patients 8 weeks post-transcatheter aortic valve implantation or surgical aortic valve replacement. Eur J Echocardiogr. 2011;12:603–11.
22. Roshanali F, Yousefnia M, Mandegar M, Rayatzadeh H, Alinejad S. Decreased right ventricular function and coronary artery bypass grafting. Tex Heart Inst J. 2008;35:250–5.
23. Lindqvist P, Holmgren A, Zhao J, Henein MY. Effect of pericardial repair after aortic valve replacement on septal and right ventricular function. Int J Cardiol. 2012;155:388–93.
24. Jasinski M, Kadziola Z, Bachowski R, et al. Comparison of retrograde versus anterograde cold blood cardioplegia: randomized trial in elective coronary artery bypass patients. Eur J Cardiothorac Surg. 1997;12:620–6.
25. Zanobini M, Saccocci M, Tamborini G, et al. Postoperative echocardiographic reduction of right ventricular function: is pericardial opening modality the main culprit? Biomed Res Int. 2017;2017:4808757. https://doi.org/10.1155/2017/4808757.

23

Epicardial infrared ablation to create a linear conduction block on a beating right atrium

Hiroshi Kubota[*] ⓘ, Hidehito Endo, Hikaru Ishii, Hiroshi Tsuchiya, Yusuke Inaba, Yu Takahashi and Katsunari Terakawa

Abstract

Background: It is still difficult to create a secure linear conduction block on a beating heart from the epicardial side. To overcome this drawback we developed an infrared coagulator equipped with a cuboid light-guiding quartz rod. This study was designed to electrophysiologically confirm the efficacy of a new ablation probe using infrared energy in a clinical case.

Methods: The infrared light from a lamp is focused into the newly developed cuboid quartz rod, which has a rectangular distal exit-plane that allows 30 mm × 10 mm linear photocoagulation. Two pairs of electrodes were attached to the right atrium of a patient who was undergoing surgery. Each pair of electrodes was placed 10 mm from an ablation line. The change in conduction time between the two pairs of electrodes was measured during ablation. The predicted conduction time delay ratio was 1.54.

Results: The actual conduction time after ablation was 1.38–1.43 times longer than the pre-ablation conduction time.

Conclusions: The infrared ablation using a newly developed cuboid probe made it possible to create a linear conduction block on the beating right atrial free wall clinically.

Keywords: Atrial fibrillation, Ablation, Coagulator, Energy source, Electrophysiology, Arrhythmia treatment, Infrared, Minimally invasive surgery, Maze procedure, Photocoagulation

Background

The newly developed infrared coagulator, named the "Kyo-Co (Photon incorporation, Saitama, Japan)", contains a reflector that focuses light from a tungsten-halogen lamp into a light-conducting 30 mm × 10 mm cuboid quartz rod, and the light emerges as 35 W/cm^2 of near-infrared light energy (wavelength: 400 nm to approximately 1600 nm; peak wavelength: 850 nm). The distal exit-plane of the light-conducting rod has a rectangular plane surface (30 × 10 mm) (Fig. 1).

Methods

In a preliminary experiment, the probe applied to a specimen of chicken muscle tissue, and the muscle tissue was ablated for a total of 28 s (4 s × 5 times at

2 s intervals) ($n = 5$). Tissue temperature with time was measured with a thermometer Ti480® (Fluke Corporation, WA, U.S.A.). The maximum temperature of muscle tissue was measured. After ablation of the chicken muscle the depth of the lesion was measured macroscopically.

The maximum temperature of the chicken muscle was 97.9 + 2.1 °C, and the depth of the lesion was 8.7 + 0.8 mm (Fig. 2).

Clinical experience

In 2014, the ethics committee of Kyorin University approved a clinical and epidemiologic study entitled, Surgical treatment of arrhythmias, infectious endocarditis, infected aortic aneurysms, and cardiac tumors with an infrared coagulator. Written consent was obtained from the patient.

We hypothesized that when a rectangular transmural lesion is created in the same shape as the exit plane of

* Correspondence: kub@ks.kyorin-u.ac.jp
Department of Cardiovascular Surgery, Kyorin University, 6-20-2, Shinkawa, Mitaka, Tokyo 181-8611, Japan

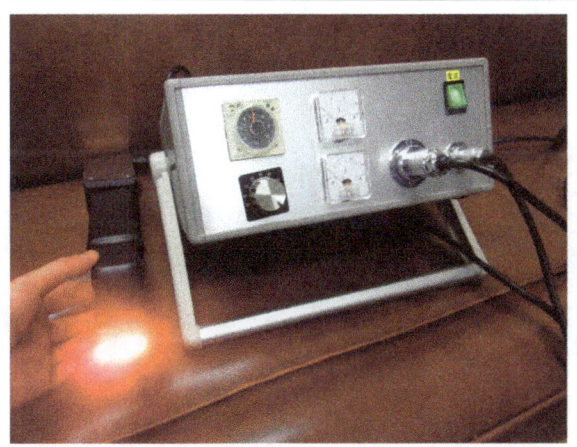

Fig. 1 Infrared coagulator "Kyo-co". The cuboid quartz rod exit plane has a rectangular (30 mm × 10 mm) surface designed to enable creation of a linear lesion. Light from a tungsten-halogen lamp emerges as 35 W/cm² of near-infrared light energy (wavelength: 400 to approximately 1600 nm; peak wavelength: 850 nm)

the cuboid quartz rod, the translesion conduction time would be prolonged. We predicted that the conduction time prolongation ratio (post-ablation conduction time/pre-ablation conduction time) would be directly proportional to the conduction distance prolongation ratio (post-ablation conduction distance/pre-ablation conduction distance). The predicted conduction prolongation ratio was 46.1/30.0 mm = 1.54 (Fig. 3). After obtaining written informed consent from the patient, in August 2016 mitral and tricuspid valve plasty and a maze procedure were performed on a 64-year-old man with infectious endocarditis, severe mitral regurgitation, moderate tricuspid regurgitation, and paroxysmal atrial fibrillation. After a median sternotomy, the pericardium was opened, and the epicardial atrial ablation and electrophysiological study were performed before

commencing the cardiopulmonary bypass. Two pairs of alligator clip electrodes were attached to the right atrium 10 mm from the expected ablation line. The pair of electrodes attached on the dorsal side of the ablation line was used to pace the right atrium, and the pair of electrodes attached on the ventral side of the ablation line was used as sensing electrodes to record the atrial potential. The cuboid 30 mm long 10 mm wide quartz rod of the infrared coagulator was applied epicardially to create a linear lesion on the free wall of the beating right atrial free wall as part of the incision line of the maze procedure (Fig. 3). The total duration of each ablation was 28 s applied in a 5 series of 4.0 s each at 2.0 s intervals. The pacing rate was set to 90 bpm. An electrocardiogram (ECG) and atrial potentials were recorded with an HPM 4500 polygraph (Fukuda Denshi, Tokyo, Japan).

Because the atrial potential was biphasic in shape, conduction times were measured as the interval between stimulation (S) and each peak of the atrial potential (A1 and A2, Fig. 4), and plotted. After the experiment, a square specimen with a side length of 5 mm of coagulated right atrial wall was excised, stained with Masson trichrome, and examined microscopically.

Results

From 1st to 4th infrared application, both S-A1 conduction time and S-A2 conduction time were prolonged and incompletely reversed each time (Fig. 5).

After 4th infrared application, both S-A1 and S-A2 conduction time plateaued, and the 5th infrared application did not affect either conduction time.

S-A1 conduction time was prolonged from 7.2 ms to 10.3 ms. The conduction prolongation ratio was 10.3/7.2 = 1.43.

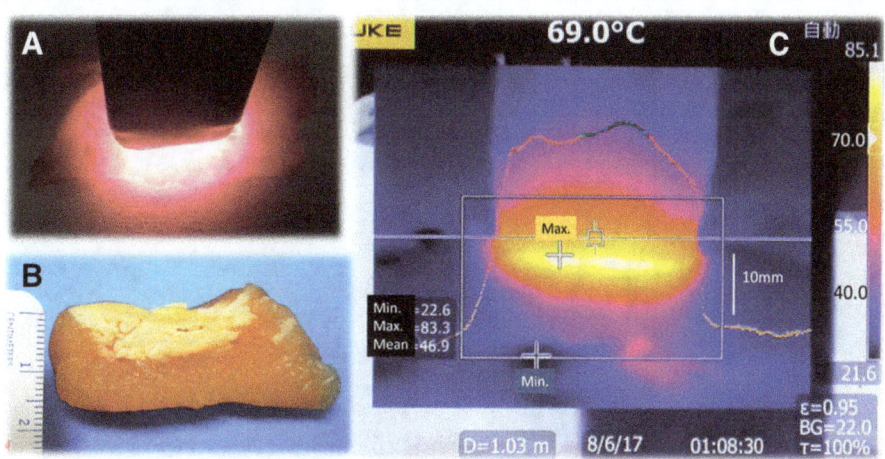

Fig. 2 Preliminary experiment on chicken muscle tissue. **a** The probe was pressed against the muscle tissue. **b** The mean depth of the lesion was 8.7 + 0.8 mm. **c** The maximum temperature was 97.9 + 2.1 ℃

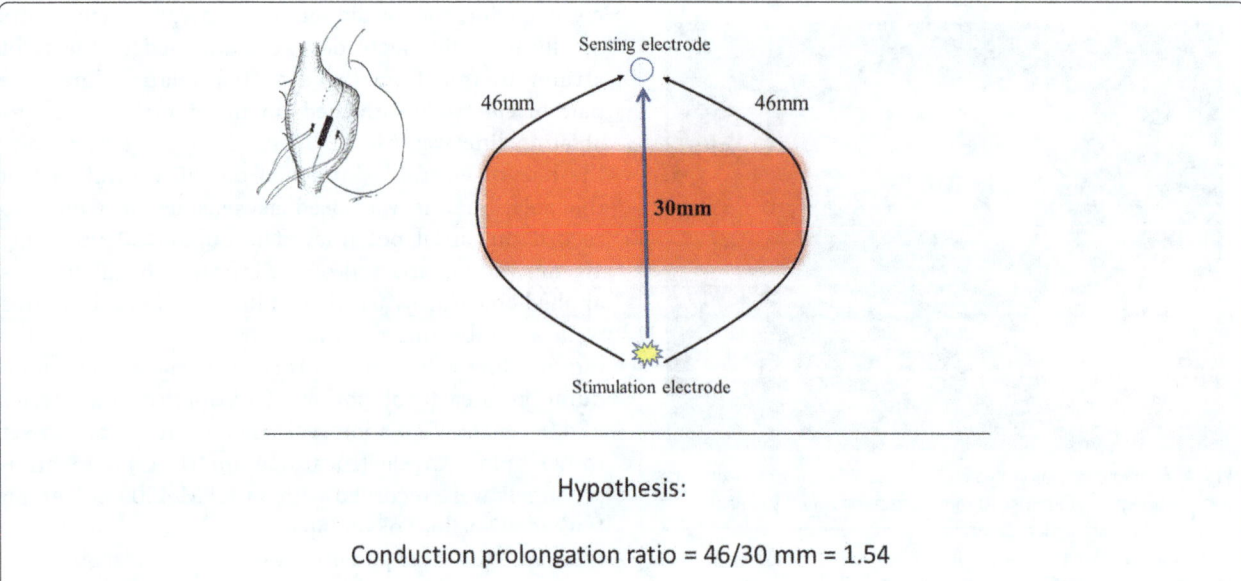

Hypothesis:

Conduction prolongation ratio = 46/30 mm = 1.54

Fig. 3 Prediction. Because the conduction distance prolongation ratio is directly proportional to the conduction time prolongation ratio, when a linear transmural lesion is created in the same shape as the rectangular exit plane, the conduction time prolongation ratio is predicted to be 1.54

S-A2 conduction time was prolonged from 8.6 ms to 11.9 ms. The conduction prolongation ratio was 11.9/8.6 = 1.38.

Histopathologic examination of the ablated right atrium showed preservation of both the endocardium and epicardium of the coagulated lesion (Fig. 6). Severely degenerated myocardium was observed from the epicardial side to mid-portion of the atrial wall. Swelling and hyperchromatosis of the nuclei, acidophilic change in the cytoplasm, and deformity of the myocardium were observed in the myocardium on the endocardial side.

Discussion

To realize the epicardial maze procedure, the major drawback is how to make the transmural lesion on the beating atrial free wall under the condition of existence of inner warm blood flow which weakens heating/cooling effect of the ablation device.

Nath et al. demonstrated that hyperthermia induced by radiofrequency energy causes significant changes in the electrophysiological properties of myocardiocytes, including membrane depolarization, reversible and irreversible loss of excitability, and abnormal automaticity, in an in vitro isolated guinea pig right ventricular papillary muscle

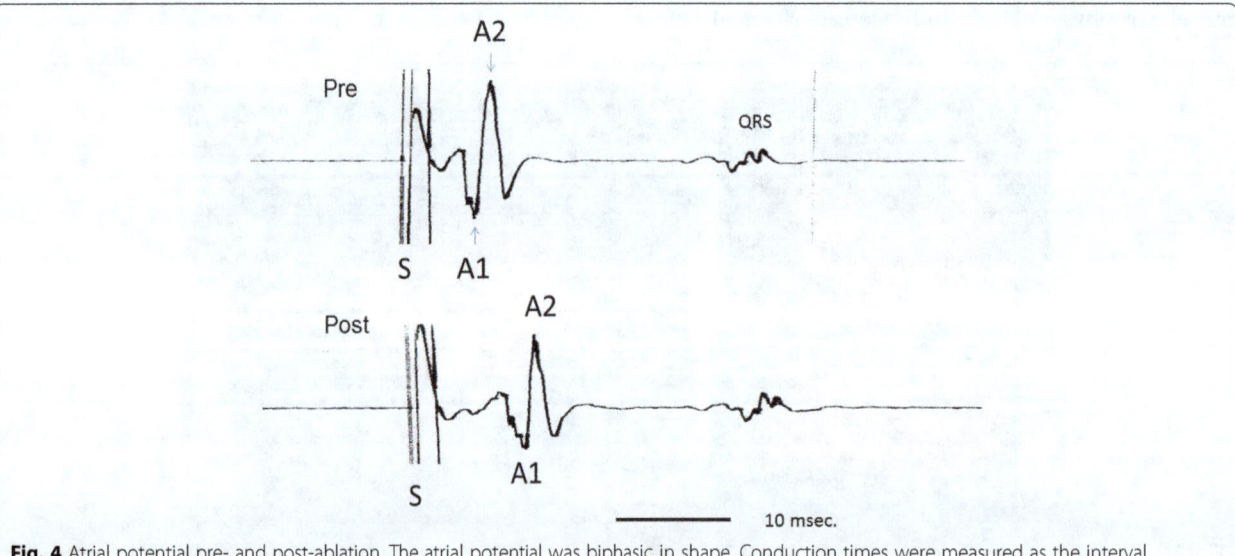

Fig. 4 Atrial potential pre- and post-ablation. The atrial potential was biphasic in shape. Conduction times were measured as the interval between stimulation (S) and each peak of the atrial potential (A1 and A2)

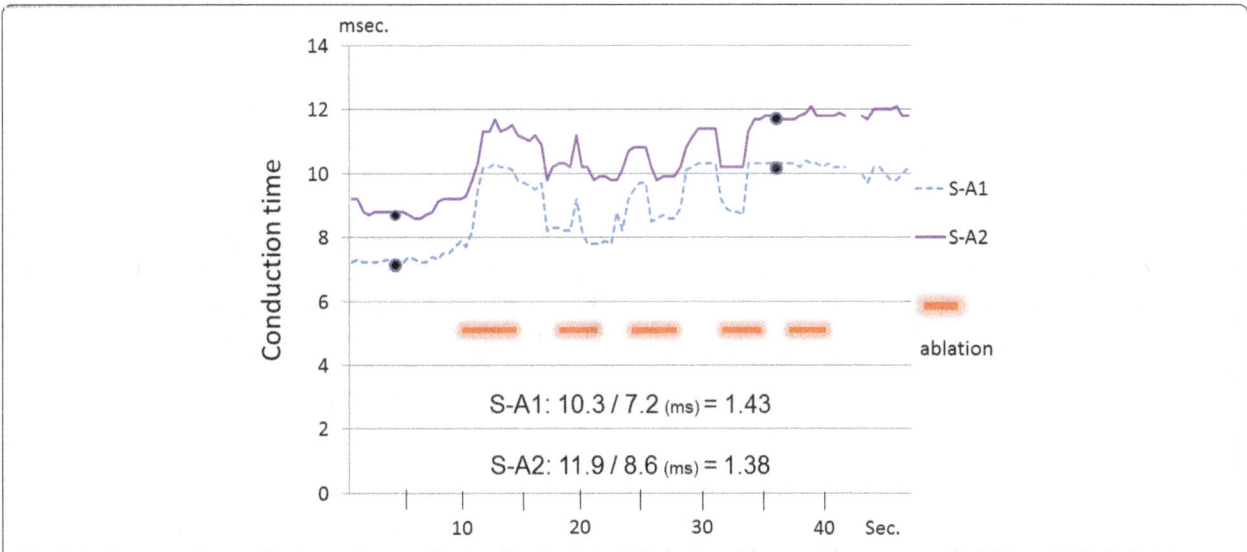

Fig. 5 Atrial potentials pre-ablation and post- ablation (S: stimulation). Biphasic atrial potentials were recorded (A1 and A2). Both S-A1 conduction time and S-A2 conduction time were prolonged after the 28 s of ablation, and the conduction prolongation ratios were 1.43 and 1.38, respectively

model. They observed reversible loss of cellular excitability and tissue injury after exposure to temperatures in the 42.7 °C to 51.3 °C range (median, 48.0 °C) for 60 s and irreversible loss of cellular excitability and tissue injury after exposure to temperatures > 50 °C for 60 seconds [1].

Bulava et al. assessed the efficacy of epicardially created lesions produced with bipolar radiofrequency (RF) energy in 70 patients who had persistent, longstanding atrial fibrillation [2] and reported achieving complete isolation of the posterior left atrial wall in only 22.9% of the patients. The success rates for creating conduction

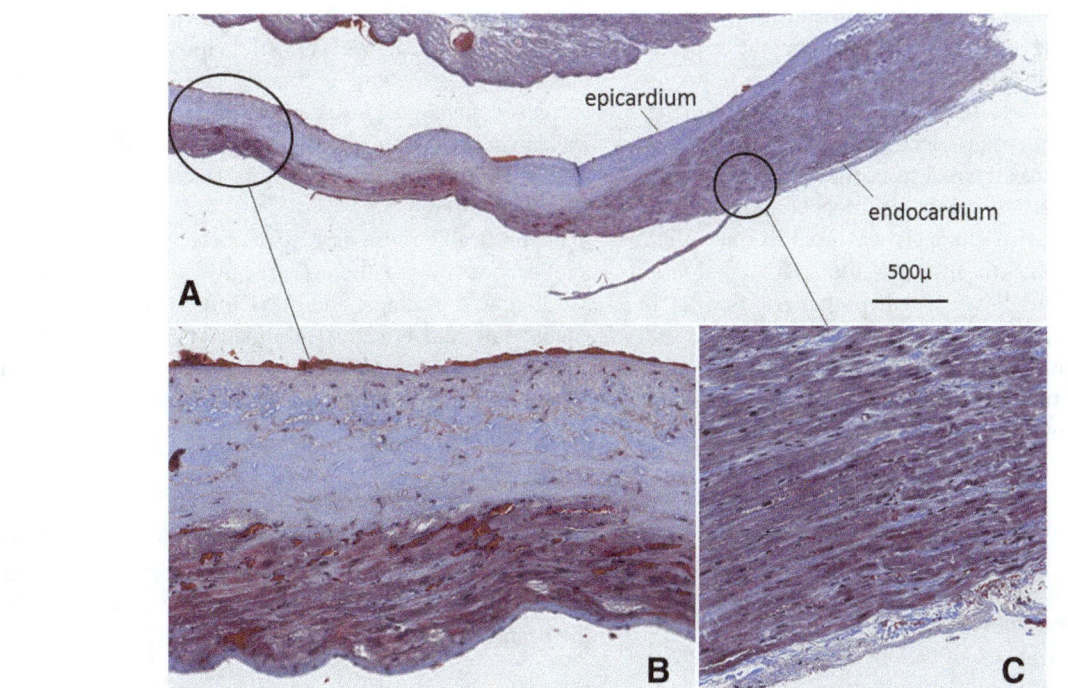

Fig. 6 Histopathologic changes in the ablated right atrium. **a** Histologic examination showed preservation of both the endocardium and epicardium of the coagulated lesion. Both the endocardium and the epicardium were intact. **b** Severely degenerated myocardium was observed from the epicardial side to the mid-portion of the atrial wall. The endocardial side showed swelling and hyperchromatosis of the nuclei, acidophilic change in the cytoplasm, and deformity of the myocardium. **c** Myocardium was intact at the endocardial side of the marginal legion

block across the inferior pulmonary veins (PVs) and across the roof line connecting the two superior PVs were only 58.0 and 24.3%, respectively. Right PVs were found to have been isolated in a significantly higher proportion of patients (91.4%) than the left PVs (75.7%) were. The low efficacy of epicardial RF ablations in creating a transmural irreversible electrophysiological block, especially on the "unclampable free wall" of the atrium, represent that heat sinking effect of the inner blood flow that weaken the thermal effect of the RF.

We previously reported the fundamental results of using an infrared coagulator in animal models [3–5]. The results of the series of experiments in animal models revealed that an infrared coagulator enables creation of a transmural lesion on the canine beating right ventricle to a maximum depth of 10.3 mm, a conduction block on an arrested heart, and a conduction block on a beating right atrium. A successful epicardial maze procedure and successful electrical isolation of the right atrial appendage with an infrared coagulator and concomitant on-pump beating coronary artery bypass grafting have been reported in a clinical case [6, 7].

A cuboid probe was newly developed to create a linear lesion and conduction block on the atrial free wall. To demonstrate the conduction block on the beating heart, encircled lesions e.g. the both atrial appendage, PV cuffs, or box lesion are easy because the ineffective overdrive pacing from inside the lesion can prove the exit block. By contrast, it is difficult to demonstrate a conduction block on a beating atrial free wall. Intraoperative epicardial mapping with multi-electrodes is in common use, but it requires a large-scaled mapping system. Furthermore, because the multi-electrodes are just placed on the epicardium, not attached to it, they slip, and it is difficult to be estimate the exact electrical conduction time. A polygraph with two channels was used in our patient, and it was possible to measure the exact conduction time in every heart beats. We hypothesized that an increase in the translesion stimulus-excitation delay indicates a continuous, transmural, linear lesion, and that the translesion stimulus-excitation delay is directly proportional to path length in the viable tissue around the lesion. Himel et al. demonstrated that complete lesions with RF in rabbit hearts increase translesion stimulus-excitation delay, whereas incomplete lesions do not increase the delay [8]. As far as we investigated, there is no report that proved the stimulus excitation delay on the ablated epicardial atrial free wall in a clinical case. The right atrial free wall was selected for examination. It is easy to apply the cuboid-shaped probe to the right atrial free wall, and it was thought that it would be more difficult to make a transmural lesion in the right atrium than in the left atrium, because the right atrium has a complicated inner structure due to its thick trabecular muscle.

In our patient the myocardium was ablated intermittently at 2-s intervals. Intermittent ablations are more effective than long continuous ablations, because the intervals prevent rapid temperature rise, and prevent to make charring that blocks the photo-energy radiation deep inside the myocardium.

The actual conduction prolongation ratios in the present study were smaller than the predicted ratios, and the main reason for the smaller ratios is thought to be that it was difficult to determine the exact distance between the ablation line and alligator clip electrodes. To determine the more acculate distance, using small bipolar needle electrodes is better. Marginal non-transmural lesions and atrial tissue shrinkage are considered to be other factors that affect conduction time; both factors may shorten the conduction distance and reduce the prolongation ratio.

Pathological examination of the tissue obtained from our patient confirmed the presence of transmural degeneration, however, it was not homogeneous. It may represent the heat sinking effect of the inner blood flow. Considering the result of the presented electrophysiologocal study, there may be a discrepancy between the histopathological transmurality of the lesion and its electrophysiological transmurality. The histopathological change may not exactly represent the electrophysiological change but instead underestimate it by overlooking the pathologically normal but electrophysiologically remodeled lesion of the myocardium. Chronic reversibility of the prolonged conduction time was not investigated in this study. However, in a previous animal study we verified hemosiderin deposition, macrophage invasion, increased capillary vessels, and increased juvenile elastic fibers in the right atrial free wall 3 months after ablation. The myocardium did not revive, the endocardium became thickened, and elastic fibers appeared.

Theoretically, same as RF, this new technology can be applied not only to the atrium but also to the ventricle. Modifying the shape and flexibility of the probe may enable safe and effective minimally invasive endoscopic ablation to create a box lesion on the beating left atrium and to treat ventricular tachycardia based on the same tissue photocoagulation principle as described above.

Conclusions

The newly developed cuboid probe of the Kyo-co infrared coagulator may have the potential to serve as a reliable device for performing the epicardial maze procedure on the beating atrial free wall clinically.

Abbreviations

ECG: Electrocardiogram; RF: Radiofrequency

Acknowledgments

The authors wish to thank Ms. Yuki Matsumoto for her assistance with the data analysis in this study.

Funding

This study was supported by funding from the "Leading-edge Industry Design Project, Medical Innovation, Saitama Prefecture, Japan, 2016."

Authors' contributions

HK designed and drafted the MS. HE, HI, HT, and YI drafted and revised the MS. YT, and KT analyzed and interpreted the measured data. All authors have approved to the submission of the MS.

Competing interests

The authors declare that they have no competing interests.

References

1. Nath S, Lynch C III, Whayne JG, Haines DE. Cellular electrophysiological effects of hyperthermia on isolated Guinea pig papillary muscle. Implications for catheter ablation. Circulation. 1993;88:1826–31.
2. Bulava A, Mokracek A, Kurfirst V. Delayed electroanatomic mapping after surgical ablation for persistent atrial fibrillation. Ann Thorac Surg. 2017; 104(6):2024–9.
3. Kubota H, Furuse A, Takeshita M, Kotsuka Y, Takamoto S. Atrial ablation with an IRK-151 infrared coagulator. Ann Thorac Surg. 1998;66:95–100.
4. Kubota H, Takamoto S, Takeshita M, Miyaji K, Kotsuka Y, Furuse A. Atrial ablation using an IRK-151 infrared coagulator in canine model. J Cardiovasc Surg. 2000;41:835–47.
5. Kubota H, Kenichi S, Takamoto S, et al. Clinical result of epicardial pulmonary vein isolation (LAVIE) by cryoablation as concomitant cardiac operation and clinical application of new device (KIRC-119 infrared coagulator) to treat atrial fibrillation. In: Choi JI, editor. Atrial fibrillation-basic research and clinical applications. Croatia: Intech; 2011. p. 267–90.
6. Kubota H, Takamoto S, Furuse A, et al. Epicardial maze procedure on the beating heart with an infrared coagulator. Ann Thorac Surg. 2005;80:1081–6.
7. Kubota H, Sudo K, Takamoto S, et al. Epicardial electrical isolation of the right atrial appendage on the beating heart with an infrared coagulator. Ann Thorac Surg. 2009;87:1592–5.
8. Himel IV, Dumas HJ III, Kiser AC, Knisley SB. Translesion stimulus-excitation delay indicates quality of linear lesions produced by radiofrequency ablation in rabbit hearts. Physiol Meas. 2007;28:611–23.

24

The EZ-blocker for one-lung ventilation in patients undergoing thoracic surgery: clinical applications and experience in 100 cases in a routine clinical setting

Andreas Moritz[1*], Andrea Irouschek[2], Torsten Birkholz[3], Johannes Prottengeier[4], Horia Sirbu[5] and Joachim Schmidt[6]

Abstract

Background: In certain clinical situations the insertion of a double-lumen tube (DLT) for one-lung ventilation (OLV) is not feasible or unfavorable. In these cases, the EZ-Blocker (EZB) may serve as an alternative. The aim of our analysis was to report on the clinical applications and our experience with the EZB for one-lung ventilation in 100 patients undergoing thoracic surgery.

Methods: All anesthetic records from patients older than 18 years of age undergoing general anesthesia in the department of thoracic surgery with intraoperative use of an EZB for OLV at the University Hospital of Erlangen in four consecutive years were analyzed retrospectively.

Results: Most frequently, EZB was used in difficult airway (27%) and for surgical procedures with high risk for left recurrent laryngeal nerve injury (21%), followed by application in intubated (12%) or tracheostomized (11%) patients. 11% of the patients had an increased risk of gastric regurgitation. Almost all EZBs were placed free of complications (99%). Clinically sufficient lung collapse was achieved in all patients. No serious airway injuries or immediate complications were documented.

Conclusions: The EZB is an efficient, easy-to-use and safe airway device and enables OLV in several clinical situations, when conventional DLTs are not feasible or less favorable. Three major applications were depicted from the data: expected difficult airway, surgical procedures with necessity of intraoperative recurrent laryngeal nerve monitoring and already intubated or tracheostomized patients.

Keywords: One-lung ventilation, Bronchial blocker, EZ-blocker, Thoracic surgery

Background

Thoracic surgery often requires lung separation and one-lung ventilation (OLV) to perform certain surgical procedures and to provide optimal site exposure. The most commonly used device is the double-lumen tube (DLT) [1]. However, the DLT is more rigid and has a larger outer diameter compared with a single-lumen tube (SLT). The placement of a DLT for one-lung ventilation may be technically difficult and has an increased risk for trauma to the trachea and the mainstem bronchi [2, 3].

Therefore the DLT should be avoided for rapid sequence induction. It is not feasible in patients with a difficult airway or tracheostomy, in patients who require unplanned OLV during an ongoing surgery or who might need prolonged mechanical ventilation after surgery, including already intubated critically ill patients [4]. To achieve lung isolation in these settings, bronchial blockers (BBs), such as Cohen Flex-tip Blocker (Cook Critical Care, Bloomington, IN) [5], the Univent Torque Control Blocker (Vitaid, Lewiston, USA) [6] and the wire-guided Arndt Endobronchial Blocker (Cook Critical Care, Bloomington, USA) [7] can be used.

The BB is a balloon-tipped semirigid catheter and can be positioned bronchoscopically into a bronchus through

* Correspondence: andreas.moritz@kfa.imed.uni-erlangen.de
[1]Department of Anesthesiology, University Hospital of Erlangen, Krankenhausstrasse 12, 91054 Erlangen, Germany
Full list of author information is available at the end of the article

the inner diameter of a single-lumen tube (SLT) via a multiport adapter. It allows lung collapse distal to the occlusion. BBs cause less postoperative sore throat and hoarseness compared with DLTs [2, 8]. Campos and Kernstine demonstrated that for elective thoracic surgery the efficacy to achieve lung isolation is comparable between the DLT and the BB [9]. However, potential disadvantages include longer placement time and difficulties in device positioning, higher incidences of dislocation during surgical manipulation and very limited suctioning through the blocker [10, 11]. Another disadvantage of the BB is the difficulty of alternating OLV to either lung for bilateral procedures.

The EZ-Blocker (EZB; AnaesthetIQ, Rotterdam, The Netherlands) (Fig. 1), a 7-French, 75-cm, 4-lumina Y-shaped semirigid endobronchial blocker, combines some of the advantages of the DLT and the BB. This device has two different colored distal extensions, both with an inflatable cuff and a small central lumen. Two pilot balloons at the proximal part of the device serve to inflate/deflate the cuffs. Two additional lumina are available for suction or oxygen insufflation. The EZB is inserted through the designated port on the enclosed multiport adapter attached to a conventional SLT (minimum 7 mm inner diameter (I.D.)). The multiport adapter is designed to connect to a ventilation device and contains two additional upper ports, one for the blocker itself and the other for the bronchoscope. The blocker is introduced and positioned under direct bronchoscopic vision with the extensions in the left and the right mainstem bronchi (Fig. 2). However, proper deployment of the Y-shaped distal part requires a minimum of 4 cm distance between the distal end of the SLT and the carina. The Y-shape of the distal portion allows the blocker to anchor on the carina. Thus, the EZB is less prone to secondary malposition than other devices [10, 12]. The cuffs can be inflated

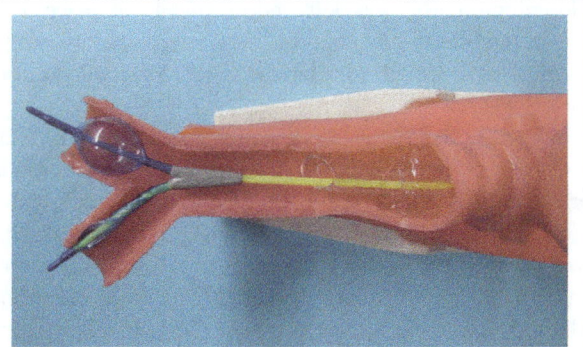

Fig. 1 Close-up view of the EZB placed through a single-lumen tube in a manikin. The Y-shape of the distal portion facilitates the anchorage of the blocker to the carina. The two distal extensions are colored differently, both with an inflatable cuff and a central lumen. One of the polyurethane high-pressure balloons is inflated, allowing lung collapse distal to the occlusion

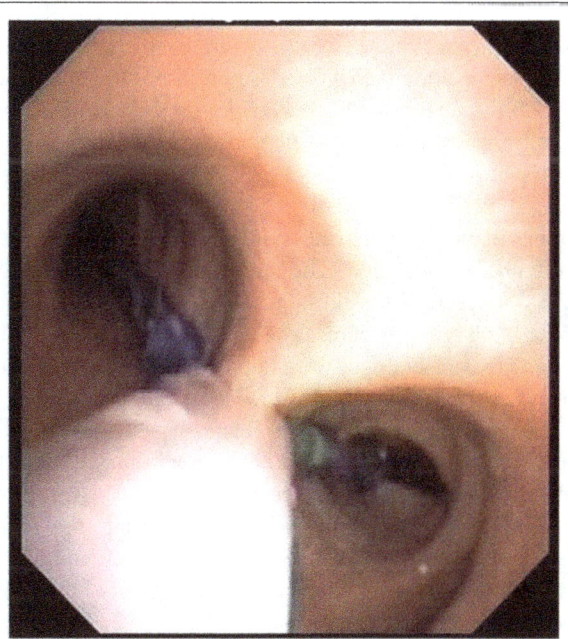

Fig. 2 Bronchoscopic view of an EZB situated in the trachea and bronchi of a patient. The differently colored extensions are positioned in the left and the right mainstem bronchi

separately, allowing OLV in either lung during the same procedure [13].

Rispoli and colleagues demonstrated that the EZB can also be used via tracheostomy [14]. Furthermore, in combination with an electromyographic endotracheal tube system (NIM EMG Endotracheal Tube, Medtronic Xomed, Jacksonville, FL) the EZB, as well as other BBs, enables recurrent laryngeal nerve monitoring during single lung ventilation [15]. This method is routinely used in our hospital in surgical procedures with necessity of OLV and high risk for left recurrent laryngeal nerve (RLN) injury.

Only a few clinical reports have assessed routine clinical performance of the EZB. In the present analysis we therefore report on the clinical applications and our experience with the intraoperative use of the EZB for OLV in 100 patients undergoing thoracic surgery in a routine clinical setting.

Methods

All anesthetic records from patients older than 18 years of age undergoing general anesthesia in the department of thoracic surgery with intraoperative use of an EZB for OLV at the University Hospital of Erlangen in four consecutive years (January 2009 to December 2012) were analyzed retrospectively. The analysis included patient demographics, Mallampati score, Cormack and Lehane (CML) classification, surgical procedure, site of surgery, time-span of clinical experience of the responsible anesthesiologist, anesthesia drugs used for induction and maintenance, airway management, type of airway devices used, indications for the use of an EZB, difficulty with EZB placement, adequacy and duration of OLV, incidence of EZB dislocation and bronchial injury, possible decrease of oxygen saturation, ventilation parameters, need for postoperative ventilation and finally adverse events during anesthesia. The data were retrieved from the electronic patient data management system (NarkoData; IMESO, Hüttenberg, Germany). The indications for the use of an EZB were recorded at the time of insertion. The adequacy of lung collapse was clinically assessed by the thoracic surgeon. All available data were anonymized and transferred to an Excel datasheet (Microsoft, Redmond, USA).

The University Hospital of Erlangen provides the full spectrum of thoracic surgery. For thoracic anesthesia with OLV standard operation procedures (SOPs) were well established and remained unchanged during the study period. The SOPs included induction and maintenance of anesthesia, as well as the clinical management of OLV and the use of different devices for OLV (DLT, EZB, BB). Standard monitoring for thoracic surgery with OLV included electrocardiogram, pulse oximetry, capnography and invasive blood pressure (SC9000XL System; Siemens, Erlangen, Germany). The DLT represents the standard device for OLV. During the reported time period, the Arndt Endobronchial Blocker and the EZB served as an alternative. EZB use in routine clinical practice was provided as follows: After induction of anesthesia and insertion of a SLT (Rüschelit Super Safety Clear, Rüsch GmbH, Kernen, Germany; Mallinckrodt Lo-Contour Oral/Nasal Tracheal Tube Cuffed Reinforced, Covidien, Tullamore, Ireland; in case of RLN monitoring: NIM EMG Endotracheal Tube, Medtronic Xomed, Jacksonville, FL) the patients were placed in a right or left decubitus position for the surgical procedure. After verifying under direct bronchoscopic vision that the distal end of the SLT is at least 4 cm above the carina, the EZB was lubricated with silicone spray and introduced through one of the two proximal ports of the multiport adapter with its cuffs completely deflated. Further advance was guided with a fiberoptic bronchoscope (FOB), placing the distal EZB ends into the right and left mainstem bronchi under direct bronchoscopic vision. If there was less than 4 cm distance between the distal end of the SLT and the carina, the SLT was retracted more proximal. With the EZB finally properly placed, the SLT was readvanced into the trachea as necessary. Both movements required a deflated SLT cuff. To test the bronchial sealing, the cuff of the EZB was inflated under FOB guidance with an appropriate volume and deflated again. The insertion technique described was used for all patients from the commencement of the study period and all EZBs were placed under supervision of an attending physician in accordance with the standard operation procedure (SOP). To facilitate unilateral lung

collapse, a specific sequence of action was used after the surgeon breaks the pleural vacuum: First, disconnection of the tube from the ventilator allows the operated lung to collapse. After 20 s, reinflation of the blocker cuff with the same volume of air as used before and reconnection of the tube to the ventilator establishes ventilation of the dependent lung. In case of ventilation problems as an increased peak pressure or total/subtotal ventilation of the non-dependent lung, the SOP ordered immediate FOB examination to check and eventually reposition the EZB. According to the SOP, after removing the EZB at the end of surgery, the mucosa of the tracheobronchial system was observed with the FOB for possible damage due to the EZB.

For surgical procedures with high risk for left RLN injury, e. g. resection of the left upper lobe and lymph node dissection in the aortopulmonal window, a ready-made EMG endotracheal tube system (NIM EMG Endotracheal Tube, Medtronic Xomed, Jacksonville, USA) was used for RLN monitoring during single lung ventilation [15].

In case of an expected difficult airway, awake fiberoptic intubation was performed initially via the nasotracheal route using a flexible fiberoptic bronchoscope. To prevent potential trauma to the nasal turbinates, the septum or the posterior nares, a smaller SLT (size 6.5 to 7.0 mm I.D.) was primarily inserted. However, for the EZB a SLT with a minimum I.D. of 7 mm is necessary. Moreover, sinusitis and local abscesses as a complication of nasotracheal intubation have been reported in critically ill patients who needed prolonged mechanical ventilation after surgery [16]. Thus, after induction of general anesthesia, the patients received video laryngoscopy (Glidescope, Verathon Medical, Rennerod, Germany or C-MAC Karl Storz, Tuttlingen, Germany) or flexible orotracheal fiberoptic bronchoscopy to change the airway to an orotracheal SLT of 7 mm I.D. (female patients) to 8 mm I.D. (male patients). To maintain airway access at any time, a Cook Airway Exchange Catheter (CAEC, Cook Medical Inc., Bloomington, IN) was left endotracheally in place after the nasotracheal tube has been removed. Before placement of the orotracheal tube, the CAEC was pulled out of the trachea.

In case of a difficult airway and the necessity of RLN monitoring awake fiberoptic nasotracheal intubation was primarily performed. The patients were then reintubated orotracheally with the Xomed EMG endotracheal tube size 7.0 mm I.D. (female patients) to 8.0 mm I.D. (male patients), using video laryngoscopy (Glidescope, Verathon Medical, Rennerod, Germany or C-MAC Karl Storz, Tuttlingen, Germany) or flexible orotracheal fiberoptic bronchoscopy and a CAEC.

Data were anonymized for statistical analysis. Descriptive statistical analysis was done using Statistica version 6 (StatSoft (Europe) GmbH, Hamburg, Germany). Categorical variables were given as absolute numbers and percentages of their occurrence. Continuous variables were presented as medians (interquartile range, IQR).

Results

Over the study period the electronic data records from 100 patients undergoing general anesthesia in the department of thoracic surgery with intraoperative use of an EZB for OLV were analyzed. In the same period 1208 DLTs were used for lung isolation. Characteristic data of the patients included in the analysis and surgical procedures are summarized in Table 1.

The involved anesthesiologists had a median clinical experience of 5 years (IQR: 3.5–7.8) and worked under close supervision of attending physicians.

Anesthesia induction was performed with etomidate (46%), propofol (44%), thiopentone (9%) or ketamine and midazolam (1%). Fentanyl (88%), sufentanil (8%) or remifentanil (4%) were used as intravenous anesthetic agents for induction. Rocuronium (83%), cis-atracurium (10%), succinylcholine (5%) or mivacurium (1%) were used as neuromuscular blocking agents. Anesthesia was maintained by total intravenous anesthesia (TIVA) using propofol in combination with fentanyl, remifentanil or sufentanil.

After induction of general anesthesia, most of the patients with EZB for OLV were intubated orotracheally (64%). In case of difficult airway, fiberoptic bronchoscope-guided awake nasotracheal intubation was performed (13%). Tracheostomized (11%) or already intubated patients from the intensive care unit (12%) were also enrolled in this retrospective analysis. The size of the SLTs used in this study varied from 6.5 to 7.0 mm I.D. for nasotracheal and from 7.0 to 8.0 mm I.D. for orotracheal intubation. The tracheostomy tubes had an internal diameter from 8.0 mm to 10.0 mm. The mean cumulative time of OLV was 67 min (IQR: 43–85 min). During OLV, pressure-controlled ventilation (91%) or volume-controlled ventilation (9%) was used on the dependent lung.

Difficult airway (27%) or surgical procedures with necessity of OLV and high risk for left RLN injury (21%) were the most frequent preconditions. The EZB was also used in already intubated (12%) or tracheostomized (11%) patients. 11% of our patients had an increased risk of gastric regurgitation. The clinical applications of the EZB are summarized in Table 2. In one case, a DLT was not feasible because the endobronchial portion of the DLT, placed in the left mainstem bronchus, applied too much pressure to the carina. Thus, the patient had to be reintubated with a SLT and an EZB was placed for OLV.

No complications were reported in 99% of patients. In a single case, the EZB got stuck with the FOB inside the SLT. However, the patient was reintubated and the EZB was introduced and positioned without any problems. Clinically sufficient lung collapse was achieved in all

Table 1 Characteristics of patients, distribution of surgical procedures and site of surgery

Patient characteristics	n (%) or median (IQR)
Gender, n (%)	
Female	32 (32)
Male	68 (68)
Age (y), median (IQR)	65.5 (53–70.5)
BMI (kg/m^2), median (IQR)	25.3 (21.8–29)
ASA physical status, n (%)	
I	3 (3)
II	33 (33)
III	52 (52)
IV	12 (12)
Mallampati score, n (%)	
I	18 (18)
II	38 (38)
III	14 (14)
IV	6 (6)
not specified	24 (24)
CML classification, n (%)	
I	41 (41)
II	8 (8)
III	7 (7)
IV	0 (0)
not specified	44 (44)
Surgical procedures, n (%)	
VATS procedure	36 (36)
Wedge resection	12 (12)
Segment resection	3 (3)
Ligation of thoracic duct	3 (3)
Pleural decortication	3 (3)
Lobectomy	1 (1)
Other surgical procedures	14 (14)
Thoracotomy	64 (64)
Lobectomy	17 (17)
Wedge resection	12 (12)
Pleural decortication	7 (7)
Segment resection	6 (6)
Pneumonectomy	2 (2)
Bilobectomy	1 (1)
Ligation of thoracic duct	1 (1)
Other surgical procedures	18 (18)
Site of surgery, n (%)	
Right	51 (51)
Left	46 (46)
Bilateral	2 (2)
Median sternotomy	1 (1)

Data are presented as absolute number of patients (%) or as median (IQR)

Table 2 Clinical applications of the EZB

Documented indications	n (%)
Difficult airway	27 (27)
Oral cancer	12 (12)
Vocal cord dysfunction	4 (4)
Mediastinal mass syndrome	1 (1)
Subcutaneous emphysema	1 (1)
Limited mouth opening	1 (1)
Tracheal dislocation	1 (1)
Other reasons	7 (7)
RLN monitoring	21 (21)
Intubated patients	12 (12)
Tracheostomized patients	11 (11)
Rapid sequence induction	11 (11)
Not fasting	3 (3)
Obesity	2 (2)
Gastroesophageal reflux disease	1 (1)
Other reasons for increased risk of gastric regurgitation	5 (5)
Difficult airway and RLN monitoring	5 (5)
Rapid sequence induction and RLN monitoring	1 (1)
Other reasons	4 (4)
DLT cuff leak	1 (1)
DLT not placeable	1 (1)
DLT applied too much pressure to the carina	1 (1)
Ailing teeth	1 (1)
Medical education	8 (8)

Data are presented as absolute number (%)

patients. In one patient OLV had to be abandoned due to severe desaturation (oxygen saturation < 90%) on initiation of lung collapse. In two cases, the EZB had to be repositioned under FOB guidance due to lung isolation failure during surgical manipulations.

No serious airway injuries or immediate complications from EZB placement or FOB were documented. In a single patient with pleural empyema, the EZB had to be removed intraoperatively due to an unplanned bilobectomy of the right lung. The distal extension of the EZB in the right mainstem bronchus interfered with the surgical procedure and was at risk of being caught in the sutures.

92% of the patients received postoperative intensive care, whereof 29% required ventilatory support. 8% were transferred to the intermediate care unit or the thoracic surgery ward after a minimum of one hour in the anesthesia recovery room.

Discussion

In several clinical situations, lung separation and OLV are essential. The choice of airway device for OLV depends on the experience of the anesthesiologist and the requirements of the surgical procedure. The DLT is still the most commonly used device to enable single lung ventilation [1]. However, in some situations conventional DLTs for one-lung ventilation are not feasible [4]. In these cases, a BB or an EZB serve as valuable alternatives. There have been relatively few reports that have assessed the effectiveness of the EZB in a routine clinical setting. It has been shown that the EZB can be positioned quickly and easily during OLV [17, 18]. As previous reports mainly focused on the performance of the device, the aim of our analysis was to report on the clinical applications and our experience with the EZB in a routine clinical setting.

The successful use of the EZB has been reported in patients with a difficult airway or tracheostomy, in those with increased risk of gastric regurgitation or who have unplanned OLV requirements during an ongoing surgery and who might need prolonged mechanical ventilation after surgery including critically ill intubated patients [4]. We could confirm these findings. In our analysis the most common indication for the use of the EZB was an expected difficult airway. The EZB enables OLV after awake fiberoptic intubation and thus improves the safety of these patients. Tracheostomized or already intubated patients were represented in almost equal numbers. As airway exchange in these critically ill patients is associated with an increased risk of clinically important procedural complications [19], BBs and especially the EZB might pose significant advantages in the management of these patients.

About one-tenth of our patients had an increased risk of gastric regurgitation. As the placement of a DLT for OLV may be technically difficult and may require too much time the EZB serves as a safe and easy alternative in patients with the necessity of a rapid sequence induction. Moreover, we could demonstrate another indication for the use of an EZB. In combination with a Xomed EMG endotracheal tube the EZB enabled recurrent laryngeal nerve monitoring during left upper lobe surgery or aortopulmonary window lymph node dissection, with high risk for left RLN injury and necessity of OLV, in twenty-one patients. The advantages of this method are as follows: RLN monitoring is possible even in cases of difficult airway or rapid sequence induction, and it allows repositioning of the SLT at any time in case of lacking EMG signal maintaining OLV [15]. RLN monitoring in patients requiring OLV could also be performed with any other BB. However, the main advantage of an EZB compared to other BBs is its Y-design, which shows similarities with the anatomic structure of the tracheobronchial tree. Based on our clinical experience the Y-shaped distal part allows the blocker to anchor on the carina and leads to positional stability. The EZB is secured between the carina and the seal at the proximal end of the tracheal tube. Thus, the two distal extensions, which are positioned in the left and the right mainstem bronchi, mutually stabilize each other by applying counter pressure on the bronchial mucosa in case of surgical manipulation. This is according to the findings of Kus and colleagues, who described that the EZB had a lower incidence of malpositioning than the Cohen Flex-Tip Blocker [12]. In addition, the Arndt Endobronchial Blocker is even less stable than the Cohen Flex-Tip and other BBs [10]. Mourisse and colleagues observed, that the EZB causes less injury to the tracheal and bronchial mucosa, when compared with the DLT. Furthermore, the quality of lung deflation is equally good and the EZB stays equally well in place during OLV [18]. Our findings confirm the positional stability. During OLV, the EZB had to be repositioned in two cases only. Kus and colleagues also demonstrated that the EZB had a shorter time to correct positioning compared with the Cohen Flex-tip Blocker [12]. Another advantage of the EZB is the possibility to alternate OLV to either lung during bilateral procedures in already intubated or tracheostomized patients. During the study period the EZB enabled OLV during bilateral VATS (Video Assisted Thoracoscopic Surgery) procedure and bilateral thoracotomy in two critically ill intubated patients. In contrast to the DLT, there is also no need to change the SLT in cases where postoperative ventilation is mandatory.

Regarding the cost-effectiveness, the EZB is almost four times more expensive than a DLT. Therefore the EZB should be used efficiently in the depicted applications. However, compared to other BBs, based on our purchase price, the EZB is marginally cheaper than the Arndt Endobronchial Blocker.

Despite of the described advantages and the almost equal cost when compared with other BBs, the EZB has some limitations which have to be mentioned. First, the EZB is initially designed for adult patients and thus only available in one size. Although extraluminal placement of an EZB can be successfully used to provide lung isolation in children down to 6 years of age [20], we use an Arndt Endobronchial Blocker for pediatric patients. The 5-French Arndt Endobronchial Blocker can be used as a consistent, safe method of single lung ventilation in most young children. The smallest tracheal tube recommended for use with this BB is 4.5 mm I.D. [21]. Second, in one case the EZB had to be removed due to an unplanned resection of the right mainstem bronchus. Thus, in some clinical situations, such as pneumonectomy or bronchial sleeve resection, where the presence of the distal tip of an EZB or any other BB would interfere with the surgical procedure or would be at risk of being stuck in the sutures, DLTs may be more suitable. Third, an EZB cannot be used for selective lobar blockade, which can be performed with other BBs. We therefor also use the Arndt Endobronchial Blocker. Fourth, a minimum of 4 cm distance between the distal end of the SLT and the carina

is mandatory to permit the Y-shaped distal part to be deployed properly. Finally, another important limitation of the EZB is the smaller suction channel, when compared with a DLT. The EZB has a 7-French outer diameter, which is split into two lumens leaving a minimal diameter for each lumen. Thus, it is nearly impossible to apply any effective suction or oxygen insufflation to the nondependent lung in case of hypoxemia [22].

Vegh and colleagues found that the use of the EZB was safe and easy [23]. We can confirm these findings. No complications were reported in 99% of patients. Clinically sufficient lung collapse was achieved in all patients. However, the use of FOB guidance for initial placement and for repositioning must be considered as mandatory, but this also applies for the DLT and other BBs. No serious tracheobronchial injuries or immediate complications from EZB placement or FOB were documented. Only in one case the EZB got stuck with the FOB inside the SLT due to an overly fast FOB advancement. This could be avoided by carefully advancing the FOB in a safe distance to the Y-shaped distal part of the EZB.

The present analysis has certain limitations, mainly related to its retrospective character. First, as in every retrospective analysis, the clinical circumstances were not uniform for every case. Second, the retrospective nature of the study implies a high dependency on the quality and completeness of documentation. Finally, in this study OLV was performed by anesthesiologists with a median clinical experience of 5 years and under supervision of an attending physician. Thus, results may differ in the hands of less experienced anesthesiologists.

Conclusions

The EZB is an efficient, easy-to-use and safe airway device to allow single lung ventilation and to provide optimal surgical exposure. The EZB combines the advantages of the DLT and the BB and enables OLV in several clinical situations, when conventional DLTs are not feasible or less favorable. Three major applications were depicted from the data: expected difficult airway, surgical procedures with necessity of RLN monitoring and already intubated or tracheostomized patients.

Abbreviations

BB: Bronchial blocker; CAEC: Cook Airway Exchange Catheter; CML: Cormack and Lehane; DLT: Double-lumen tube; EZB: EZ-Blocker; FOB: Fiberoptic bronchoscope; I.D.: Inner diameter; IQR: Interquartile range; OLV: One-lung ventilation; RLN: Recurrent laryngeal nerve; SLT: Single-lumen tube; SOP: Standard operation procedures; TIVA: Total intravenous anesthesia; VATS: Video assisted thoracoscopic surgery

Acknowledgements

The authors thank the entire anesthesiology staff of the University Hospital Erlangen for the disciplined documentation throughout the last years.

Authors' contributions

AM conceived the study, analyzed the results and drafted the manuscript. JP contributed to the data analyses. AI, TB and HS critically reviewed the manuscript and offered guidance. JS helped to analyze the anesthesia records and to draft the manuscript. All authors read and approved the final manuscript.

Competing interests

The authors declare that they have no competing interests.

Author details

[1]Department of Anesthesiology, University Hospital of Erlangen, Krankenhausstrasse 12, 91054 Erlangen, Germany. [2]Department of Anesthesiology, University Hospital of Erlangen, Krankenhausstrasse 12, 91054 Erlangen, Germany. [3]Department of Anesthesiology, University Hospital of Erlangen, Krankenhausstrasse 12, 91054 Erlangen, Germany. [4]Department of Anesthesiology, University Hospital of Erlangen, Krankenhausstrasse 12, 91054 Erlangen, Germany. [5]Department of Thoracic Surgery, University Hospital of Erlangen, Krankenhausstrasse 12, 91054 Erlangen, Germany. [6]Department of Anesthesiology, University Hospital of Erlangen, Krankenhausstrasse 12, 91054 Erlangen, Germany.

References

1. Lewis JW, Serwin JP, Gabriel FS, Bastanfar M, Jacobsen G. The utility of a double-lumen tube for one-lung ventilation in a variety of noncardiac thoracic surgical procedures. J Cardiothorac Vasc Anesth. 1992;6:705–10.
2. Knoll H, Ziegeler S, Schreiber JU, et al. Airway injuries after one-lung ventilation: a comparison between double-lumen tube and endobronchial blocker: a randomized, prospective, controlled trial. Anesthesiology. 2006;105:471–7.
3. Fitzmaurice BG, Brodsky JB. Airway rupture from double-lumen tubes. J Cardiothorac Vasc Anesth. 1999;13:322–9.
4. Campos JH. An update on bronchial blockers during lung separation techniques in adults. Anesth Analg. 2003;97:1266–74.
5. Cohen E. The Cohen flexitip endobronchial blocker: an alternative to a double lumen tube. Anesth Analg. 2005;101:1877–9.
6. Inoue H, Shohtsu A, Ogawa J, Kawada S, Koide S. New device for one-lung anesthesia: endotracheal tube with movable blocker. J Thorac Cardiovasc Surg. 1982;83:940–1.
7. Arndt GA, DeLessio ST, Kranner PW, Orzepowski W, Ceranski B, Valtysson B. One-lung ventilation when intubation is difficult–presentation of a new endobronchial blocker. Acta Anaesthesiol Scand. 1999;43:356–8.
8. Zhong T, Wang W, Chen J, Ran L. Story DA sore throat or hoarse voice with bronchial blockers or double-lumen tubes for lung isolation: a randomised prospective trial. Anaesth Intensive Care. 2009;37:441–6.
9. Campos JH, Kernstine KH. A comparison of a left-sided Broncho-Cath with the torque control blocker univent and the wire-guided blocker. Anesth Analg. 2003;96:283–9. table of contents
10. Narayanaswamy M, McRae K, Slinger P, et al. Choosing a lung isolation device for thoracic surgery: a randomized trial of three bronchial blockers versus double-lumen tubes. Anesth Analg. 2009;108:1097–101.
11. Campos JH. Which device should be considered the best for lung isolation: double-lumen endotracheal tube versus bronchial blockers. Curr Opin Anaesthesiol. 2007;20:27–31.
12. Kus A, Hosten T, Gurkan Y, Gul Akgul A, Solak M, Toker K. A comparison of the EZ-blocker with a Cohen flex-tip blocker for one-lung ventilation. J Cardiothorac Vasc Anesth. 2014;28:896–9.
13. Brodsky JB, Tzabazis A, Basarb-Tung J, Shrager JB. Sequential bilateral lung isolation with a single bronchial blocker. A A Case Rep. 2013;1:17–8.
14. Rispoli M, Nespoli MR, Salvi R, Corcione A, Buono S. One-lung ventilation in tracheostomized patients: our experience with EZ-blocker. J Clin Anesth. 2016;31:288–90.
15. Schmidt J, Irouschek A, Heinrich S, Oster O, Klein P, Birkholz T. Recurrent laryngeal nerve monitoring during esophagectomy and mediastinal lymph node dissection: a novel approach using a single-lumen endotracheal EMG tube and the EZ-blocker. World J Surg. 2012;36:2946–7. author reply 8
16. O'Reilly MJ, Reddick EJ, Black W, et al. Sepsis from sinusitis in nasotracheally intubated patients A diagnostic dilemma. Am J Surg. 1984;147:601–4.
17. Ruetzler K, Grubhofer G, Schmid W, et al. Randomized clinical trial comparing double-lumen tube and EZ-blocker for single-lung ventilation. Br J Anaesth. 2011;106:896–902.
18. Mourisse J, Liesveld J, Verhagen A, et al. Efficiency, efficacy, and safety of EZ-blocker compared with left-sided double-lumen tube for one-lung ventilation. Anesthesiology. 2013;118:550–61.
19. Elmer J, Lee S, Rittenberger JC, Dargin J, Winger D, Emlet L. Reintubation in critically ill patients: procedural complications and implications for care. Crit Care. 2015;19:12.
20. Templeton TW, Templeton LB, Lawrence AE, Sieren LM, Downard MG, Ririe DG. An initial experience with an Extraluminal EZ-blocker. Paediatr Anaesth. 2018;28:347–51.
21. Wald SH, Mahajan A, Kaplan MB, Atkinson JB. Experience with the Arndt paediatric bronchial blocker. Br J Anaesth. 2005;94:92–4.
22. Cohen E. Back to blockers?: the continued search for the ideal endobronchial blocker. Anesthesiology. 2013;118:490–3.
23. Végh T, Juhász M, Enyedi A, Takács I, Kollár J, Fülesdi B. Clinical experience with a new endobrochial blocker: the EZ-blocker. J Anesth. 2012;26:375–80.

25

Long-term performance of an external stent for saphenous vein grafts: the VEST IV trial

David P. Taggart[1†], Carolyn M. Webb[2,3*†] (iD), Anthony Desouza[4], Rashmi Yadav[4], Keith M. Channon[5], Fabio De Robertis[6] and Carlo Di Mario[3]

Abstract

Background: Externally stenting saphenous vein grafts reduces intimal hyperplasia, improves lumen uniformity and reduces oscillatory shear stress 1 year following surgery. The present study is the first to present the longer-term (4.5 years) performance and biomechanical effects of externally stented saphenous vein grafts.

Methods: Thirty patients previously implanted with the VEST external stent in the randomized, within-patient-controlled VEST I study were followed up for adverse events; 21 of these were available to undergo coronary angiography and intravascular ultrasound.

Results: Twenty-one stented and 29 nonstented saphenous vein grafts were evaluated by angiography and ultrasound at 4.5 ± 0.3 years. Vein graft failure rates were comparable between stented and nonstented grafts (30 and 23% respectively; $p = 0.42$). All failures were apparent at 1 year except for one additional nonstented failure at 4.5 years. In patent vein grafts, Fitzgibbon perfect patency remained significantly higher in the stented versus nonstented vein grafts (81 and 48% respectively, $p = 0.002$), while intimal hyperplasia area ($4.27 \, mm^2 \pm 1.27 \, mm^2$ and $5.23 \, mm^2 \pm 1.83 \, mm^2$ respectively, $p < 0.001$) and thickness ($0.36 \, mm \pm 0.09 \, mm$ and $0.42 \, mm \pm 0.11 \, mm$ respectively, $p < 0.001$) were significantly reduced. Intimal hyperplasia proliferation correlated with lumen uniformity and with the distance between the stent and the lumen ($p = 0.04$ and $p < 0.001$ respectively).

Conclusions: External stenting mitigates saphenous vein graft remodeling and significantly reduces diffuse intimal hyperplasia and the development of lumen irregularities 4.5 years after coronary artery bypass surgery. Close conformity of the stent to the vessel wall appears to be an important factor.

Keywords: Coronary artery bypass graft surgery, Saphenous vein graft, Intimal hyperplasia, External stent

Background

Saphenous vein grafts (SVG) remain the most commonly used conduit in coronary artery bypass grafting (CABG). However, despite significant advances in understanding SVG pathophysiology post implantation, relatively little progress has been made in the clinical setting - current vein graft failure rates range from 35 to 50% 5 to 10 years following CABG surgery [1]. SVG failure is attributed to the onset of structural changes in the conduit immediately post implantation due to its exposure to the hemodynamics of the arterial circulation [2]. SVG remodeling includes an inflammatory response accompanied by the development of intimal hyperplasia (IH) that serves as the foundation for graft thrombosis and occlusive atherosclerosis [2, 3]. Attempts to mitigate IH in vein grafts have been the focus of intense clinical research. However, most of the pharmacological therapeutic modalities have had a limited effect in the clinical setting, except for statins and beta-blockers [4–6].

* Correspondence: c.webb@imperial.ac.uk
†David P. Taggart and Carolyn M. Webb contributed equally to this work.
²National Heart & Lung Institute, Imperial College London, London, UK
³Department of Cardiology, Royal Brompton Hospital, Sydney Street, London SW3 6NP, UK
Full list of author information is available at the end of the article

External stenting of SVGs has long been postulated to have the potential to lessen adverse mechanical and structural changes that contribute to SVG deterioration. In 2015 we reported our first in human experience with a new cobalt chrome external stent for SVGs (VEST, Vascular Graft Solutions, Israel) [7]. At 1 year, externally stented SVGs showed significant reduction in IH, improved lumen uniformity and reduced oscillatory shear stress compared to non-stented SVGs [7]. Conversely, a notable limitation was the lower patency rate of externally stented SVGs to the right compared to the left coronary vessels at 1 year [7]. As recently reported in the VEST II trial in this journal, avoidance of both metal clip ligation of SVG side branches and of fixation of the stent to the anastomoses significantly improved early patency rates of SVGs to the right coronary territory from 55 to 86% [8]. Currently two larger trials of external stenting are underway. VEST III (NCT02511834) is a European multicentre study that completed recruitment of 180 patients in January 2017. The study endpoints are major cardiovascular and cerebral events (MACCE) and graft patency as assessed by CT angiography at 6 months and 2 years. In the USA a similar 224 patient trial has recently started recruiting under the auspices of the Cardiothoracic Surgical Trials Network (VEST Pivotal, NCT 03209609). In the meantime, while several groups have reported 1-year patency rates there are no data in the literature regarding patency rates beyond this. The objective of the current VEST IV study was to investigate the effects of mechanical external stents 4–5 years after CABG.

Methods

Patients and design

The VEST I study prospectively enrolled 30 CABG patients with multi-vessel disease who were implanted with the VEST external stent (Vascular Graft Solutions, Tel Aviv, Israel) in a within-patient randomized controlled design, from October 2011 to September 2012 [7]. Eligible patients were scheduled for on-pump multi-vessel CABG including a left internal mammary artery to the left anterior descending coronary artery and SVGs to right and circumflex territories. Eligibility required a target vessel diameter ≥ 1.5 mm with a coronary stenosis > 75% and with an adequate distal vascular bed, as assessed by preoperative angiography. Each patient received one external stent device to a single SVG, randomly assigned intra-operatively by the opening of a sealed envelope only after all distal anastomoses were performed, to either the right or the circumflex coronary territories. One or more SVG remained non-stented and served as the control group. All SVGs were harvested in an open technique. Transit Time Flow Measurement (TTFM) was determined in all grafts. There was no

significant difference in baseline grafting variables between stented and control groups (Table 2 of reference [7]). The primary effectiveness endpoint compared intimal hyperplasia area between groups, assessed by intravascular ultrasound (IVUS) at 12 months.

In the current extended follow-up study (VEST IV), MACCE data were collected for all patients. MACCE was defined as the composite occurrence of all-cause mortality, myocardial infarction (MI), revascularization, and/or stroke. Only patients who were alive and last known to have at least one patent vein graft were invited to return for a coronary angiogram and IVUS. Patients who did not have angiography underwent telephone follow-up. The study protocol conformed to the Declaration of Helsinki and was approved by a UK Research Ethics Committee. Each patient gave their informed consent to participate in the study.

Angiography and IVUS

Contrast angiography was attempted for all grafts using the same camera angles as in VEST I, and using an identical method of analysis by the same core laboratory. Quantitative coronary angiography (QAngio XA®, Medis, The Netherlands) was performed for all patent grafts. Fitzgibbon grade I, II, or III was assigned to each graft to determine lumen uniformity: I, no intimal irregularity; II/III, irregularity of the intimal surface of < 50 and > 50% respectively [9].

IVUS examination was performed along the entire length of patent vein grafts (40 MHz IVUS catheter with automated 1.0 mm/s pullback, Boston Scientific, Hemel Hempstead, UK). Individual cross sectional IVUS images, approximately 10 mm apart over the entire vein graft length, were analyzed using QIVUS software (QIVUS® Medis, The Netherlands). Lumen and external elastic membrane (EEM) were identified and marked in accordance with convention [10] by an independent observer. IH area was calculated for every cross-section as the area between the EEM and the lumen perimeters. The IH thickness was calculated as the mean EEM radius minus the mean lumen radius. The VEST was identified and marked in the stented grafts and its distance from the lumen was calculated by subtracting the mean lumen radius from the mean VEST radius. To assess IVUS intra-observer variability, 11 pullbacks from 6 vein grafts (3 stented and 3 nonstented) were measured 1 month apart. IVUS intra-observer variability for EEM cross sectional area was $- 0.02 +/- 0.6 mm^2$ ($r = 0.99$, $p = 0.99$), and for lumen was $0.03 +/- 0.24 mm^2$ ($r = 0.99$, $p = 0.97$).

The primary efficacy endpoint compared IH area and thickness between stented and nonstented groups. Graft occlusion and Fitzgibbon perfect patency rates were also compared between the groups. The interaction between various disease markers obtained from the two imaging modalities was quantified by comparing the cross-sectional parameters derived from IVUS across angiographically perfectly patent (Fitzgibbon I) and patent with irregularities (Fitzgibbon II/III) graft groups. The effect of external stent dimensional conformity to the vessel wall was assessed by computing the correlation between stent distance from the lumen and IH thickness for the stented grafts.

Statistical analysis

Descriptive statistics are provided as mean, standard deviation, minimum, median and maximum for continuous variables and as count and percent for non-continuous variables. Statistical testing was done using a mixed-effect model repeated measures, using measures taken at 1 and 4.5 year follow-ups. Continuous variables were analyzed using a linear regression model with ordinal variables analyzed using logistic regression. In both cases, subject was included as a random variable in the model. P-values of the device effect were obtained based on least squares mean estimates over both time points, since no interaction with

time was obtained. Missing values at 4.5 years were inputed by using last observation carried forward from 1 year and included in the model. Pearson correlations were computed between wall thickness and plaque-thickness/area at 1 and 4.5 years separately within the stented grafts group; time points were not combined for this analysis due to the same subjects providing data in each, while Pearson assumes between-subject independence.

Results

Patient characteristics

Of the 30 patients who underwent randomization and treatment with the VEST in the original trial, MACCE data were available for all patients, and angiography and IVUS measurements were available for 21 patients (70%) at a mean (±SD) 4.5 ± 0.3 year follow-up. Of the 9 patients that did not return for angiographic follow-up, 2 had both vein grafts previously known to be occluded and were not asked to return, 3 were deceased, and 4 refused the procedure. Demographic and medical history data are provided in Table 1.

Table 1 Clinical characteristics of all patients at randomization and those who underwent follow-up angiography

Characteristic	All patients ($n = 30$)	Angiographic follow-up ($n = 21$)
Age (years)	65 ± 8	65 ± 9
Male	27 (90)	16 (89)
Smoking status:		
Current	3 (10)	2 (10)
Ex-smoker	22 (73.3)	15 (71)
Never	5 (16.7)	4 (19)
Diabetes:		
IDDM	5 (17)	3 (14)
NIDDM	6 (20)	5 (24)
No history	19 (63)	13 (62)
Hypertension:	20 (66.7)	14 (67)
Hyperlipidemia	29 (96.7)	20 (95)
Prior stroke (non-debilitating)	1 (3.3)	1 (5)
COPD	1 (3.3)	0
NYHA class:		
I	11 (36.7)	6 (29)
II	13 (43.3)	9 (43)
III	4 (13.3)	4 (19)
IV	2 (6.7)	2 (9)
LVEF (%)	56 ± 10	55 ± 10
Creatinine (umol/L)	85 ± 18.9	81.7 ± 18.1
Pre-op Logistic EuroSCORE (%)	1.58 ± 1.29	1.7 ± 1.4
Total number grafts/patient	3.3 ± 0.5	3.4 ± 0.5
Days of follow up	1601 ± 102	1601 ± 113

Mean (±SD) or n (%). *IDDM* insulin dependent diabetes, *NIDDM* non-insulin dependent diabetes, *COPD* chronic obstructive pulmonary disease, *NYHA* New York Heart Association, *LVEF* left ventricular ejection fraction

Clinical outcomes

Three patients (10%) had died since surgery; one was a cardiac-related death and two were due to cancer. Overall 3 patients (10%) experienced one or more MACCE events. Of 3 revascularization events, one was triggered by the protocol-mandated angiographic control, one was to the nonstented territory, and one was to both stented and nonstented territories. One myocardial infarction (3.3%) and no strokes were reported.

Vein graft disease markers

Figure 1 shows angiographic images of a within-patient comparison of stented and nonstented SVGs at 1 and 4.5 year follow-up. Vein graft failure rates at 4.5 years were comparable between the stented and non-stented graft groups (Fig. 2). In the stented group, all grafts that were patent at the 1 year follow up, maintained their patency at the 4.5 year follow up, however in the non-stented group there was one additional graft occlusion between 1 and 4.5 years. At 4.5 years, stented vein grafts maintained perfectly-patent lumens without irregularities at significantly higher proportions than non-stented grafts (Fig. 2).

Fig. 3 illustrates IVUS images of a within-patient comparison of stented and nonstented SVGs at 1 and 4.5 year follow-up. IH area and thickness at 4.5 years did not change significantly compared to 1 year but both were significantly reduced in the stented versus the nonstented grafts (Fig. 4). Lumen diameters did not significantly differ between the two groups (3.38 ± 0.50 mm vs. 3.45 ± 0.54 mm stented vs. nonstented; $p = 0.585$).

Grafts with Fitzgibbon I classification had significantly lower plaque area compared to grafts with Fitzgibbon II/III ($p = 0.04$, Table 2). Figure 5 illustrates IVUS images of a constrictive- and a loose-fitting external stent. The distance of the stent to SVG wall was positively correlated with IH thickness both at 1 year (correlation coefficient 0.76, $p < 0.001$) and at 4.5 years (correlation coefficient 0.84, $p < 0.001$; Fig. 6).

Discussion

VEST IV is a unique study, presenting for the first time the long-term follow-up of a randomized controlled trial evaluating the impact of external stenting of SVGs used in CABG surgery. Our key finding is that the benefits of external stents on improving Fitzgibbon perfect patency and reducing IH that was demonstrated at 1 year are maintained at 4.5 years. Similarly, with the exception of an additional vein graft occlusion in the nonstented group, there was little further deterioration at longer-term follow up. A second key finding, as discussed subsequently, is that the distance of the VEST stent from the SVG lumen was an important determinant of the degree of IH. The MACCE rate of 18% in this study was comparable to that reported by the SYNTAX trial group for their 3-vessel disease subgroup at 4 years and at 5 years post CABG at 19 and 24% respectively [11, 12].

This study strengthens and corroborates previous pre-clinical and clinical reports suggesting a protective biomechanical effect of a braided cobalt chrome external stent on vein graft remodeling [7, 8, 13, 14]. A particular

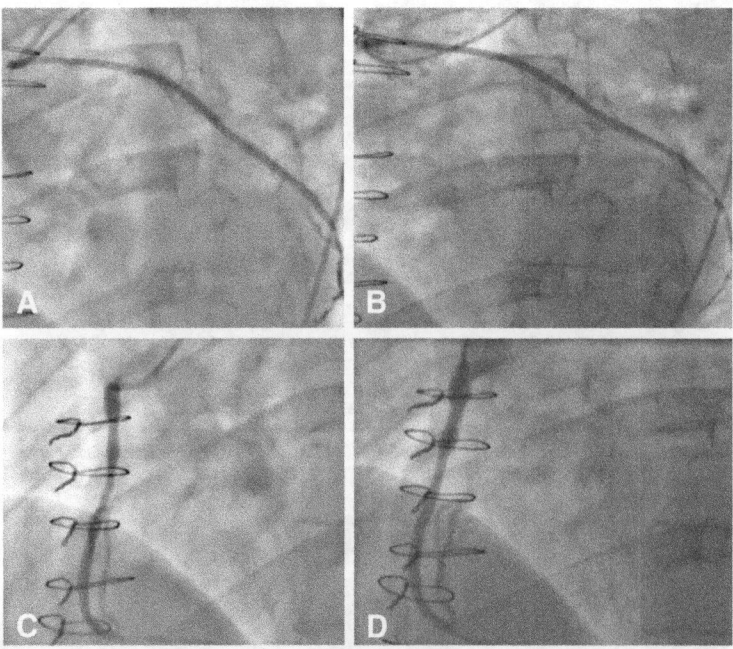

Fig. 1 Angiographic images showing a within-patient comparison of stented and nonstented SVGs at 1 and 4.5 year follow-up. Stented SVG to obtuse marginal artery at 1 year (**a**) and after 4.5 years (**b**). Nonstented SVG to right coronary artery at 1 year (**c**) and 4.5 years (**d**)

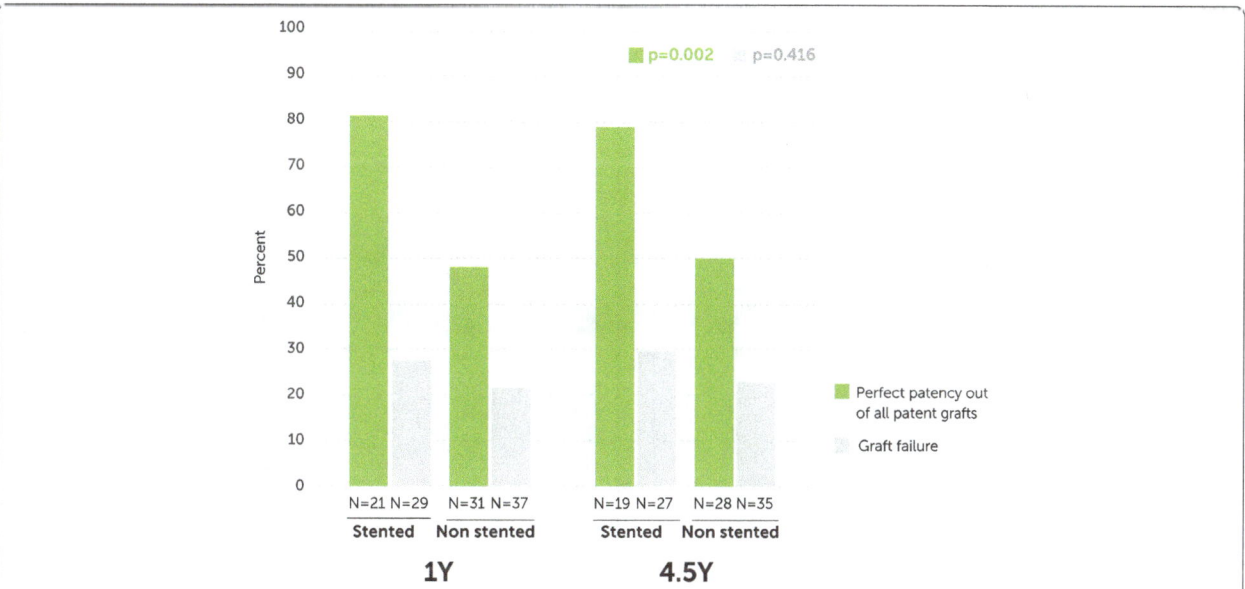

Fig. 2 Perfect patency and graft failure rates of stented and nonstented vein grafts at 1 and 4.5 years post CABG. Green bars - perfect patency rates within each arm of stented (*n* = 40) and nonstented (*n* = 59) grafts (*p* = 0.002). Grey bars - graft failure rates within each arm of stented (*n* = 56) and nonstented (*n* = 72) grafts (*p* = 0.416)

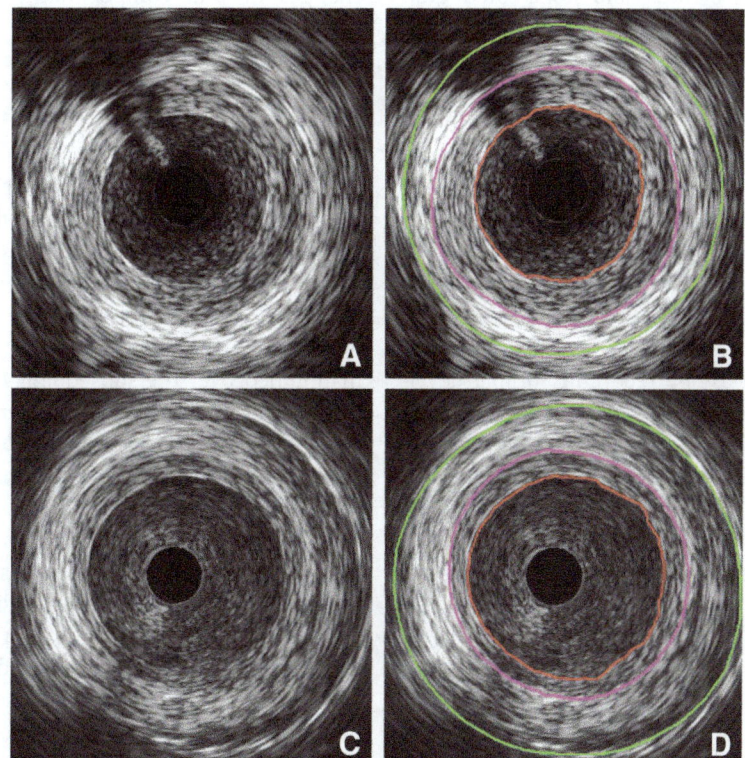

Fig. 3 Within-patient comparison of intimal hyperplasia using IVUS. Segment of a nonstented SVG to the first obtuse marginal 4.5 years after implantation without (**a**) and with (**b**) marking of the lumen (red), EEM (purple) and outer vessel (green). Segment of externally stented SVG to the second obtuse marginal 4.5 years after implantation without (**c**) and with (**d**) marking of the lumen (red), EEM (purple) and stent (green)

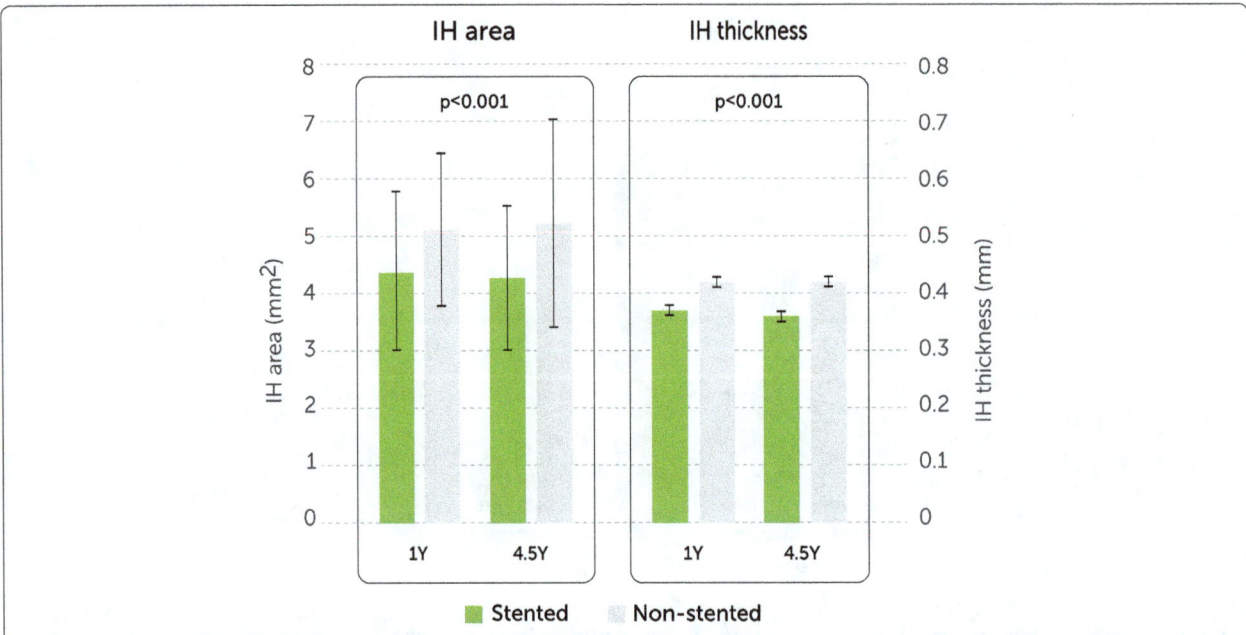

Fig. 4 Comparison of intimal hyperplasia proliferation markers at 1 and 4.5 year follow-up. Data are mean ± SD. IH, intimal hyperplasia; 1Y, 1 year follow-up; 4.5Y, 4.5 year follow-up. Green square Stented grafts, grey square Non-stented grafts

strength of our trial was the paired study design with each patient acting as their own control, thereby eliminating many of the potential factors that could affect SVG disease progression. The stented and nonstented graft groups were well balanced with respect to baseline anatomical and physiological parameters that might contribute to the development of IH, including the diameter of the native coronary artery and the severity of the proximal coronary artery stenosis. This was also evidenced by the similarity of measured graft flows in both the stented and nonstented SVGs, intraoperatively by TTFM and at 1-year by angiography [7]. Furthermore, while previous IVUS studies on SVGs were limited only to the proximal part of the grafts at one time point [15], our study provides, for the first time, new insight into the diffuse nature of the disease by recording intimal development along the entire SVG length at both 1 and 4.5 years.

The early phase of vein graft remodeling is dominated by luminal enlargement followed by a later phase of vein graft thickening and IH. Luminal enlargement is generated mainly by the exposure to the high shear stress of

Table 2 Cross sectional IVUS parameters for Fitzgibbon grade vein graft groups

Variable	Fitzgibbon I	Fitzgibbon II & III	P value
IH area [mm^2]	4.5 (3.9, 5.0)	5.2 (4.5, 5.8)	0.04
IH thickness [mm]	0.4 (0.3, 0.4)	0.4 (0.4, 0.5)	0.09
Lumen diameter [mm]	3.4 (3.2, 3.6)	3.5 (3.3, 3.8)	0.38

Data are mean (95% CI). *IH* intimal hyperplasia

the arterial circulation [3]. During the first months post implantation, as a reaction to the elevated wall tension, there is a proliferative thickening of the venous wall and changes in wall composition [3]. Hozumi et al. have shown that between 1 to 12 months post implantation, intimal area was significantly increased from 0.90 mm^2 to 5.26 mm^2 ($p < 0.001$) [15]. Our findings concur with Hozumi et al., suggesting that most SVG remodeling occurs over the first year after grafting and, consequently, that early intervention is crucial in order to effectively lessen the pathological changes which serve as the foundation for occlusive atheromatous lesions 5–10 years following surgery [15]. The mitigation of IH and lumen deformation achieved by external stenting was most pronounced in the first year after implantation and was maintained over the subsequent 3.5 years. This observation is also in line with experimental data on biodegradable external stents which demonstrated that the majority of the inhibitory effect on SVG remodeling was achieved 6 months post implantation [16].

In both arteries and veins, lumen irregularities generate low and oscillatory shear stress that is directly correlated with accelerated vascular disease [13, 17]. A high proportion of SVGs, mainly from the upper leg, demonstrate caliber irregularities even during harvesting while > 25% of SVG show severe segmental ectasia with > 50% dilatation at 1 year [7]. In their landmark publication, Fitzgibbon and colleagues described the progression of SVG disease over the course of 15 years [9]. At 5, 10 and 15 years, only 52, 23 and 19% of the patent grafts respectively demonstrated "perfect" patency with no

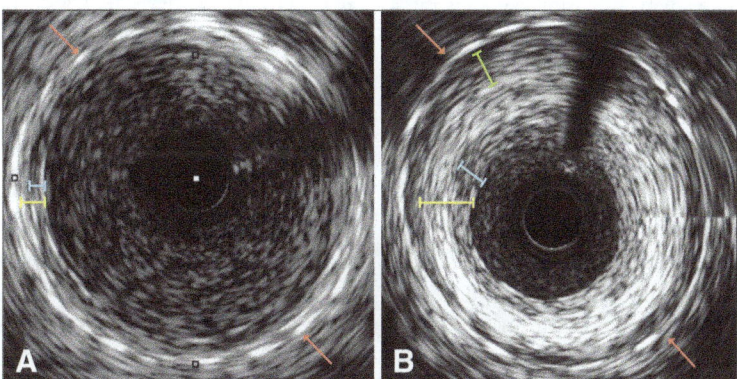

Fig. 5 IVUS images showing **a** constrictive versus **b** loose fitting external stent (red arrows). Difference in wall thickness (yellow) and intima layer (blue) can be observed. In addition, there is formation of "neo-adventitia" between the loose-fitting stent and the original vessel wall

lumen irregularities. The diffuse progressive nature of vein graft disease was further supported by contemporary studies that demonstrate that only 12–25% of SVG are perfectly patent 10 years after surgery [18]. We found that reduced SVG lumen irregularity is associated with decreased intimal area and thickness, most probably due to the improved hemodynamics and reductions in oscillatory shear stress provided by external stents [13, 17]. External stenting prevented SVG deformation early after implantation and mitigated development of further lumen irregularities at 4.5 years.

Mechanical external support of SVGs has been a focus of intense research, with their use intended to reduce well-documented pathophysiological changes that occur in the SVG following implantation. These devices have developed substantially over recent years, and there is now a large body of data in both animal models and human patients related to their biomechanical effects [17, 19, 20]. External stenting targets some of the key factors initiating the pathological cascade in SVG post implantation such as high circumferential wall stress and disturbed flow patterns due to luminal irregularities [13, 14, 17]. The rationale and the physiological basis for mechanical external stents is further supported by the reported benefits of the "no touch" technique, in which the saphenous vein is harvested with a pedicle of surrounding tissue that serves as an external support with both mechanical and biological roles [21]. Randomized prospective studies showed that no

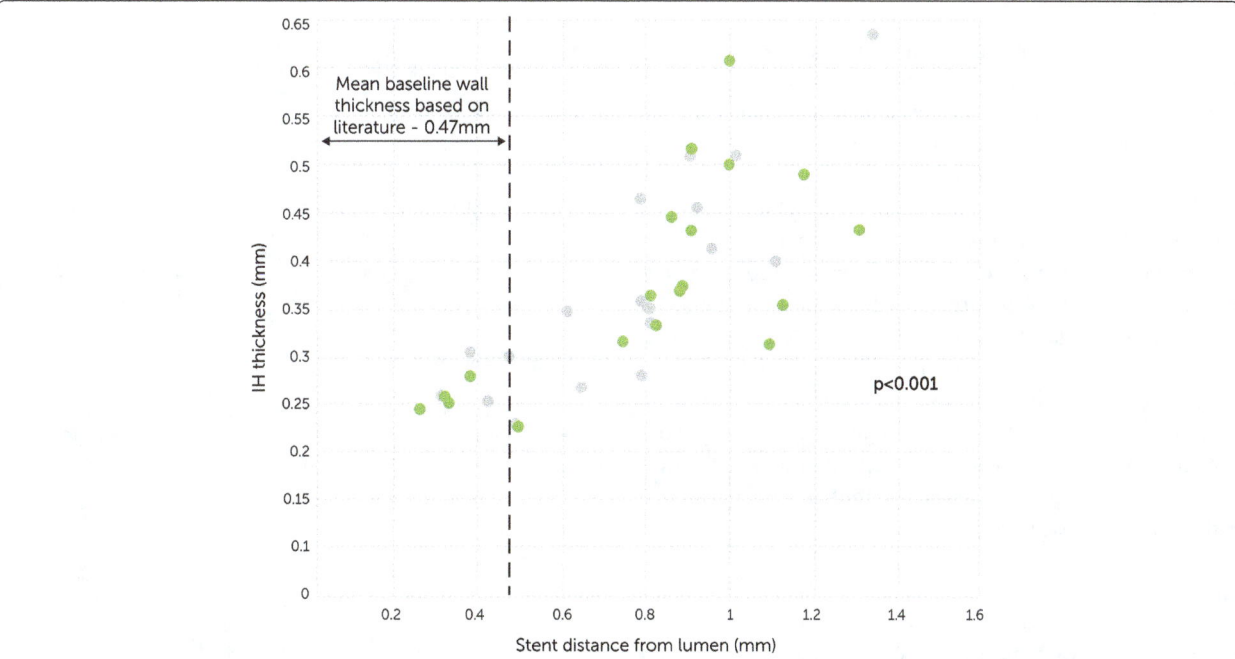

Fig. 6 Intimal hyperplasia thickness correlated with distance of the external stent from the lumen. grey circle 1 year (correlation coefficient 0.76, $p < 0.001$), green circle 4.5 years (correlation coefficient 0.84, $p < 0.001$). Baseline saphenous vein wall thickness (---) is derived from relevant literature [30, 31]

touch technique is associated with superior patency rates compared with conventionally prepared vein grafts both in the short-term (18 months) and long-term (8.5 years) at angiographic follow-up [22, 23].

Early clinical experience with external stents showed conflicting data with early patency rates ranging from 28 to 92% at 6–12 months [24, 25]. High SVG failure rates were attributed to the design of the first generation of external stents that required incorporation of the device into the anastomoses, constriction of the graft and fixation of the stent to the SVG with fibrin glue [25]. Several studies have shown that fibrin glue on the external surface of vein grafts lead to aneurysmal degeneration and excessive IH which may jeopardize vein graft patency [25–27]. Second generation technologies which did not require the use of fibrin glue or incorporation to the anastomoses site showed comparable patency rates to non-stented SVG at 1 year [7].

The appropriate size of external stents for vein grafts has been a focus of controversy and another possible confounding factor for success of external stenting. Zilla and colleagues concluded that constrictive external stents, which reduce diameter mismatch with the target artery, are more effective in mitigating IH compared to non-restrictive stents [28]. In contrast, Izzat and colleagues have shown that loose-fitting external stents are more effective in suppressing intimal proliferation [29]. The rationale behind using oversized external supports was to provide sufficient space to promote adventitial neovascularization, which was potentially interrupted by constrictive stents [20]. The distance of the external stent from the lumen is equivalent to the SVG wall thickness. The closer this measure is to the vein baseline wall thickness, the better the conformity of the VEST to the vein. We postulated that a closer conformity would improve VEST performance in mitigating IH, and indeed we found that the correlation between the distance of the VEST from the lumen and the IH thickness was indeed significant in our study. As shown in Fig. 6, the closer the value is to the baseline literature reported vein wall thickness, the lesser the proliferation of IH [30, 31]. This finding suggests that mildly constricting the vein has a beneficial effect on intimal proliferation, most probably due to more effective reduction in wall tension, SVG dilatation, and lumen irregularities. It is expected that future studies, in which appropriate model selection will ensure a mildly constrictive stent, a more effective reduction in IH will be achieved.

Limitations
Together with the small sample size, a further limitation of our study is that the study cohort was based on a first in human trial and exhibited learning curve effects of both the technology and the implantation technique (which

were largely resolved in VEST II [8]). The technical failures and inappropriate model selection, with suboptimal dimensional match between the SVG and the stent, likely have adversely affected the stent's ability to even more effectively mitigate IH. VEST III, a large randomized trial that is currently underway (NCT02511834), will address both the population size and learning curve issues.

Conclusion
Improving SVG longevity may have a direct impact on the clinical outcome of CABG and patients' quality of life. Our study provides novel insights into the biomechanical effects of external stenting of SVGs and their long-term performance – to our knowledge, the only long-term follow-up of external stenting to SVGs to date. If the beneficial effect of external stenting that we observed at one and 4.5 years is maintained over a 10–15 year period, it may have a substantial impact on improving clinical outcomes. Future and ongoing large randomized trials with long-term follow up will further determine the role of external stents in CABG surgery.

Abbreviations
CABG: Coronary artery bypass graft; EEM: External elastic lamina; IH: Intimal hyperplasia; IVUS: Intravascular ultrasound; MACCE: Major cardiovascular and cerebral events; MI: Myocardial infarction; SD: Standard deviation; SVG: Saphenous vein graft

Acknowledgements
Not applicable.

Funding
This work was supported by Vascular Graft Solutions Ltd. (Tel Aviv, Israel) and the Victor Phillip Dahdaleh Charitable Foundation (Guernsey, UK).

Authors' contributions
All authors made substantial contributions to the conception and design, or/and acquisition of data, or/and analysis and interpretation of the data. CW and DT drafted the manuscript, all authors revised it critically for important intellectual content and have given approval of the final version of the manuscript. All authors agree to be accountable for all aspects of the work.

Competing interests
Prof Taggart serves as a consultant to Vascular Graft Solutions, has stock ownership and receives consulting fees. Prof Taggart has received travel support and speaking honoraria from Vascular Graft Solutions. The remaining authors have no disclosures relating to this study.

Author details
[1]Nuffield Department of Surgery, University of Oxford, John Radcliffe Hospital, Oxford, UK. [2]National Heart & Lung Institute, Imperial College London, London, UK. [3]Department of Cardiology, Royal Brompton Hospital, Sydney Street, London SW3 6NP, UK. [4]Department of Cardiothoracic Surgery, Royal Brompton Hospital, Sydney Street, London, UK. [5]Department of Cardiovascular Medicine, University of Oxford, John Radcliffe Hospital, Oxford, UK. [6]Department of Cardiothoracic Surgery, Harefield Hospital, Middlesex, London, UK.

References

1. Harskamp RE, Lopes RD, Baisden CE, de Winter RJ, Alexander JH. Saphenous vein graft failure after coronary artery bypass surgery: pathophysiology, management, and future directions. Ann Surg. 2013;257:824–33.
2. Motwani JG, Topol EJ. Aortocoronary saphenous vein graft disease: pathogenesis, predisposition, and prevention. Circulation. 1998;97:916–31.
3. Owens CD, Gasper WJ, Rahman AS, Conte MS. Vein graft failure. J Vasc Surg. 2015;61:203–16.
4. Alexander JH, Hafley G, Harrington RA, et al. Efficacy and safety of edifoligide, an E2F transcription factor decoy, for prevention of vein graft failure following coronary artery bypass graft surgery: PREVENT IV: a randomized controlled trial. JAMA. 2005;294:2446–54.
5. Kulik A, Le May MR, Voisine P, et al. Aspirin plus clopidogrel versus aspirin alone after coronary artery bypass grafting: the clopidogrel after surgery for coronary artery disease (CASCADE) trial. Circulation. 2010;122:2680–7.
6. Une D, Kulik A, Voisine P, Le May M, Ruel M. Correlates of saphenous vein graft hyperplasia and occlusion 1 year after coronary artery bypass grafting: analysis from the CASCADE randomized trial. Circulation. 2013;128:S213–8.
7. Taggart DP, Ben-Gal Y, Lees B, et al. A randomized trial of external stenting for saphenous vein grafts in coronary artery bypass grafting. Ann Thorac Surg. 2015;99:2039–45.
8. Taggart DP, Amin S, Djordjevic J, et al. A prospective study of external stenting of saphenous vein grafts to the right coronary artery: the VEST II study. Eur J Cardiothorac Surg. 2017;51:952–8.
9. FitzGibbon GM, Kafka HP, Leach AJ, Keon WJ, Hooper GD, Burton JR. Coronary bypass graft fate and patient outcome: angiographic follow-up of 5,065 grafts related to survival and reoperation in 1,388 patients during 25 years. J Am Coll Cardiol. 1996;28:616–26.
10. Mintz GS, Nissen SE, Anderson WD, et al. American College of Cardiology Clinical Expert Consensus Document on standards for acquisition, measurement and reporting of intravascular ultrasound studies (IVUS). A report of the American College of Cardiology Task Force on clinical expert consensus documents. J Am Coll Cardiol. 2001;37:1478–92.
11. Head SJ, Davierwala PM, Serruys PW, et al. Coronary artery bypass grafting vs. percutaneous coronary intervention for patients with three-vessel disease: final five-year follow-up of the SYNTAX trial. Eur Heart J. 2014;35:2821–30.
12. Mohr FW, Morice MC, Kappetein AP, et al. Coronary artery bypass graft surgery versus percutaneous coronary intervention in patients with three-vessel disease and left main coronary disease: 5-year follow-up of the randomised, clinical SYNTAX trial. Lancet. 2013;381:629–38.
13. Meirson T, Orion E, Di Mario C, et al. Flow patterns in externally stented saphenous vein grafts as related to the development of intimal hyperplasia. J Thorac Cardiovasc Surg. 2015;150:871–8.
14. Webb CM, Orion E, Taggart DP, Channon KM, Di MC. OCT imaging of aorto-coronary vein graft pathology modified by external stenting: 1-year post-surgery. Eur Heart J Cardiovasc Imaging. 2016;17:1290–5.
15. Hozumi T, Yoshikawa J, Yoshida K, et al. Use of intravascular ultrasound for in vivo assessment of changes in intimal thickness of angiographically normal saphenous vein grafts one year after aortocoronary bypass surgery. Heart. 1996;76:317–20.
16. Vijayan V, Shukla N, Johnson JL, et al. Long-term reduction of medial and intimal thickening in porcine saphenous vein grafts with a polyglactin biodegradable external sheath. J Vasc Surg. 2004;40:1011–9.
17. Chiu JJ, Chien S. Effects of disturbed flow on vascular endothelium: pathophysiological basis and clinical perspectives. Physiol Rev. 2011;91:327–87.
18. Gaudino M, Tondi P, Benedetto U, et al. Radial artery as a coronary artery bypass conduit: 20-year results. J Am Coll Cardiol. 2016;68:603–10.
19. Hu J, Wan S. External support in preventing vein graft failure. Asian Cardiovasc Thorac Ann. 2012;20:615–22.
20. Jeremy JY, Gadsdon P, Shukla N, et al. On the biology of saphenous vein grafts fitted with external synthetic sheaths and stents. Biomaterials. 2007;28:895–908.
21. Johansson BL, Souza DS, Bodin L, et al. Slower progression of atherosclerosis in vein grafts harvested with 'no touch' technique compared with conventional harvesting technique in coronary artery bypass grafting: an angiographic and intravascular ultrasound study. Eur J Cardiothorac Surg. 2010;38:414–9.
22. Souza DS, Dashwood MR, Tsui JC, et al. Improved patency in vein grafts harvested with surrounding tissue: results of a randomized study using three harvesting techniques. Ann Thorac Surg. 2002;73:1189–95.
23. Souza DS, Johansson B, Bojo L, et al. Harvesting the saphenous vein with surrounding tissue for CABG provides long-term graft patency comparable to the left internal thoracic artery: results of a randomized longitudinal trial. J Thorac Cardiovasc Surg. 2006;132:373–8.
24. Klima U, Elsebay AA, Gantri MR, Bangardt J, Miller G, Emery RW. Computerized tomographic angiography in patients having eSVS mesh(R) supported coronary saphenous vein grafts: intermediate term results. J Cardiothorac Surg. 2014;9:138.
25. Schoettler J, Jussli-Melchers J, Grothusen C, et al. Highly flexible nitinol mesh to encase aortocoronary saphenous vein grafts: first clinical experiences and angiographic results nine months postoperatively. Interact Cardiovasc Thorac Surg. 2011;13:396–400.
26. Stojanovic T, El-Sayed AA, Didilis V, et al. Extravascular perivenous fibrin support leads to aneurysmal degeneration and intimal hyperplasia in arterialized vein grafts in the rat. Langenbecks Arch Surg. 2009;394:357–62.
27. Wan S, Arifi AA, Chan MC, et al. Differential, time-dependent effects of perivenous application of fibrin glue on medial thickening in porcine saphenous vein grafts. Eur J Cardiothorac Surg. 2006;29:742–6.
28. Zilla P, Human P, Wolf M, et al. Constrictive external nitinol meshes inhibit vein graft intimal hyperplasia in nonhuman primates. J Thorac Cardiovasc Surg. 2008;136:717–25.
29. Izzat MB, Mehta D, Bryan AJ, Reeves B, Newby AC, Angelini GD. Influence of external stent size on early medial and neointimal thickening in a pig model of saphenous vein bypass grafting. Circulation. 1996;94:1741–5.
30. Human P, Franz T, Scherman J, Moodley L, Zilla P. Dimensional analysis of human saphenous vein grafts: implications for external mesh support. J Thorac Cardiovasc Surg. 2009;137:1101–8.
31. Owens CD, Ho KJ, Conte MS. Lower extremity vein graft failure: a translational approach. Vasc Med. 2008;13:63–74.

26

Atrial fibrillation after transhiatal esophagectomy with transcervical endoscopic esophageal mobilization: one institution's experience

Elizabeth M. Colwell[1]*⦿, Carlos O. Encarnacion[2], Lisa E. Rein[3], Aniko Szabo[4], George Haasler[5], Mario Gasparri[6], William Tisol[7] and David Johnstone[5]

Abstract

Background: There have been numerous studies regarding atrial fibrillation (AF) associated with cardiac and pulmonary surgery; however, studies looking at esophagectomy and atrial fibrillation are sparse. The goal of this study was to review our institution's atrial fibrillation rate following esophagectomy in order to better define the incidence and predisposing factors in this patient population.

Methods: A retrospective chart review of all patients undergoing esophagectomy with transcervical endoscopic mobilization of the esophagus (TEEM) at the Medical College of Wisconsin and Affiliated Hospitals from July 2009 through December 2012.

Results: Seventy-one patients underwent TEEM esophagectomy during the study period. Of those, 23 (32.4%) patients developed new atrial fibrillation postoperatively. ICU (Intensive Care Unit) length of stay was 7.1 days for those that did not receive amiodarone, compared to 5.3 days for those that did receive amiodarone ($p < 0.025$). Those that went into AF spent on average 9.3 days in the ICU compared to 4.7 days for their counterparts that did not go into AF ($p < 0.006$). Total length of stay was not statistically different between populations [15.1 +/− 11.3 days compared to 13.5 +/− 9.4 days for those who did not go into AF ($p < 0.281$)]. Receiving preoperative amiodarone was found to reduce the overall incidence of AF. There was a trend towards decreased risk of going into AF in those who received preoperative amiodarone with an adjusted hazard ratio of 0.555 ($p = 0.057$).

Conclusion: Similar to data reported in previous literature, postoperative atrial fibrillation was found to increase ICU length of stay as well as overall length of hospital stay. Preoperative amiodarone administration displayed a trend toward decreasing the rates of atrial fibrillation in patients undergoing TEEM.

Keywords: Esophagectomy, Atrial Fibrillation, Amiodarone

Background

Atrial fibrillation (AF) after thoracic surgery is a common event. Its incidence, risk factors, and consequences have been extensively studied in patients undergoing cardiac surgery. More recently many authors have looked at AF after noncardiac thoracic surgery, reporting its occurrence between 12 and 44% [1] as well as showing an increase in morbidity and mortality in patients developing AF [2–4]. The few reports on postoperative AF after esophageal surgery have found that AF is common. It has been reported in up to 45% of patients following esophagectomy [5]. In 2003 Murthy et al. found AF in 22% of their esophagectomy patients and found it to be a marker for postoperative morbidity and mortality. They reported increased rates of pulmonary complications, anastomotic leak rates, as well as sepsis in patients who had AF [6].

Our study looks at the incidence and treatment of atrial fibrillation in our institution since the implementation of

---
* Correspondence: ecolwell@stanford.edu
[1]Cardiothoracic Surgery, Stanford University, 300 Pasteur Dr. Falk Cardiovascular Research Bldg, Stanford, CA 94305-5407, USA
Full list of author information is available at the end of the article

a novel transhiatal esophagectomy technique with endoscopic mobilization of the esophagus (TEEM) and the routine use of perioperative amiodarone.

Methods

Patients

A retrospective chart review of all patients undergoing TEEM esophagectomy at the Medical College of Wisconsin and Affiliated Hospitals from July 2009 through December 2012 was performed. This included 80 patients who had an operation performed at Froedtert Hospital or Zablocki VA Hospital in Milwaukee, Wisconsin. Seventy-one patients were included in the final data as one patient from the VA Hospital was excluded due to being unable to obtain a thorough chart review and 8 patients that had pre-operative atrial fibrillation were also excluded from the cohort. Our cohort consisted of a variety of diagnoses such as adenocarcinoma ($n = 65$), squamous cell carcinoma ($n = 9$), achalasia ($n = 3$), GE junction disruption ($n = 1$) and enterocaval fistula (n = 1).

Data collection

Recorded data included patient demographics, length of stay, length of ICU stay, diagnosis requiring surgery, clinical as well as pathological stage of cancer, medical comorbidities, preoperative chemoradiation status, lymph node dissection, atrial fibrillation during hospital stay, prophylactic amiodarone status, length of surgery, and estimated blood loss. Chart review included extensive review of patient records in EPIC and CPRS (electronic medical records used at our institutions) including preoperative notes, operative records, physician and support staff progress notes, pathology reports and medication administration records. Data collection was approved for use in research by the institutional review board both at Froedtert Hospital and Zablocki VA Hospital.

Technique

The only surgical approach used in our cohort was a transhiatal esophagectomy with transcervical endoscopic mobilization of the esophagus. Once the abdomen is opened, inspected, and found to be free of any metastatic disease, the left neck is opened in standard fashion medial to the carotid sheath, and the esophagus is encircled with a penrose drain. An endoscopic vein harvest scope is then passed in a posterior plane in order to mobilize the posterior aspect of the esophagus from the thoracic inlet down to the diaphragmatic hiatus. This process is repeated in the anterior and lateral planes as well. Lymph nodes encountered during the dissection are biopsied and sent as specimens to pathology. Tissue division is done with either a Ligasure or Harmonic device (the latter used exclusively in the later portion of this cohort). The esophagus is then divided in the neck.

Concurrently, the stomach is mobilized and tubularized in a standard fashion for a transhiatal esophagectomy. The conduit is then passed through the posterior mediastinum and an esophagastric anastomosis is made at the cervical incision, with either a stapled or handsewn anastomosis, or combination of both, depending on patient details and surgeon preference.

Our institution's therapy of choice for new onset atrial fibrillation for the last several years has been amiodarone. Typically, we have treated our patients who go into stable atrial fibrillation with a 150 mg bolus of amiodarone followed by initiation of an amiodarone drip starting at 1 mg/min for 6 h followed by 0.5 mg/min for 18 h. They are then typically transitioned to j-tube amiodarone as soon as deemed appropriate.

However, starting in January 2011 at Froedtert Hospital we began routinely starting amiodarone the evening before surgery. Patients were admitted for initiation of an amiodarone drip starting at 0.5 mg/min as well as a bowel prep. This amiodarone drip was continued through surgery and transitioned to j-tube dosing once appropriate post-operatively. However, at our other institution, the Zablocki VA Hospital patients did not get admitted the evening before and thus did not get prophylactic amiodarone administration. At this institution, they would only receive amiodarone if they experienced post-operatively AF. All of our patients, at both institutions, generally remained on telemetry throughout their hospital stay.

Statistical analysis

Statistical analysis was performed by the Biostatistics Division at the Medical College of Wisconsin. The dataset includes 71 patients without pre-op atrial fibrillation, who underwent TEEM esophagectomy from 2009 to 2012. All outcomes (except 30-day survival) were measured during the post-op hospitalization (length of stay varies). All patients except 1 were discharged alive. All patients have adequate follow-up to assess 30-day survival; the minimum follow-up among surviving patients was 33 days.

Predictors and outcomes were compared by pre-op amiodarone status using Wilcoxon rank-sum tests for continuous variables and Fisher's exact tests for categorical variables.

Predictors and outcomes were compared by post-op day 3 atrial fibrillation status using Wilcoxon rank-sum tests for continuous variables and Fisher's exact tests for categorical variables. Post-op day 3 status was used because all patients were monitored for atrial fibrillation in hospital at least 3 days (there is no censoring at day 3).

Cox proportional hazards regression analysis (unadjusted and adjusted) was performed for the primary outcome, post-op atrial fibrillation. The cause-specific hazard of atrial fibrillation was modeled using Cox proportional hazards regression. Patients were censored at discharge/death. *P*-values less than 5% were considered significant.

Results

Seventy-one patients whose ages ranged from 31 to 89 years (mean 61.5 +/− 10.7) were included in the study. There were 63 men and 8 women.

Twenty-eight patients (39.4%) went into atrial fibrillation postoperatively. Sixty-eight percent of our patients underwent preoperative radiation. Of those who had postoperative AF, 67.6% had undergone preoperative radiation; and thus preoperative radiation was not found to be a significant risk factor for atrial fibrillation.

Those who went into AF had a mean age of 66.2 compared with 59.3 in those who did not (p-value of < 0.004). The average BMI of our patients was 27.8. We found no difference in the BMI of patients who went into atrial fibrillation and those that did not.

During post-operative follow up, none of the patients who had AF during their hospital stay had AF at their post-operative visit.

Those who went into atrial fibrillation were found to spend 9.3 [1.0–9.0] days in the ICU, compared to 4.7 [0.0–27.0] days in the ICU for those who did not go into AF (p < 0.006), however, their overall length of stay was not significantly different, 15.1 [8.0–33.0] days vs. 13.9 [3.0–65.0] days.

Thirty-five (49.3%) of our patients received preoperative amiodarone. Receiving preoperative amiodarone was found to reduce the overall incidence of AF. There was a trend towards decreased risk of going into AF in those who received preoperative amiodarone with an adjusted hazard ratio of 0.555 [95% CI 0.302–1.018 (p = 0.057)].

Discussion

Risk factors for atrial fibrillation following thoracic surgery have spurred much discussion in the literature. Studies have shown male sex, older age, pneumonectomy, esophagectomy, history of smoking, history of congestive heart failure, preoperative supraventricular arrhythmias, and postoperative increase in white blood cell count as risk factors for postoperative arrhythmias [7, 8]. A study by Hahm and colleagues in 2007, looking specifically at esophagectomy patients, found cardiac disease, poor PFTs, cervical anastomosis, elevated CVP, and higher ephedrine doses to be predictors for the occurrence of arrhythmia during surgery [9]. Pneumonia, pleural effusions and elevated c-reactive protein post operative have been associated with increased risk of atrial fibrillation [10].

We found the incidence of new onset postoperative atrial fibrillation in our patient population (all patients undergoing the TEEM approach) to be 39.4%, which is within the wide range reported by other studies [5, 6, 11].

In our group of patient's arrhythmia most commonly presented on postoperative day 2 or 3. This is consistent with arrhythmia onset after other types of thoracic surgery [2, 8]. Although the reason for a delayed presentation is likely multifactorial, some have speculated that the onset of the arrhythmia is due in part to the resolution of an inflammatory response following surgical trauma which alters the ability of the atrial myocardial cells to respond to catecholamine [11].

Thirty-five of our patients (49.2%) received preoperative amiodarone in attempts to decrease the postoperative AF rate. The use of prophylactic antiarrhythmic medications in thoracic surgery has been highly documented in both cardiac as well as pulmonary surgery. The efficacy of amiodarone for atrial fibrillation prophylaxis has been widely documented in cardiac surgery [12–14]. Guarnieri and colleagues published a trial showing the safe and effective use the use of IV amiodarone in patients undergoing open heart surgery. They found a significant (p = 0.01) decrease in the occurrence of postoperative AF in these patients: 35% in patients on amiodarone and 47% in the placebo group. Other groups have found oral amiodarone to be effective as well [12, 14]. Its use has also been documented in lung surgery. Lanza and colleagues showed a decrease in AF rates in patients receiving prophylactic low dose oral amiodarone following pulmonary resections. They found 33% of patients without prophylaxis and 9.7% with prophylaxis (p = 0.0253) to have postoperative atrial fibrillation [15]. Even those in whom prophylaxis failed still appeared to benefit as the duration of AF and length of hospital stay were shortened in this group [15]. Although many are concerned about the side effects of amiodarone use, Lanza found no significant complications from prophylactic use in their group of patients.

Tisdale and colleagues published a study in 2010 looking at the efficacy and safety of amiodarone for prevention of atrial fibrillation after transthoracic esophagectomy. They found the incidence of atrial fibrillation requiring treatment was lower in the amiodarone group than in the control group; however there were no significant differences between the groups in terms of overall or ICU length of stay [16]. Our data agrees with Tisdale in that the rate of atrial fibrillation does appear to decrease with prophylactic use of amiodarone. However, our study also suggests that decreasing the rate of AF will decrease the length of stay in the ICU as well as the overall hospital stay. More recently one paper addressed atrial fibrillations affect on long term mortality. Chin et al. showed a significantly lower survival rate in the atrial fibrillation group compared to those who did not have atrial fibrillation p = 0.045 via Kaplan Meier survival analysis [17].

There are limitations to this study. The fact that it is a retrospective study brings inherent biases into the study. Being a tertiary care center brings with it a probable patient selection bias as many patients referred to our center are more ill than those receiving care from non-tertiary care centers. In addition, our study size is relatively small as we had only 71 patients undergoing the TEEM approach at the time of data analysis. It may prove beneficial to look at the data again in the near future as many more patients could now be included.

Conclusion

It is well established that postoperative AF is common in noncardiac thoracic surgery, and it has also been shown to be associated with increased morbidity and mortality as well as increased costs. In our study this is shown by the increased ICU length of stay for patients who go into atrial fibrillation. We found prophylactic amiodarone trended towards a reduction in rates of atrial fibrillation in our patient population, although the rates still remain high. It will be important to continue to investigate ways to recognize those at risk for atrial fibrillation as well as discover ways to continue to decrease the incidence of this arrhythmia in the postoperative period.

Abbreviations

AFA: Trial fibrillation; TEEM: Transcervical endoscopic mobilization of the esophagus; ICU: Intensive Care Unit

Authors' contributions

EC Data collection, analysis and interpretation of the data, and manuscript preparation; CE Data collection, analysis and interpretation of the data, and manuscript preparation; LR Performed statistical analysis of the data. AS Performed statistical analysis of the data; GH Analysis and interpretation of the data and manuscript preparation; MG Analysis and interpretation of the data and manuscript preparation; WT Analysis and interpretation of the data and manuscript preparation; DJ Analysis and interpretation of the data and manuscript preparation. All authors read and approved the final manuscript.

Competing interests

The authors declare that they have no competing interests.

Author details

¹Cardiothoracic Surgery, Stanford University, 300 Pasteur Dr. Falk Cardiovascular Research Bldg, Stanford, CA 94305-5407, USA. ²University of Maryland, Division of Cardiac Surgery, 110 S. Paca St. 7th floor, Baltimore, MD 21201, USA. ³Medical College of Wisconsin, 8701 Watertown Plank Road, PO Box 26509, Milwaukee, WI 53226, USA. ⁴Division of Biostatistics, Institute for Health & Equity, Medical College of Wisconsin, 8701 W. Watertown Plank Road, Milwaukee, WI 53226, USA. ⁵Division of Cardiothoracic Surgery, HUB for Collaborative Medicine, Medical College of Wisconsin, 8701 Watertown Plank Road, Milwaukee, WI 53226, USA. ⁶Division of Cardiovascular and Thoracic Surgery, SSM Heath – St. Mary's Madison, Madison, WI 53715, USA. ⁷Aurora Medical Group CVTS, 2901 W Kinnickinnic River Pkwy Suite 501, Milwaukee, WI 53125, USA.

References

1. Fernando HC, Jaklitsch MT, Walsh GL, Tisdale JE, Bridges CD, Mitchell JD, Shrager JB. The society of thoracic surgeons practice guideline on the prophylaxis and management of atrial fibrillation associated with general thoracic surgery: executive summary. Ann Thorac Surg. 2011;92:1144–52.
2. Roselli EE, Murthy SC, Rice TW, Houghtaling PL, Pierce CD, Karchmer DP, Blackstone EH. Atrial fibrillation complicating lung cancer resection. J Thorac Cardiovasc Surg. 2005;130:438–44.
3. Irshad K, Feldman LS, Chu VF, Dorval JF, Baslaim G, Morin JE. Causes of increased length of hospitalization on a general thoracic surgery service: a prospective observational study. Can J Surg. 2002;45:264–8.
4. Brathwaite D, Weissman C. The new onset of atrial arrhythmias following major noncardiothoracic surgery is associated with increased mortality. CHEST. 1998;114(2):462–8.
5. Konno O, Tezuka T, Muto A, et al. Postoperative arrhythmia after operation for esophageal cancer. J Jpn Assoc Thorac Surg. 1993;41:45–51.
6. Murthy SC, Law S, Whooley BP, et al. Atrial fibrillation after esophagectomy is a marker for postoperative morbidity and mortality. J Thorac Cardiovasc Surg. 2003;126(4):1162–7.
7. Vaporciyan AA, Correa AM, Rice DC, Roth JA, Smythe WR, Swisher SG, Walsh GL, Putnam JB. Risk factors associated with atrial fibrillation after noncardiac thoracic surgery: analysis of 2588 patients. J Thorac Cardiovasc Surg. 2004; 127:779–86.
8. Amar D, Goenka A, Zhang H, Park B, Thaler HT. Leukocytosis and increased risk of atrial fibrillation after general thoracic surgery. Ann Thorac Surg. 2006; 82:1057–62.
9. Hahm TS, Lee JJ, Yang MK, Kim JA. Risk factors for an intraopertive arrhythmia during esophagectomy. Yonsei Med Journal. 2007;48:474–9.
10. McCormack O, Zaborowski A, Sinead K, Healy L, Daly C, et al. New-onset atrial fibrillation post-surgery for esophageal and junctional Cancer: Incidence, Management, and Imact on Short and Long-term Outcomes. Ann Surg. 2014;260:772–8.
11. Amar D, Burt ME, Bains MS, Leung DH. Symptomatic tachyarrhythmias after esophagectomy: incidence and outcome measures. Ann Thorac Surg. 1996; 61:1506–9.
12. Daoud EG, Strickberger SA, Man KC, et al. Preoperative amiodarone as prophylaxis against atrial fibrillation after heart surgery. N Engl J Med. 1997; 337:1785–91.
13. Guarnieri T, Nolan S, Gottlieb SO, Dudek A, Lowry DR. Intravenous amiodarone for the prevention of atrial fibrillation after open heart surgery: the amiodarone reduction in coronary heart (ARCH) trial. J Am Coll Cardiol. 1999;34:343–7.
14. Katariya K, DeMarchena E, Bolooki H. Oral amiodarone reduces incidence of postoperative atrial fibrillation. Ann Thorac Surg. 1999;68:1599–604.
15. Lanza LA, Visbal AI, DeValeria PA, Zinsmeister AR, Diehl NN, Trastek VF. Low-Dose Oral Amiodarone Prophylaxis Reduces Atrial Fibrillation After Pulmonary Resection. Ann Thorac Surg. 2003;75:223–30.
16. Tisdale JE, Wroblewski HA, Wall DS, et al. A randomized, controlled study of amiodarone for prevention of atrial fibrillation after transthoracic esophagectomy. J Thorac Cardiovasc Surg. 2010;140:45–51.
17. Chin JH, Moon Y, Jo J, Han Y, Kim H, et al. Association between postoperatively developed atrial fibrillation and long-term mortality after Esophagectomy in esophageal Cancer patients: an observational study. PLoS One. 11(5):e0154931.

27

Role of pulmonary hemodynamics in determining 6-minute walk test result in atrial septal defect: an observational study

Supomo Supomo[1]* (iD), Handy Darmawan[2] and Adika Zhulhi Arjana[2]

Abstract

Background: The presence of altered pulmonary hemodynamics in adult patients with atrial septal defect (ASD) is common. However, there are no observational studies which evaluate the impact of altered pulmonary hemodynamics on the 6-min walk test (6MWT) result. This study aimed to investigate the role of pulmonary hemodynamics in determining 6MWT result of patients with ASD.

Method: Forty-six consecutive adult patients with ASD were included in this study. Right heart catheterization was performed to obtain the pulmonary hemodynamics profile. Meanwhile, 6MWT was presented as high or low with cut-off point 350 m. Receiver operating characteristic (ROC) was used for analytical methods.

Result: Abnormal functional capacity was indicated by ROC result of mPAP cut-off value of > 24 mmHg ($p = 0.0243$; AUC = 0.681). The value of PVR > 3.42 woods unit (WU) showed high specificity in determining abnormal functional capacity ($p = 0.0069$; AUC = 0.713). Flow ratio with cut-off point ≤4.89 had the highest sensitivity (100%) ($p = 0.8300$; AUC = 0.520).

Conclusion: Pulmonary hemodynamics can serve as an indicator of 6MWT result in adult ASD patients with values of mPAP> 24 mmHg and PVR > 3.42 WU.

Keywords: Atrial septal defect, Cardiac catheterization, Hemodynamic, Pulmonary hypertension

Background

Atrial septal defect (ASD) is a common congenital heart disease (CHD) with 1.64 per 1000 living birth prevalence and female predominance [1]. Ninety percent of the patients were reported to survive into adulthood and 35% of them developed secondary pulmonary hypertension (PH) [2, 3], which is defined as increased mean pulmonary artery pressure (mPAP) ≥25 mmHg in right heart catheterization (RHC) [4].

The presence of altered pulmonary hemodynamics due to secondary PH in adult patients with ASD is associated with reduced survival and high hospital utilization [5, 6]. Previous studies had presented the impact of altered pulmonary hemodynamics due to primary PH to functional capacity of the patient, which was measured by the 6-min walk test (6MWT) [7, 8]. The 6MWT result represents the functional capacity and predicts the outcome of the patient with PH. Values of 6MWT distance less than 350 m are a predictor of worse outcome [9].

In our knowledge, there has not been any observational studies which evaluate the impact of altered pulmonary hemodynamics due to secondary PH on adult patients with ASD on the 6MWT result. We conducted this study to investigate the role of each of the components of pulmonary hemodynamics in determining the 6MWT result.

Methods

Study participants and ethical consideration

Between January 2014 and March 2017, 46 consecutive patients with ASD in Dr. Sardjito General Hospital were included in this study. The inclusion criteria were: adults above 18 years of age, who were diagnosed with ASD. The diagnosis of ASD was confirmed by either transthoracic echocardiography or transesophageal echocardiography.

* Correspondence: supomo.tkv@mail.ugm.ac.id
[1]Department of Thoracic and Cardiovascular Surgery, Dr. Sardjito General Hospital, Faculty of Medicine, Public Health and Nursing, Universitas Gadjah Mada, Kesehatan St. Number 1, Sleman, Yogyakarta 55281, Indonesia
Full list of author information is available at the end of the article

This study included subjects who had not underwent ASD closure or vasodilator therapy to decrease PAP. This study was approved by the Institutional Ethics Committee of Faculty of Medicine, Public Health and Nursing of Universitas Gadjah Mada, Indonesia and the need for individual informed consent was waived.

Study protocols and definitions

All of the subjects underwent RHC to obtain their pulmonary hemodynamic profile. Pulmonary hemodynamic profile components analyzed in this study were mPAP, pulmonary vascular resistance (PVR), and flow ratio. Flow ratio is defined as ratio of Qp and Qs taken from RHC data.

$$Q_p = \frac{O_2 \text{ consumption (mL/ min)}}{\text{PV } O_2 \text{ content (mL/L)-PA } O_2 \text{ content (mL/L)}}$$

$$Q_s = \frac{O_2 \text{ consumption (mL/ min)}}{\text{SA } O_2 \text{ content (mL/L)-PA } O_2 \text{ content (mL/L)}}$$

PV (pulmonary vein); PA (pulmonary artery); SAO2 (blood oxygen saturation); MVO2 (myocardial volume oxygen).

High flow ratio is defined as Qp/Qs > 2.36 [10]. The PH was diagnosed when mPAP was ≥25 mmHg in RHC. The 6MWT was performed after RHC to obtain the information regarding the functional capacity of the patients according to American Thoracic Society guidelines [11]. It was performed indoors on a long, flat, straight, and hard surface. This test measures the distance in meters which a patient can quickly reach unassisted in 6 min. The abnormal functional capacity was defined as 6MWT distance less than 350 m. All patients were not provided supplemental oxygen while

Table 1 Baseline characteristic of the patients

Variables	N (%)	Mean ± SD	Median (min-max)
PH	25 (54.3)		
Non-PH	21 (45.7)		
Systolic Pressure (mmHg)			110 (84–150)
Diastolic Pressure (mmHg)			70 (60–104)
Age (years)[a]			33 (18–58)
mPAP (mmHg)		28.91 ± 11.41	
PVR (WU)[a]			1.90 (0.20–16.90)
Flow Ratio[a]			2.93 (1.27–9.00)
6MWT (m)[a]			366 (119–800)
Oxygen Saturation (%)			98 (88–99)
Normal 6MWT	20 (43.5)		
Abnormal 6MWT	26 (56.5)		

[a]Non-parametric data

Table 2 Difference characteristic between PH and non-PH

Variables	PH	Non-PH	p
ASD diameter (mm)	2.84 ± 0.82	2.47 ± 0.78	0.1154
LA dimension (mm)	34.52 ± 5.3	31.86 ± 5.03	0.0727
RA dimension (mm)[a]	48 (38–69)	45 (30–50)	0.0081
LV dimension (mm)	37.45 ± 5.37	34.55 ± 4.91	0.0495
RV dimension (mm)	46.3 ± 7.8	42.41 ± 4.15	0.0384
mPAP (mmHg)	36.42 ± 9.69	19.42 ± 4.19	< 0.0001
PVR (WU)[a]	3.05 (0.99–16.90)	1.05 (0.20–3.42)	< 0.0001
Flow Ratio[a]	2.70 (1.27–4.89)	3.12 (1.50–9.00)	0.3157
6MWT (m)[a]	326 (200–462)	391 (119–800)	0.0119
High Flow	332.67 ± 73.76	357.87 ± 83.41	0.2288[b]
Low Flow	373.5 (118.2–800)[a]	357 ± 25.06	

[a]Non-parametric data; [b]Analyzed by Kruskal Wallis

undergoing the 6MWT. Echocardiography data was used as a baseline data for further ASD evaluation.

Statistical analysis

Baseline characteristics of the patients are shown in Table 1. Continuous variables were presented as mean ± standard deviation (SD) and categorical variable was presented as percentage. Continuous variables with non-parametric data were presented in median. On bivariate analysis, difference between PH and non-PH is presented on Table 2. The results are considered to be significant if $p < 0.05$. The relationship between PH and functional capacity was analyzed using chi-square test (Table 3). In addition, correlations between each pulmonary hemodynamics component and 6MWT were analyzed using Spearman's rank correlation test due to their non-parametric data (Fig. 1). The ROC analysis was used for analyzing capability of mPAP, PVR, and flow ratio in determining functional capacity of the patient, which was presented as binary data of normal or abnormal (Fig. 2). Statistical review of the study was performed by a biomedical statistician. The data were analyzed using Medcalc software.

Results

Twenty-five (54.3%) patients had PH with mean mPAP 28.91 ± 11.41 mmHg (Table 1). On bivariate analysis, there were significant differences of 6MWT

Table 3 Relationship between PH and functional capacity of the patient

Variables	Abnormal functional capacity	Normal functional capacity	p
	(6MWT < 350 m)	(6MWT ≥350 m)	
PH	15	10	0.0302
Non-PH	5	16	

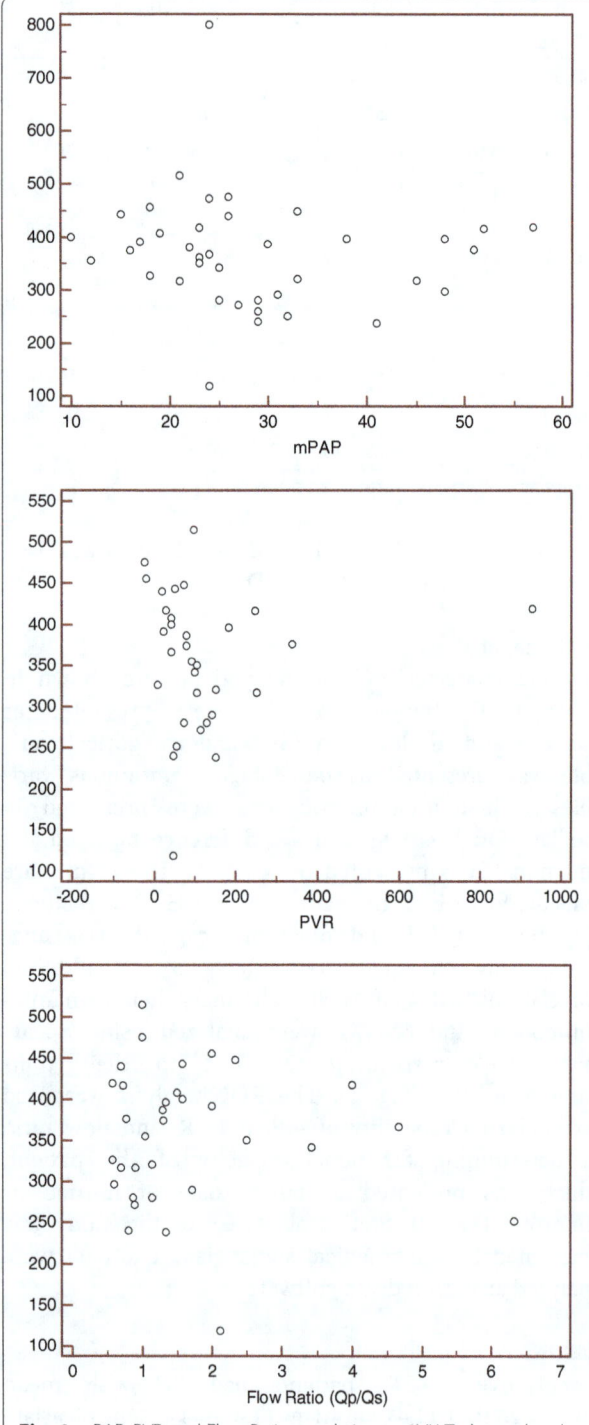

Fig. 1 mPAP, PVR, and Flow Ratio correlating to 6MWT plot analyzed with Spearman's rank correlation test ($r = -0.329$ $p = 0.0238$; $r = -0.339$ $p = 0.0212$; $r = -0.002$ $p = 0.9850$)

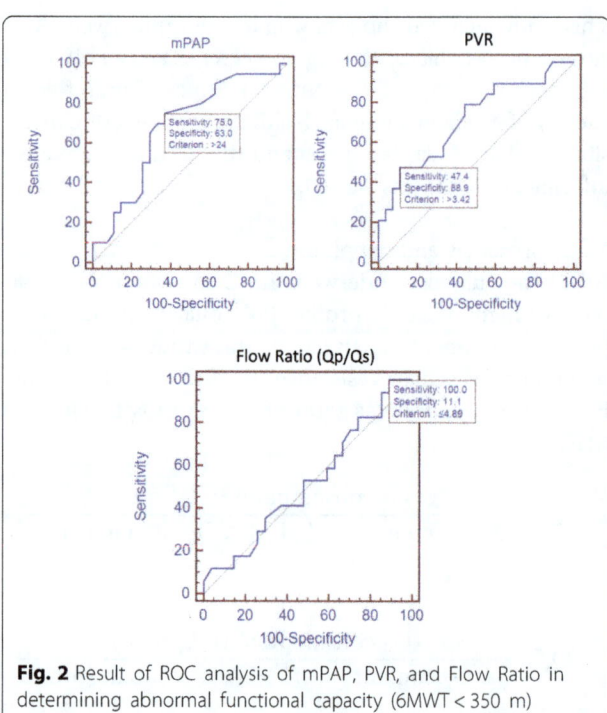

Fig. 2 Result of ROC analysis of mPAP, PVR, and Flow Ratio in determining abnormal functional capacity (6MWT < 350 m)

Relationship between PH and abnormal functional capacity of the patient was significant in chi-square analysis with $p = 0.0302$ (Table 3). Figure 1 shows the correlations between pulmonary hemodynamics and 6MWT distance. Increased mPAP and pulmonary vascular resistance (PVR) were significantly correlated with decline in 6MWT distance ($p = 0.0238$ and 0. 0212, respectively). However, the correlation between increased flow ratio and declined 6MWT distance was not significant ($p = 0.9850$).

ROC analysis results are shown in Fig. 2. The mPAP cut-off value of > 24 mmHg had 63% of specificity and 75% of sensitivity in determining abnormal functional capacity ($p = 0.0243$; AUC = 0.681). The value of PVR > 3.42 woods unit (WU) was shown to have 88.9% of specificity and 47.4% of sensitivity in determining abnormal functional capacity ($p = 0.0069$; AUC = 0.713). Flow ratio had the highest sensitivity (100%) in determining abnormal functional capacity with cut-off point ≤4.89. However, this result was not significant ($p = 0.8300$; AUC = 0. 520) and had a very low specificity (11.11%).

Discussion

In adult patients with ASD, the presence of PH was reported to have association with high mortality and hospital utilization [5, 6]. The presence of PH itself is determined using the value of mPAP, which is one of the pulmonary hemodynamic components. The value of mPAP≥25 mmHg is defined as PH [4]. However, whether this abnormal value also correlates with

distance between PH and non-PH patients with $p = 0.$ 0119 (Table 2). Mann Whitney analysis on 6MWT for high flow ratio and low ratio group showed a significant result ($p = 0.048$). Kruskal Wallis analysis for all flow ratio group showed no significant result.

functional limitation of the patient or not has previously not been studied. This study strengthens the link between altered pulmonary hemodynamics and functional capacity in adult patients with ASD.

This study used 6MWT as an indicator of functional capacity. Earlier studies showed that 6MWT could substitute cardiopulmonary exercise testing to measure functional capacity in low resources setting [12–14]. Several studies demonstrated the impact of altered pulmonary hemodynamics on functional capacity of the patient, which was determined using 6MWT [7, 8]. Minai et al. [7] found that patients with PH had significantly lower 6MWT compared to non-PH patients and mPAP was the best predictor of declined 6MWT distance in multivariate analysis. On the other hand, Miyamoto et al. [8] found that 6MWT significantly correlated with PVR, but was not significantly correlated with mPAP. These studies were conducted in patients with unexplained or primary PH.

In the case of altered pulmonary hemodynamics in secondary PH due to ASD, our study showed significant difference in 6MWT distance between PH and non-PH patients (Table 2). After 6MWT distance was divided into normal and abnormal functional capacity, chi-square analysis also revealed a significant relationship between those variables (Table 3). Both increased mPAP and PVR were significantly correlated with declined 6MWT distance (Fig. 1). These results demonstrated that altered pulmonary hemodynamics have an impact on functional capacity of the adult patients with ASD.

Significant difference of 6MWT results between high and low flow ratio PH patients showed that functional capacity is correlated with shunt severity. Results from ROC analysis showed flow ratio of pulmonary to systemic circulation had the highest sensitivity (100%) in determining abnormal functional capacity, but this result was not significant and had a very low specificity (11.1%).

In addition, this study also analyzed the capability of each of the pulmonary hemodynamic components in determining abnormal functional capacity of the patients using ROC analysis. Significant result was shown by mPAP and PVR. The value of mPAP> 24 mmHg (sensitivity 75%, specificity 63%) and PVR > 3.42 WU (sensitivity 47.4%, specificity 88.9%) were determined to be predictors of this abnormal condition (Fig. 2).

Limitations

Our study has the limitation of using a cross-sectional design, which only provides the outcome and factors associated to it at a specific point of time. In addition, patients included in this study were only adult ASD patients with more than 18 years of age. Therefore, the results of this study may not be applicable for pediatric ASD patients.

Conclusion

The presence of altered pulmonary hemodynamic on secondary PH due to ASD in adult patients is associated with abnormal functional capacity. Values of mPAP> 24 mmHg and PVR > 3.42 WU were found to be indicators of this abnormal condition.

Abbreviations
6MWT: 6-min walk test; ASD: Atrial septal defect; CHD: Congenital heart disease; mPAP: Mean pulmonary artery pressure; PH: Pulmonary hypertension; PVR: Pulmonary vascular resistance; RHC: Right heart catheterization; SD: Standard deviation

Acknowledgements
The authors give thanks to all ASD patients in Dr. Sardjito General hospital, who participated in this study.

Funding
This study used authors' personal funds.

Authors' contributions
S, HD, and AZA contributed to study conception and design; HD and AZA contributed to data acquisition, analysis, and interpretation; S and HD contributed to article writing; S, HD, and AZA contributed to editing, reviewing, and final approving of article.

Competing interests
The authors declare that they have no competing interests.

Author details
[1]Department of Thoracic and Cardiovascular Surgery, Dr. Sardjito General Hospital, Faculty of Medicine, Public Health and Nursing, Universitas Gadjah Mada, Kesehatan St. Number 1, Sleman, Yogyakarta 55281, Indonesia.
[2]Faculty of Medicine, Universitas Islam Indonesia, Yogyakarta, Indonesia.

References
1.　Van Der Linde D, Konings EEM, Slager MA, Witsenburg M, Helbing WA, Takkenberg JJM, Roos-Hesselink JW. Birth prevalence of congenital heart disease worldwide: a systematic review and meta-analysis. J Am Coll Cardiol. 2011;58:2241–7 PMID: 22078432. https://doi.org/10.1016/j.jacc.2011.08.025.
2.　Kuijpers JM, Mulder BJM, Bouma BJ. Secundum atrial septal defect in adults: a practical review and recent developments. Neth Heart J. 2015;23:205–11 PMID: 25884091. https://doi.org/10.1007/s12471-015-0663-z.
3.　Engelfriet P, Meijboom F, Boersma E, Tijssen J, Mulder B. Repaired and open atrial septal defect type II in adulthood: an epidemiological study of a large european cohort. Int J Cardiol. 2008;126:379–85 PMID: 17586067. https://doi.org/10.1016/j.ijcard.2007.04.044.
4.　Badesch DB, Champion HC, Sanchez MAG, Hoeper MM, Loyd JE, Manes A, McGoon M, Naeije R, Olschewski H, Oudiz RJ, Torbicki A. Diagnosis and assessment of pulmonary arterial hypertension. J Am Coll Cardiol. 2009;54: s55–66 PMID: 19555859. https://doi.org/10.1016/j.jacc.2009.04.011.
5.　Lowe BS, Therrien J, Ionescu-Ittu R, Pilote L, Martucci G, Marelli AJ. Diagnosis of pulmonary hypertension in the congenital heart disease adult population. J Am Coll Cardiol. 2011;58:538–46 PMID: 21777753. https://doi.org/10.1016/j.jacc.2011.03.033.
6.　Rodriguez FH 3rd, Moodie DS, Parekh DR, Franklin WJ, Morales DL, Zafar F, Graves DE, Friedman RA, Rossano JW. Outcomes of hospitalization in adults in the United States with atrial septal defect, ventricular septal defect, and

atrioventricular septal defect. Am J Cardiol. 2011;108:290–3 PMID: 21545985. https://doi.org/10.1016/j.amjcard.2011.03.036.

7. Minai OA, Santacruz JF, Alster JM, Budev MM, McCarthy K. Impact of pulmonary hemodynamics on 6-min walk test in idiopathic pulmonary fibrosis. Respir Med. 2012;106:1613–21 PMID: 22902266. https://doi.org/10.1016/j.rmed.2012.07.013.

8. Miyamoto S, Nagaya N, Satoh T, Kyotani S, Sakamaki F, Fujita M, Nakanishi N, Miyatake K. Clinical correlates and prognostic significance of six-minute walk test in patients with primary pulmonary hypertension. Am J Respir Crit Care Med. 2000;161:487–92 PMID: 10673190. https://doi.org/10.1164/ajrccm.161.2.9906015.

9. Lai YC, Potoka KC, Champion HC, Mora AL, Gladwin MT. Pulmonary arterial hypertension: the clinical syndrome. Circ Res. 2014;115:115–30 PMID: 24951762. https://doi.org/10.1161/CIRCRESAHA.115.301146.

10. Farouk A, Algowhary M, Hassan MH, et al. Circulating B-type natriuretic peptide levels and its correlation to Qp/Qs ratio among children undergoing congenital heart surgery. J Egypt Soc Cardio-Thoracic Surg. 2017;25(1):58–63. https://doi.org/10.1016/j.jescts.2017.03.002.

11. ATS Committee on Proficiency Standards for Clinical Pulmonary Function Laboratories. ATS statement: guidelines for the six-minute walk test. Am J Respir Crit Care Med. 2002;166:111–7 PMID: 12091180. https://doi.org/10.1164/ajrccm.166.1.at1102.

12. de Assis Ramos R, Guimarães FS, Dionyssiotis Y, Tsekoura D, Papathanasiou J, de Sá Ferreira A. Development of a multivariate model of the six-minute walked distance to predict functional exercise capacity in hypertension. J Bodyw Mov Ther. 2018:1–7. https://doi.org/10.1016/j.jbmt.2018.01.010.

13. Omar HR, Guglin M. The longitudinal relationship between six-minute walk test and cardiopulmonary exercise testing, and association with symptoms in systolic heart failure: analysis from the ESCAPE trial. Eur J Intern Med. 2017;40:e26–8. https://doi.org/10.1016/j.ejim.2016.12.017.

14. Burr JF, Bredin SSD, Faktor MD, Warburton DER. The 6-minute walk test as a predictor of objectively measured aerobic fitness in healthy working-aged adults. Phys Sports Med. 2011;39(2):133–9. https://doi.org/10.3810/psm.2011.05.1904.

28

Preoperative determinants of quality of life a year after coronary artery bypass grafting: a historical cohort study

Lisa Verwijmeren[1], Peter Gerben Noordzij[1]*[iD], Edgar Jozeph Daeter[2], Bas van Zaane[3], Linda Margaretha Peelen[3,4] and Eric Paulus Adrianus van Dongen[1]

Abstract

Background: Health related quality of life (HRQL) is an important patient related outcome measure after cardiac surgery. Preoperative determinants for postoperative HRQL have not yet been identified, but could aid in preoperative decision making. The aim of this article is to identify associations between preoperative determinants and change in HRQL 1 year after coronary artery bypass grafting (CABG).

Methods: Single centre retrospective cohort study in 658 patients. Change in HRQL was defined as a decrease or increase of ≥5 points on the physical or mental domain of the Short Form 12 (SF-12) questionnaire. Patients were stratified in three groups according to worse, unchanged, or better HRQL. Multinomial logistic regression analysis was used to investigate the association between preoperative risk factors and postoperative change in HRQL.

Results: Physical HRQL improved in 22.8% of patients, did not change in 61.2% of patients and worsened in 16.0% of patients. Comorbidities associated with change in physical HRQL were a history of stroke, atrial fibrillation, vascular disease or pulmonary disease. Most important risk factor for change in physical HRQL was preoperative HRQL. Higher preoperative SF-12 score decreased the odds for worse physical HRQL and increased the odds for better physical HRQL. Mental HRQL improved in 49.8% of patients, remained unchanged in 34.5% of patients and worsened in 15.7% of patients. Preoperative HRQL was an important risk factor for a change in mental HRQL. Higher preoperative physical HRQL increased the odds for improved mental HRQL. Lower preoperative mental HRQL increased the odds for better mental HRQL.

Conclusions: One year after CABG the majority of patients experiences equal or improved HRQL compared to before surgery. Most important preoperative risk factor for change in HRQL is preoperative HRQL.

Keywords: Quality of life, Coronary artery bypass graft surgery, Risk factors

Background

In the past years the population of patients referred for coronary artery bypass grafting (CABG) changed to an older and more complex population [1–3]. Assumed causes are an increased life expectancy and improvements in surgical and anaesthetic techniques, making it possible for elderly high risk patients to undergo surgery [1, 2]. Even though CABG is considered safe for elderly patients, a considerable risk for complications or mortality remains [4]. Especially in more complex patients a tailored approach is needed in which health benefits are weighed against risk of complications. Risk stratification tools like the European System for Cardiac Operative Risk Evaluation (euroSCORE), Parsonnet score or the American College of Surgeons Risk Calculator can aid in estimating outcome after surgery [5–7]. However, these tools were developed to predict morbidity or mortality, not health related quality of life (HRQL) [8]. In general, HRQL improves after cardiac surgery, but it is known that 8–19% of patients experiences a decrease in HRQL [9]. In addition to the traditional outcome parameters of major morbidity or mortality, information on patient-perceived postoperative HRQL is crucial for full informed consent

---

* Correspondence: p.noordzij@antoniusziekenhuis.nl
[1]Anesthesiology, Intensive Care and Pain Medicine, St. Antonius Hospital, Koekoekslaan 1, Nieuwegein 3430 EM, The Netherlands
Full list of author information is available at the end of the article

prior to surgery. To optimize preoperative risk-assessment and facilitate shared decision making, more accurate data on risk factors that influence postoperative HRQL are needed. This study aims to identify which preoperative determinants are associated with a clinically relevant change in HRQL 1 year after CABG.

Materials and methods
Design
This was a single centre retrospective cohort study. Since patients were not subjected to investigational actions and were treated according to standard guidelines the need for informed consent was waived by the local review board of the ethical committee (Medical research Ethics Committee United, number W15.069). The study was conducted in accordance with the principles of the Declaration of Helsinki.

Population
All patients older than 18 years who underwent elective isolated CABG between the first of July 2011 and the first of May 2014 were eligible for inclusion. Inclusion criteria were a completed medical outcomes study Short Form (SF) 12 version 2 questionnaire at baseline and at 12 months after CABG. Surgical procedures were performed by multiple cardiothoracic surgery consultants and their supervised trainees in a tertiary referral hospital (St. Antonius Hospital, Nieuwegein, The Netherlands). Perioperative care was carried out according to standard clinical practice and based on international guidelines for all patients [10].

Clinical characteristics and data collection
As potential determinants for postoperative HRQL patient characteristics, medical history and comorbidities, preoperative laboratory tests and preoperative HRQL were considered.

Data on age, gender, body mass index and preoperative laboratory tests were collected from the routine preoperative anaesthesia visit. Medical history, additive euroSCORE and postoperative complications were collected from the hospital's electronic database for cardiac surgery patients. Registration of postoperative complications was conducted in the context of a national registry of cardiac interventions in The Netherlands (Supervisory Committee for Cardiac Interventions (Begeleidingscommissie Hartinterventies Nederland) [11]. Intraoperative data was collected from the computerized medical record (MetaVision 5.46.44, iMDsoft®, Düsseldorf, Germany). A manual review of the data was performed to check for accuracy and missing values by a member of the research team (LV). Missing data on laboratory values, medication use and surgical characteristics were fully completed by manually checking electronic patient records.

Outcomes
Primary outcome was change in HRQL 12 months after surgery measured with the SF-12 before surgery and at 1 year after surgery. The SF-12 is derived from the SF-36, a widely validated questionnaire including 36 questions on physical and mental well-being [12]. The SF-12 is a validated shorter version with 12 questions [13]. Questions include, but are not limited to items relating to overall health perception, being able to exercise, feeling at ease or feeling full of energy. Answers on these 12 items are converted into two norm-based scores ranging from 0 to 100, representing physical and mental HRQL [14]. Higher scores represent better HRQL. Additional file 1: Table S1 presents reference scores for the Dutch population.

Secondary outcome was a composite endpoint of any complication and defined as one or more of the following; new atrial fibrillation defined as rhythm disturbance requiring treatment including reanimation, defibrillation or medication; re-sternotomy, defined as reoperation requiring opening of the sternum; myocardial infarction, defined as presence of ≥2 of the following symptoms: prolonged typical chest pain, ≥ten-fold increase of cardiac enzyme levels, and new wall motion abnormalities and/or changes in two or more leads in at least two consecutive ECGs; deep sternal wound infection, defined as requiring surgical drainage or fixation, positive wound cultures or antibiotic therapy; and ischemic stroke, defined as an acute episode of cerebral, spinal or retinal dysfunction caused by infarction of the central nervous system lasting > 72 h.

Procedures
As part of routine care, SF-12 questionnaires were sent by mail to all patients before surgery and were collected at the time of hospital admission. Twelve months after the operation a questionnaire was sent by email to each surviving patient. This study was carried out as a retrospective analysis of data collected for quality assessment purposes. In this process no second request was made to retrieve a missing questionnaire when a patient did not respond.

Statistical analysis
Data are presented as frequencies and percentages of total for categorical data, as mean ± standard deviation (SD) for normally distributed continuous data and as median and interquartile range (IQR) for non-normally distributed continuous data. Normality was tested using visual inspection of histograms and Kolmogorov-Smirnov test. Scores for preoperative HRQL were compared to the Dutch population mean using a one sample t-test. A paired sample t-test was used to compare preoperative HRQL to scores at 1 year after surgery. A delta score was calculated for change in HRQL by subtracting preoperative SF-12

scores from postoperative SF-12 scores. A positive delta score represents an improvement in HRQL.

To study the clinical relevance of the difference in HRQL a threshold value was used to compare groups. As standard threshold values are lacking in CABG surgery for the SF-12 questionnaire, we based our threshold value on two articles using the SF-36 in elderly patients undergoing CABG or aortic valve surgery. Welke et al. defined a clinically relevant change as a difference of ≥5.42 points in physical or ≥ 6.33 in mental HRQL [15]. Jansen-Klomp et al. used a cut-off point of ≥2.5 points [16]. As with the SF-12 questionnaire the HRQL could increase or decrease as much as four points by changing the results of a single question, we set the threshold value at 5 or more points decrease or increase to ensure a clinically relevant change. Subsequently, the study cohort was stratified in three groups according to change in HRQL: worse, no change or better HRQL. Differences between the three groups were tested using Chi square test for dichotomous or categorical variables and one way ANOVA or Kruskal Wallis test for continuous data depending on normality.

To analyse the independent effects of all risk factors a multivariable model was built using multinomial logistic regression analysis. This analysis allows for a dependent variable with more than two categories. Patients with no clinically relevant change in HRQL were used as reference category to which the outcomes 'worse HRQL' and 'better HRQL' were compared. No variable selection took place and all variables were added simultaneously. To prevent multicollinearity, correlations between all variables were tested using Pearson's correlation coefficient. Of variables with a correlation > 0.8 one variable was excluded from the model. Non-linearity of the continuous variables regarding preoperative physical and mental HRQL was investigated by adding various transformations and assessing model fit in terms of log likelihood. If model fit improved, the transformations were retained in the multivariable model. Results are presented as odds ratios with their accompanying confidence intervals. For statistical analysis IBM SPSS version 22 (IBM Corp. Released 2013. IBM SPSS Statistics for Windows, Version 22.0. Armonk, NY: IBM Corp.) was used. A p-value < 0.05 was considered as statistically significant for all analyses.

Results
Study population
In total, 2100 patients underwent elective isolated CABG. Of these patients, 1225 completed a baseline SF-12. Thirty-two patients died within 1 year. 658 (31.3% of total, 53.7% of 1225) patients returned the 12 month follow up questionnaire and were included in the final cohort (Fig. 1). Overall, non-responders had more comorbidities compared to responders. This was expressed by significant

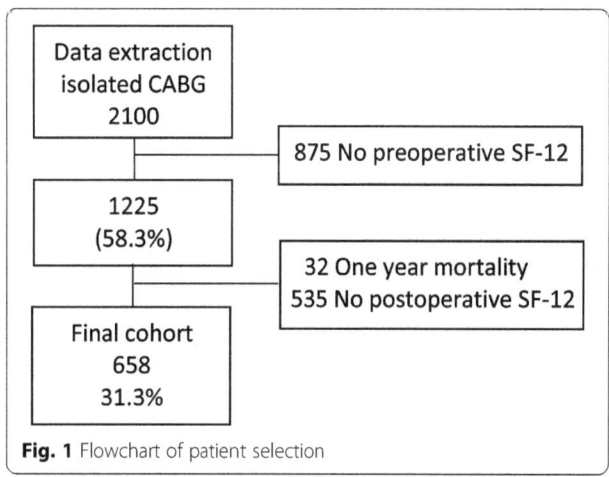

Fig. 1 Flowchart of patient selection

differences in age, incidence of male gender, diabetes mellitus, prior myocardial infarction, LVEF and euroSCORE. Additional file 2: Table S2 shows other baseline variables for responders and non-responders.

Patient characteristics and outcome
Mean age was 66 years (SD ±9) minimum age was 47 and maximum age was 87 years old. The majority of patients was male (82.4%). Baseline characteristics including preoperative HRQL are presented in Table 1. In-hospital complications occurred in 41 (6.2%) patients. Postoperative atrial fibrillation was most common and occurred in 19 (2.9%) patients. Median length of stay was 6 (IQR 4–7) days. Mean preoperative physical HRQL in the study cohort was lower compared to the Dutch population mean (39.2 (SD ±5.4) vs 50.6 (SD ±9.2) $p < 0.001$ respectively, difference: -11.4; 95% CI -11.8 to − 11.0). One year after surgery mean physical HRQL increased slightly to 39.9 (SD ±4.6) ($p = 0.007$) but remained below the population mean (difference − 10.7; 95% CI -11.0 to − 10.3). Mean preoperative mental HRQL was lower compared to the population mean (48.9 (SD ±13.1) vs 50.2 (SD ±9.2) $p = 0.001$ respectively, difference: -1.7; 95% CI -2.7 to − 0.7). Mean mental HRQL improved to 54.4 (SD ±12.6) ($p < 0.001$) after surgery and rose above population mean (difference 3.8; 95% CI 2.8 to 4.8).

Determinants of a clinically relevant change in physical HRQL
Physical HRQL 1 year after surgery improved in 150 (22.8%) patients, did not change in 403 (61.2%) patients and got worse in 105 (16.0%) patients. Preoperative median EuroSCORE was 3 (IQR 1–4), 3 (IQR 1–4), and 3 (IQR 1–5) for worse, no change or better physical HRQL respectively ($p = 0.802$). Median preoperative physical HRQL was 45.3 (IQR 41.5–48.5) for patients with worse physical HRQL; 39.7 (IQR 37.1–42.1) for patients with no change in physical HRQL and 34.8 (IQR 31.3–37.2)

Table 1 Baseline

	N = 658
Age (years)	65.5 ± 9.0
Male gender	542 (82.4%)
Current smoking	191 (29.0%)
Body mass index (kg/m2)	26.8 (24.6–29.8)
Hypertension	338 (51.4%)
Myocardial infarction	75 (11.4%)
Stroke	54 (8.2%)
Pulmonary disease	50 (7.6%)
Atrial fibrillation	26 (4.0%)
Peripheral vascular disease	68 (10.3%)
Unstable angina	65 (9.9%)
Diabetes mellitus	133 (20.2%)
Left ventricular ejection fraction	
Good (≥50%)	546 (83.0%)
Moderate (30–50%)	94 (14.3%)
Poor (< 30%)	18 (2.7%)
Additive EuroSCORE	3 (1–4)
Preoperative hemoglobine (mmol/l)	8.8 (8.2–9.3)
Preoperative creatinine (µmol/)	82 (73–95)
Health related quality of life	
Preoperative physical HRQL	39.2 ± 5.4 39.0 (36.0–42.6)
Preoperative mental HRQL	48.9 ± 13.1 50.3 (40.2–59.0)
Surgical characteristics	
Duration of surgery (min)	189 (163–226)
Extra corporeal circulation time(min)	83 (68–101)
Mini extra corporeal circulation	485 (73.7%)
Use of internal mammary artery	626 (95.1%)
Packed red blood cell transfusion[a]	54 (8.2%)
Blood loss (ml)[b]	660 (519–850)

Data are presented as mean (±standard deviation), medians (interquartile range) or frequencies (%)
HRQL health related quality of life
[a]Intraoperative packed red blood cell transfusion
[b]Blood loss at 24 h after surgery

for patients with better HRQL ($p < 0.001$). Median preoperative mental HRQL was 47.2 (IQR 35.9–54.1); 50.5 (IQR 40.8–59.2) and 52.6 (IQR 43.1–60.8) for patients with worse, no change or better HRQL respectively ($p = 0.001$). Postoperative complications occurred in 6.7% of patients with worse physical HRQL, in 5.5% of patients with no change in physical HRQL and in 8.0% of patients with better physical HRQL ($p = 0.536$).

Table 2 shows the independent odds ratios of preoperative risk factors for a change in physical HRQL. Clinical features significantly associated with a change in physical HRQL were a history of stroke, atrial fibrillation, vascular disease or pulmonary disease. Patients with a prior stroke showed increased odds for worse physical HRQL. A history of atrial fibrillation or vascular disease decreased the odds for a worse physical HRQL and a history of pulmonary disease increased the odds for improved HRQL. Preoperative physical HRQL was significantly associated with a change in physical HRQL. A higher preoperative value on the SF-12 decreased the odds for worse HRQL and increased the odds for better HRQL.

Determinants of a clinically relevant change in mental HRQL

Mental HRQL improved in 328 (49.8%) patients at 1 year after surgery, remained unchanged in 227 (34.5%) patients and worsened in 103 (15.7%) patients. Preoperative median euroSCORE was 3 (IQR 1–5) for patients with worse mental HRQL, 3 (IQR 1–4) for patients with no change in mental HRQL, and 3 (IQR 1–4) for patients with better mental HRQL ($p = 0.887$). Prior to surgery, physical HRQL was 37.9 (IQR 35.0–41.7); 37.9 (IQR 35.1–41.4) and 40.5 (IQR 37.0–43.9) for patients with worse, no change or better HRQL respectively ($p < 0.001$). Preoperative mental HRQL was 55.2 (IQR 46.9–63.7); 55.6 (IQR 46.6–63.6) and 45.1 (IQR 34.7–53.4) for patients with worse, no change or better HRQL respectively ($p < 0.001$). Postoperative complications were seen in 8.7% of patients with worse mental HRQL, in 5.3% of patients with no change in mental HRQL and in 6.1% of patients with better mental HRQL ($p = 0.481$).

Independent odds ratios of preoperative risk factors for a change in mental HRQL are shown in Table 3. No significant associations were seen between clinical risk factors and worse or better mental HRQL 1 year after CABG. Higher preoperative physical HRQL increased the odds for improved mental HRQL. Lower preoperative mental HRQL increased the odds for better mental HRQL.

Discussion

In this study the most important determinant for a change in HRQL 1 year after CABG was preoperative HRQL. Higher preoperative physical HRQL led to improved outcomes regarding physical and mental HRQL at 1 year after surgery considering other clinical risk factors. Lower mental HRQL before surgery increased the chance to improve in mental HRQL at 1 year after surgery. The influence of preoperative HRQL on a change after surgery illustrates the vital importance of acquiring information on HRQL in the preoperative setting in order to fully inform patients on expected patient-centred outcomes.

Change in HRQL

In the majority of patients physical HRQL hardly changed, as was reflected by a mean increase of 0.7 points. Mental

Table 2 Multinomial regression analysis for change in physical HRQL

	Worse physical HRQL		Better physical HRQL	
	Beta	OR (95% CI)	Beta	OR (95% CI)
Age (per year)	−0.03	0.97 (0.92–1.01)	−0.00	1.00 (0.95–1.04)
Body mass index (per point)	0.02	1.02 (0.94–1.09)	−0.04	0.96 (0.91–1.02)
EuroSCORE (per point)	0.16	1.18 (0.95–1.46)	−0.03	0.98 (0.81–1.18)
LVEF > 50%	0	1.00	0	0
LVEF 30–50%	1.67	5.32 (0.41–69.61)	0.60	1.82 (0.43–7.65)
LVEF < 30%	1.15	3.16 (0.25–39.56)	0.66	1.94 (0.50–7.61)
Hemoglobin (per point)	−0.03	0.97 (0.65–1.44)	−0.24	0.79 (0.56–1.10)
Creatinine (per point)	−0.01	0.99 (0.98–1.01)	−0.00	1.00 (0.99–1.01)
Preoperative physical HRQL (per point)				
Singular	−1.25[***]		0.54	
Quadratic	0.02[***]	a	−0.01[*]	a
Preoperative mental HRQL (per point)	0.00	1.00 (0.98–1.03)	0.01	1.01 (0.99–1.03)
Male gender	0.07	1.07 (0.43–4.47)	0.11	1.12 (0.52–2.41)
Active smoking	0.41	1.51 (0.79–2.88)	0.45	1.57 (0.91–2.69)
Hypertension	0.51	1.67 (0.91–3.06)	−0.04	0.96 (0.60–1.55)
Myocardial infarction	0.18	1.19 (0.50–2.84)	0.37	1.45 (0.69–3.04)
Stroke	0.99[*]	2.68 (1.04–6.88)	0.47	1.60 (0.98–3.79)
Pulmonary disease	0.44	1.56 (0.55–4.43)	0.86[*]	2.36 (1.05–5.31)
Atrial fibrillation	−3.17[*]	0.04 (0.00–0.97)	−1.50	0.22 (0.05–1.10)
Peripheral vascular disease	−1.23[*]	0.29 (0.10–0.90)	0.20	1.23 (0.57–2.64)
Unstable angina	−0.47	0.62 (0.24–1.63)	0.22	1.25 (0.57–2.75)
Diabetes mellitus	0.22	0.25 (0.59–2.65)	−0.13	0.88 (0.49–1.60)

Unchanged HRQL was the reference category. Worse and Better HRQL were defined as ≥5 points change in delta HRQL

LVEF left ventricular ejection fraction, *HRQL* health related quality of life

[*] = $p < 0.050$, [***] = $p < 0.001$

[a]Since clinical interpretation of odds ratios is limited for quadratic equations this is not presented

HRQL increased in half of patients, with a mean increase of 5.5 points.

Contrasting to our findings, other studies using the SF-36, showed a mean increase in physical HRQL ranging from 4.8 to 5.3 points and a mean increase in mental HRQL of 1.2 to 1.9 points [17, 18]. In a cohort of 1744 patients, Rumsfeld et al. assessed SF-36 before and 6 months after CABG surgery. Health related quality of life increased 5.3 and 1.9 points for physical and mental HRQL respectively. Comparable to our results, preoperative physical HRQL was identified as the most important risk factor for a change in HRQL after taking other preoperative cardiac and non-cardiac risk factors into account [17].

Deutsch et al. performed a study in 106 octogenarians undergoing CABG, valve surgery or CABG combined with valve surgery. They assessed HRQL by SF-36 three and 12 months after surgery and compared it to preoperative scores. At 3 months physical HRQL significantly increased with 5.1 points and mental HRQL was comparable to preoperative levels. Cardiac and non-cardiac comorbidities

and procedural data were not identified as relevant risk factors for change in HRQL. Unfortunately, baseline HRQL was not considered as possible risk factor for a change in HRQL in their study [18].

In contrast to other literature reports, physical HRQL at 1 year after surgery increased to a lesser extent in our study, while the increase in mental HRQL was more eminent [15, 17, 18].

These differences could be due to the moment of measuring HRQL. At 1 year after surgery, which was the moment of measurement in our study, HRQL could have been affected by other factors as well, resulting in lower scores.

Furthermore, CABG is mainly performed to relieve complaints of angina, which is likely to result in improved physical functioning. In our cohort less than 10% of patients suffered from unstable angina while this was present in up to 28–61% in patients in other articles [17, 19]. It is conceivable that patients in this study suffered from fewer complaints before surgery and therefore did not notice a relevant increase in physical HRQL.

Table 3 Multinomial regression analysis for change in mental HRQL

	Worse mental HRQL		Better mental HRQL	
	Beta	OR (95% CI)	Beta	OR (95% CI)
Age (per year)	−0.02	0.98 (0.93–1.02)	0.01	1.01 (0.97–1.04)
Body mass index (per point)	0.02	1.02 (0.96–1.08)	0.01	1.01 (0.96–1.06)
EuroSCORE (per point)	0.02	1.02 (0.85–1.23)	−0.07	0.94 (0.80–1.10)
LVEF > 50%	0	0	0	0
LVEF 30–50%	−0.36	0.84 (0.21–3.39)	1.13	3.09 (0.60–15.83)
LVEF < 30%	− 0.18	0.70 (0.19–2.63)	0.66	1.93 (0.40–9.36)
Hemoglobin (per point)	−0.15	0.86 (0.61–1.23)	0.03	1.07 (0.80–1.43)
Creatinine (per point)	0.01	1.01 (1.00–1.02)	−0.00	1.00 (0.99–1.01)
Preoperative physical HRQL (per point)	− 0.00	1.00 (0.95–1.05)	0.08[***]	1.08 (1.04–1.13)
Preoperative mental HRQL (per point)				
Singular	0.02		−1.07[**]	
Quadratic	−0.01		0.02[**]	
Cubic	0.00	[a]	0.00[**]	[a]
Male gender	0.15	1.17 (0.52–2.61)	−0.04	0.96 (0.50–1.85)
Active smoking	− 0.09	0.92 (0.51–1.65)	0.03	1.04 (0.65–1.65)
Hypertension	0.16	1.18 (0.71–1.95)	0.12	1.13 (0.75–1.71)
Myocardial infarction	0.20	1.23 (0.60–2.51)	−0.56	0.57 (0.29–1.11)
Stroke	− 0.03	0.97 (0.37–2.50)	0.18	1.19 (0.57–2.52)
Pulmonary disease	0.37	1.45 (0.63–3.34)	−0.62	0.54 (0.25–1.14)
Atrial fibrillation	0.39	1.48 (0.44–4.99)	−0.35	0.71 (0.23–2.15)
Peripheral vascular disease	0.00	1.00 (0.41–2.44)	0.34	1.41 (0.72–2.77)
Unstable angina	0.17	1.12 (0.52–2.74)	0.20	1.22 (0.62–2.41)
Diabetes mellitus	− 0.6	0.94 (0.49–1.81)	0.02	1.02 (0.60–1.74)

Unchanged HRQL was the reference category. Worse and Better HRQL were defined as ≥5 points change in delta HRQL respectively
LVEF Left ventricular ejection fraction, *HRQL* health related quality of life
[**]$p = < 0.005$, [***] $= p < 0.00$
[a]Since clinical interpretation of odds ratios is limited for quadratic and cubic equations this is not presented

Also, questions regarding mental HRQL in the SF-12 include items as feeling full of energy, calm and peaceful or feeling downhearted. Although patients did not report an improvement in questions on physical functioning, CABG surgery may have improved mental status by relieving anxiety and enhancing feelings of security and self-esteem. The increase in mental HRQL in our study could reflect the overall benefit of the surgery.

Risk factors for change in HRQL after cardiac surgery
Preoperative risk stratification based on patient-centered outcomes, such as HRQL, could have great additional value in cardiac surgery but remains challenging as well designed risk models are lacking. Possible risk factors for change in HRQL that are readily available such as comorbidities, laboratory values or LVEF have been considered by others but resulted in conflicting results. Female gender [20, 21], older age [22], diabetes mellitus [15, 21, 23], body mass index > 35 [15], low LVEF [21], pulmonary disease [15], vascular disease [15], EuroSCORE > 3 [8], deprived

socio-economic status [23] and smoking [23] have been associated with worse HRQL following cardiac surgery. Older age [15], high social support [23], and EuroSCORE > 6 [24] have been associated with better HRQL after cardiac surgery. However, several other studies, including ours, found no association between preoperative clinical factors and change in postoperative HRQL [17, 19]. Studies that included preoperative HRQL in their analysis concluded that HRQL prior to surgery was the most promising predictor for postoperative change in HRQL [15, 17, 19] and that routine preoperative assessment of HRQL should be incorporated in standard care to supplement current risk assessment [25, 26].

Some limitations should be addressed. First, the retrospective design limited the amount of available data. Comparison of responders versus non-responders showed that non-responders were older, more often male and showed a higher prevalence of diabetes mellitus, myocardial infarction, lower LVEF and higher euroSCORE. These factors can have a negative effect on postoperative HRQL [15, 20–23].

With inclusion of these patients likely greater differences in HRQL might have been present and possibly more preoperative predictors would have been identified. A possible reason for non-responding could be the method of approach during the follow up period, where questionnaires were sent by email without a reminder for unanswered questionnaires. Not all patients have email, which is more often the case for elderly. Second, obviously no SF-12 scores were available for deceased patients and these patients were excluded from the analysis. Mortality risk is highest for patients with more comorbidities. It is conceivable that this excluded group of patients had more comorbidities, leading to lower scores for preoperative HRQL and, subsequently different change scores. However, 1 year mortality was merely 2.6% and it seems unlikely this had a major influence on results. Third, only elective surgery patients were analysed limiting the generalisability and excluding patients with emergency CABG. However, the indication for emergency surgery is focussed on survival, while the main indication for elective CABG is to relieve angina. In elderly patients scheduled for elective surgery risk factors for postoperative HRQL are more essential for the decision making process than in patient presenting for emergency surgery.

Conclusion

In conclusion, 1 year after CABG surgery the majority of patients experiences equal or improved HRQL when compared to before surgery. Most important preoperative determinant for a change in HRQL is HRQL prior to surgery.

Abbreviations

CABG: Coronary artery bypass grafting; euroSCORE: European System for Cardiac Operative Risk Evaluation; HRQL: Health related quality of life; IQR: Interquartile range; LVEF: Left ventricular ejection fraction; OR: Odds ratio; SD: Standard deviation; SF-12: Short Form 12

Acknowledgements

Not applicable.

Funding

None of the authors received funding.

Authors' contributions

All authors contributed to the manuscript. LV acquired part of the patient data, performed the statistical analysis, and wrote the draft of the manuscript. PGN was responsible for the conception and design of the study, design of the analysis and revising the manuscript. EJD was responsible for the acquisition of the health related quality of life data and revisions of the manuscript. BvZ took part in the design of the analysis and revising the manuscript. LMP played a vital role in the design of the study, the statistical analysis and interpretation of the data and revising the manuscript. EPAvD was part of critically revising the manuscript for important intellectual content. All authors read and approved the final manuscript.

Authors' information

Not applicable.

Competing interests

The authors declare that they have no competing interests.

Author details

[1]Anesthesiology, Intensive Care and Pain Medicine, St. Antonius Hospital, Koekoekslaan 1, Nieuwegein 3430 EM, The Netherlands. [2]Cardiac Surgery, St. Antonius Hospital, Koekoekslaan 1, Nieuwegein 3430 EM, The Netherlands. [3]Anesthesiology, Intensive Care and Emergency Medicine, University Medical Center Utrecht, Utrecht University, Heidelberglaan 100, Utrecht 3584 CX, The Netherlands. [4]Epidemiology, Julius Center for Health Sciences and Primary Care, University Medical Center Utrecht, Utrecht University, Heidelberglaan 100, Utrecht 3584 CX, The Netherlands.

References

1. Pierri MD, Capestro F, Zingaro C, Torracca L. The changing face of cardiac surgery patients: an insight into a Mediterranean region. Eur J Cardiothorac Surg. 2010;38(4):407–13.
2. Buth KJ, Gainer RA, Legare J-F, Hirsch GM. The changing face of cardiac surgery: practice patterns and outcomes 2001-2010. Can J Cardiol. 2014;30:224–30.
3. Cloin ECW, Noyez L. Changing profile of elderly patients undergoing coronary bypass surgery. Neth Heart J. 2005;13(4):132–8.
4. Barsoum EA, Azab B, Patel N, Spagnola J, Shariff MA, Kaleem U, et al. Long-term outcome after percutaneous coronary intervention compared with minimally invasive coronary artery bypass surgery in the elderly. Open Cardiovasc Med J. 2016;10:11–8.
5. Nashef SAM, Roques F, Michel P, Gauducheau E, Lemeshow S, Salamon R. European system for cardiac operative risk evaluation (EuroSCORE). Eur J Cardiothorac Surg. 1999;16(1):9–13.
6. Parsonnet V, Dean D, Bernstein AD. A method of uniform stratification of risk for evaluating the results of surgery in acquired adult heart disease. Circulation. 1989;79(6 Pt 2):I3–12.
7. Bilmoria KY, Liu Y, Paruch JL, Zhou L, Kmiecik TE, Ko CYC, et al. Surgical risk calculator : a decision aide and informed consent tool for patients and surgeons. J Am Coll Surg. 2014;217(5):833–42.
8. Loponen P, Luther M, Nissinen J, Wistbacka J-O, Biancari F, Laurikka J, et al. EuroSCORE predicts health-related quality of life after coronary artery bypass grafting. Interact Cardiovasc Thorac Surg. 2008;7(4):564–8.
9. Abah U, Dunne M, Cook A, Hoole S, Brayne C, Vale L, et al. Does quality of life improve in octogenarians following cardiac surgery? A systematic review. BMJ Open. 2015;5(4):e006904.
10. Wijns W, Kolh P, Danchin N, Di Mario C, Falk V, Folliguet T, et al. Guidelines on myocardial revascularization. Eur Heart J. 2010;31:2501–55.
11. Supervisory Committee for Cardiac Interventions in The Netherlands (Begeleidingscommissie Hartinterventies Nederland, BHN) [Internet]. Geraadpleegd van: https://nederlandsehartregistratie.nl/handboeken/. [geciteerd 2 Juni 2017]
12. Gandek B, Ware JE, Aaronson NK, Apolone G, Bjorner JB, Brazier JE, et al. Cross-validation of item selection and scoring for the SF-12 health survey in nine countries: results from the IQOLA project. J Clin Epidemiol. 1998;51(11):1171–8.
13. De Smedt D, Clays E, Annemans L, Doyle F, Kotseva K, Pająk A, et al. Health related quality of life in coronary patients and its association with their cardiovascular risk profile: results from the EUROASPIRE III survey. Int J Cardiol. 2013;168(2):898–903.
14. Ware J, Kosinski M, Keller SD. A 12-item short-form health survey: construction of scales and preliminary tests of reliability and validity. Med Care. 1996;34(3):220–33.
15. Welke KF, Stevens JP, Schults WC, Nelson EC, Beggs VL, Nugent WC. Patient characteristics can predict improvement in functional health after elective coronary artery bypass grafting. Ann Thorac Surg. 2003;75(6):1849–55.
16. Jansen Klomp WW, Nierich AP, Peelen LM, Brandon Bravo Bruinsma GJ,

Dambrink J-HE, KGM M, et al. Survival and quality of life after surgical aortic valve replacement in octogenarians. J Cardiothorac Surg. 2016;11:38.

17. Rumsfeld JS, Magid DJ, O'Brien M, McCarthy M, MaWhinney S, Scd, et al. Changes in health-related quality of life following coronary artery bypass graft surgery. Ann Thorac Surg. 2001;72(6):2026–32.

18. Deutsch MA, Krane M, Schneider L, Wottke M, Kornek M, Elhmidi Y, et al. Health-related quality of life and functional outcome in cardiac surgical patients aged 80 years and older: a prospective single center study. J Card Surg. 2014;29(1):14–21.

19. Grady KL, Lee R, Subačius H, Malaisrie SC, Mcgee EC, Kruse J, et al. Improvements in health-related quality of life before and after isolated cardiac operations. Ann Thorac Surg. 2011;91(3):777–83.

20. Kendel F, Dunkel A, Müller-Tasch T, Steinberg K, Lehmkuhl E, Hetzer R, et al. Gender differences in health-related quality of life after coronary bypass surgery: results from a 1-year follow-up in propensity-matched men and women. Psychosom Med. 2011;73(3):280–5.

21. Peric V, Borzanovic M, Stolic R, Jovanovic A, Sovtic S, Dimkovic S, et al. Predictors of worsening of patients' quality of life six months after coronary artery bypass surgery. J Card Surg. 2008;23(6):648–54.

22. Järvinen O, Saarinen T, Julkunen J, Huhtala H, Tarkka MR. Changes in health-related quality of life and functional capacity following coronary artery bypass graft surgery. Eur J Cardiothorac Surg. 2003;24(5):750–6.

23. Lindsay GM, Hanlon P, Smith LN, Wheatley DJ. Assessment of changes in general health status using the short-form 36 questionnaire 1 year following coronary artery bypass grafting. Eur J Cardio-Thoracic Surg. 2000;18(5):557–64.

24. Colak Z, Segotic I, Uzun S, Mazar M, Ivancan V, Majeric-Kogler V. Health related quality of life following cardiac surgery — correlation with EuroSCORE. Eur J Cardio-Thoracic Surg. 2008;33(1):72–6.

25. Rumsfeld JS, Alexander KP, Goff DC, Graham MM, Ho PM, Masoudi FA, et al. Cardiovascular health: the importance of measuring patient-reported health status a scientific statement from the American heart association. Circulation. 2013;127(22):2233–49.

26. Spertus JA. Evolving applications for patient-centered health status measures. Circulation. 2008;118(20):2103–10.

29

Robotic lobectomy has the greatest benefit in patients with marginal pulmonary function

Peter J. Kneuertz*📍, Desmond M. D'Souza, Susan D. Moffatt-Bruce and Robert E. Merritt

Abstract

Background: Patients with limited pulmonary function have a high risk for pulmonary complications following lobectomy. Robotic approach is currently the least invasive approach. We hypothesized that robotic lobectomy may be of particular benefit in high-risk patients.

Methods: We reviewed our institutional Society of Thoracic Surgeons (STS) data on lobectomy patients from 2012 to 2017. Postoperative outcomes were compared between robotic and open lobectomy groups. High-risk patients were identified by pulmonary function test. Risk of pulmonary complication was assessed by binary logistic regression analysis.

Results: A total of 599 patients underwent lobectomy by robotic ($n = 287$), or by open ($n = 312$) approach, including 189 high-risk patients. Robotic lobectomy patients had a lower rate of prolonged air leak (6% vs. 10%, $p = 0.047$), less atelectasis requiring bronchoscopy (6% vs. 16%, $p = 0.02$), pneumonia (3% vs. 8%, $p = 0.01$), and shorter length of stay (4 vs. 6 days, $p = 0.001$). Overall pulmonary complication rate was significantly lower after robotic lobectomy in high-risk patients (28% vs. 45%, $p = 0.02$), less in intermediate or low risk patients. No significant difference was seen relative to major complication rate (12% vs. 17%, $p = 0.09$). After multivariate analysis, when adjusting for age, gender, smoking history, FEV1, DLCO, cardiopulmonary comorbidities, and prior chest surgery, the robotic approach remained independently associated with decreased pulmonary complications (odds ratio 0.54, 95% confidence interval [0.34–0.85], $p = 0.008$).

Conclusions: Robotic lobectomy has the potential to decrease the risk of postoperative pulmonary complication as compared with traditional open thoracotomy. In particular, patients with limited pulmonary function derive the most benefit from a robotic approach.

Keywords: Robotic, Lobectomy, High risk, Pulmonary function, Outcomes

Background

Posterolateral open thoracotomy has been the traditional approach to pulmonary lobectomy, which is associated with significant morbidity and a decrease in functional reserve capacity (FRC). Minimally invasive techniques using video-assisted thoracoscopic surgery (VATS) and more recently robotic assisted lobectomy have been developed to enhance recovery by decreasing complications, shorten length of stay and improve quality of life [1, 2]. Robotic lobectomy uses a completely port based approach, which is currently the least invasive technology. Despite the increased cost as compared with VATS, many surgeons have found value in the robotics due to improved three-dimensional visualization, increased freedom of instrument motion, and precise instrument movement with 3:1 motion scaling [3]. Nationally, the use of robotic lobectomy for lung cancer has tripled between 2010 and 2012 in the US from 3 to 9% [4]. In year 2015, more than 8600 pulmonary lobectomies have been performed robotically [5].

* Correspondence: Peter.Kneuertz@osumc.edu
Presented at the 13rd Annual Academic Surgical Congress, January 31th, 2018 in Jacksonville, FL
Department of Surgery, Thoracic Surgery Division, The Ohio State University Wexner Medical Center, Doan Hall N846, 410 W 10th Avenue, Columbus, OH 43210, USA

Although the overall robotic lobectomy experience is growing, less is known about the use of robotics in high-risk patients. As with any new technology, it is natural to select the easier cases in the early experience. Concerning anatomic lung resection in patients with intrinsic lung disease and poor pulmonary function, traditional thoughts may fear a higher incidence of air leaks, and possibly increased pain due to torqueing of the robotic ports. However, based on the benefit of minimally invasive lobectomy in patients with impaired pulmonary reserve in the VATS experience, we have been liberal in applying robotics in patients with increased pulmonary risk. We hypothesize, that robotic lobectomy may be of particular benefit in high-risk patients with marginal baseline pulmonary function. In this current study we aim to assess the postoperative outcomes of robotic lobectomy patients as compared with thoracotomy patients and to determine the relative impact of robotic approach on outcomes in high-risk patients undergoing lobectomy.

Methods

This is a retrospective cohort study of patients who underwent lobectomy at a single institution. The study was approved by The Ohio State Institutional Review Board (Study#2018-C0021) and granted waiver of individual patient consent. The institutional Society of Thoracic Surgery (STS) general thoracic database was queried for patients who underwent lobectomy between January 1st 2012 and August 31st 2017. Included were all patients who underwent lobectomy by either robotic-assisted or open approach using thoracotomy. Patients who underwent, bronchoplastic, sleeve resection, or bilobectomy were excluded. Patients undergoing resection of Pancoast tumors or concomitant chest wall resection were also excluded.

The selection of surgical approach was at the discretion and experience of the surgeon. Robotic lobectomy was performed with a 4-arm technique with ports placed in line in the 8th intercostal space. We used the DaVinci Si robot until 2014 and thereafter the Xi model (Intuitive Surgical, Sunnyvale, CA). Additionally a 12 mm access port was used to for manual stapling, and since 2016 we have utilized the robotic controlled endo-wrist stapler. Stapled bronchial closure was performed in all patients.

Demographics, comorbidities, smoking status, use of induction therapy, lung cancer staging and prior thoracic surgery were reviewed. The definitions of postoperative events were categorized according to the STS definitions. The primary endpoint was pulmonary complication, as defined by the presence of any perioperative pulmonary complications, including air leak > 5 days, pneumonia, atelectasis requiring bronchoscopy, pleural effusion requiring drainage, pneumothorax requiring

chest tube reinsertion, initial ventilator support > 48 h, bronchopleural fistula or tracheobronchial injury, respiratory failure, tracheostomy, acute respiratory distress syndrome (ARDS), or other pulmonary event (including pulmonary embolus). Respiratory failure was defined as impaired gas exchange, which requires reintubation and mechanical ventilation. According to the American College of Chest Physicians (ACCP) guidelines, preoperative pulmonary function tests were used to attribute surgical risk [6–8]. High risk was defined as preoperative forced expiratory volume in one second (FEV1) or diffusing capacity of the lung for carbon monoxide (DLCO) less than 60% predicted, as previously described [6]. Low risk were defined as patients with FEV1and DLCO > 80% [8], and intermediate risk patients as those with FEV1 or DLCO between 60 and 80%.

Statistical analysis

Robotic and open lobectomy patients were compared using Chi-square/Fisher's exact test for categorical variables, and Student's T-test or Mann-Whitney U test for continuous variables based on presence of normal distribution. Univariate and multivariate binary logistic regression analysis was performed to test the association of clinical factors with pulmonary complications. Variables with $p < 0.01$ on univariate analysis were included in the multivariate model. Statistical significance was defined as a p-value ≤ 0.05. Data analysis was performed using SPSS 24.0 (LEAD Technologies, Inc., Chicago, IL) statistical software package.

Results

A total of 599 patients underwent lobectomy by robotic ($n = 287$) or open approach ($n = 312$). Six patients who started with a robotic approach were converted to thoracotomy for limited visibility ($n = 4$) or restricted mobility ($n = 2$). Results were analyzed based on the approach in which the lobectomy was completed. Demographics and patient characteristics are summarized in Table 1. Patients who underwent robotic lobectomy were slightly older (mean age 65.3 ± 11.3 vs. 63.2 ± 10.1, $p = 0.02$), had better pulmonary function by spirometry (mean FEV1 82.4 ± 19.8 vs. 77.6 ± 19.7, $p = 0.003$), and had less frequent prior cardiothoracic surgery (14% vs. 20%, $p = 0.04$). Fewer patients in the robotic group underwent preoperative chemotherapy for clinical stage IIIa lung cancer (4% vs. 8%, $p = 0.03$). On final pathology, most patients had lung cancer on final pathology, with similar stage distribution between groups (Table 1).

Outcomes

Overall rate of pulmonary complication was lower following robotic as compared with open lobectomy (21% vs. 32%, $p = 0.002$), which included lower rates of

Table 1 Baseline patient demographics and clinical characteristics of patients undergoing robotic and open lobectomy

	Robotic Lobectomy	Open Lobectomy	P-value
	(n = 287)	(n = 312)	
Age [years], mean ± SD	65.3 ± 11.3	63.2 ± 10.1	0.016
Male Gender	134 (47%)	157 (50%)	0.41
Zubrod Score			
0–1	270 (94%)	291 (93%)	0.67
2+	17 (6%)	21 (7%)	
Pack years, median (IQR)	40 (21–60)	40 (23–60)	0.51
Active smoker	91 (32%)	92 (30%)	0.59
FEV1 [% predicted], mean ± SD	82.4 ± 19.7	77.6 ± 19.7	0.003
DLCO [% predicted], mean ± SD	75.5 ± 22.8	74.5 ± 20.2	0.59
COPD	128 (45%)	118 (38%)	0.09
BMI > 30 kg/m^2	88 (31%)	100 (32%)	0.80
Hypertension	180 (63%)	188 (60%)	0.56
Steroid use	9 (3%)	10 (3%)	0.96
Coronary artery disease	121 (42%)	132 (42%)	0.97
Peripheral vascular disease	29 (10%)	22 (7%)	0.19
Prior cardiothoracic surgery	40 (14%)	64 (20%)	0.040
Preoperative chemotherapy	11 (4%)	26 (8%)	0.027
Preoperative radiation therapy	13 (5%)	25 (8%)	0.10
Diabetes	45 (16%)	61 (20%)	0.22
Preoperative creatinine > 1.5 mg/dl	25 (4%)	13 (4%)	0.98
Lung cancer	240 (83%)	256 (82%)	0.61
Pathologic Stage (AJCC 7th ed.)			
Stage I-II	209 (87%)	220 (86%)	0.75
Stage III-IVa	31 (13%)	35 (14%)	
Laterality			
Left	176 (61%)	197 (63%)	0.65
Right	111 (39%)	115 (37%	

Table 2 Pulmonary complication and morbidity

Outcome	Robotic Lobectomy	Open Lobectomy	P-value
	(n = 287)	(n = 312)	
Pulmonary complication	60 (21%)	100 (32%)	0.002
Air leak (> 5 days)	16 (6%)	31 (10%)	0.047
Atelectasis (req. bronchoscopy)	18 (6%)	51 (16%)	0.001
Pleural effusion (req. drainage)	5 (2%)	9 (3%)	0.36
Pneumonia	9 (3%)	25 (8%)	0.010
Respiratory failure	22 (8%)	35 (11%)	0.14
ARDS	0	8 (2%)	0.031
Pneumothorax	12 (4%)	10 (3%)	0.52
Initial vent support > 48 h	0	2 (1%)	0.17
Tracheostomy	2 (1%)	8 (3%)	0.07
Other pulmonary event	6 (2%)	6 (2%)	1.00
Length of hospitalization [days], median (IQR)	4 (3–6)	6 (5–10)	0.001
Major Complications	34 (12%)	52 (17%)	0.09
Mortality	3 (1%)	5 (2%)	0.58

peripheral vascular disease, chronic obstructive pulmonary disease (COPD) and thoracotomy were associated with pulmonary complications (Table 3). On multivariate analysis, robotic lobectomy was the independently associated with a decreased risk for pulmonary complications (odds ratio (OR) 0.53, 95% confidence interval (CI) 0.34–0.85], Table 3). Other predictive factors in the multivariate model were FEV1 and peripheral vascular disease (Table 3).

Comparison of high risk patients

A subgroup analysis of 191 (32%) high-risk patients included 82 robotic and 107 open lobectomies. High-risk patients in the robotic group included more older patients > 75 years (22% vs. 11%, 0.05), more active smokers 46% vs. 31%, $p = 0.04$), and more patients with COPD (81% s. 54%, $p < 0.001$). There was no difference in lung cancer stage between robotic and thoracotomy groups in the high risk patients. High-risk patients undergoing robotic lobectomy were less likely to have any pulmonary complication (28% vs. 45%, $p = 0.02$). The difference in pulmonary complications between robotic and open lobectomy was greatest for high-risk patients, and less pronounced for with intermediate or intermediate or low risk patients (Fig. 1). Similarly to the entire cohort, robotic lobectomy in high-risk patients was associated with decreased rates of prolonged air leak, atelectasis and pneumonia (Table 4). In addition, none of the robotic lobotomy high-risk patients developed ARDS, needed a tracheostomy, or required initial vent support > 48 h (Table 4). Median length of stay following robotic lobectomy in high risk patients

prolonged air leak, atelectasis, pneumonia, and ARDS (Table 2). There were no intraoperative tracheobronchial injuries and one bronchopleural fistula (0.3%) in both groups. Median length of stay was two days shorter following robotic lobectomy (4 days vs. 6 days, $p = 0.001$). There was no significant difference in major complication rate or mortality (Table 2).

The regression analysis of predictors of pulmonary function is presented in Table 3. On univariate analysis, active smoking, increasing total pack year smoking history, low FEV1 and DLCO, coronary artery disease,

Table 3 Binary logistic regression analysis of factors associated with pulmonary complications

Characteristic	Univariate analysis			Multivariate analysis		
	Crude OR	95% CI	p-value	Adjusted OR	95% CI	p-value
Age	1.02	[0.99–1.03]	0.07	1.02	[0.99–1.05]	0.19
Male Gender	1.37	[0.95–1.97]	0.09	1.15	[0.73–1.82]	0.53
Active smoker	1.48	[1.01–2.17]	0.043	1.16	[0.72–1.85]	0.54
Pack Years (per year)	1.01	[1.00–1.02]	0.006	1.01	[0.96–1.01]	0.35
FEV1 (per % predicted)	0.97	[0.96–0.98]	< 0.001	0.97	0.96–0.98	< 0.001
DLCO (per % predicted)	0.99	[0.98–0.99]	0.006	1.00	[0.99–1.01]	0.60
Zubrod Score						
0–1	Reference					
2–5	1.46	[0.73–2.93]	0.28			
BMI						
20–30	Reference					
< 20	1.61	[0.85–3.07]	0.14			
> 30	0.89	[0.59–1.34]	0.58			
Steroid use	0.98	[0.35–2.76]	0.97			
Coronary artery disease	2.22	[1.51–3.14]	< 0.001	1.40	[0.87–2.23]	0.16
Peripheral vascular disease	2.69	[1.50–4.82]	0.001	1.99	[1.03–3.86]	0.042
Prior cardiothoracic surgery	1.67	[1.07–2.62]	0.026	1.62	[0.93–2.82]	0.088
Preoperative chemotherapy	1.53	[0.76–3.08]	0.24			
Preoperative radiation therapy	1.29	[0.64–2.62]	0.48			
Diabetes	1.23	[0.78–1.96]	0.37			
Last Cr > 1.5	1.87	[0.82–4.25]	0.14			
Last Hgb < 10	1.25	[0.52–2.85]	0.65			
COPD	2.42	[1.67–3.49]	< 0.001	1.62	[0.96–2.69]	0.052
Approach						
Open	Reference			Reference		
Robotic	0.56	[0.39–0.81]	0.002	0.54	[0.34–0.85]	0.008

was 4 days and significantly shorted as compared with 8 days following open lobectomy ($p < 0.001$).

Discussion

Pulmonary complications are the most common postoperative events following lung resection and can contribute to prolonged hospital length of stay and overall increased morbidity [9]. In this study of a large single institution dataset, we present that robotic lobectomy is associated with less pulmonary complication as compared with traditional open approach with thoracotomy in a high risk population. We show that while the risk of pulmonary complication increases in patients with worse pulmonary function regardless of approach, the robotic technique may serve to attenuate this risk independent of baseline pulmonary function. This study is important, because it includes a large set of patients with

marginal pulmonary function, who were found to derive the greatest benefit from robotic lobectomy.

Minimally invasive thoracic surgery aims to expedite recovery by avoiding the chest wall trauma of a thoracotomy and the associated decrease in respiratory mechanics. Minimally invasive approach to lobectomy was first performed with VATS. Studies have shown the potential of the VATS approach to reduce blood loss, duration of chest tube drainage, postoperative pain, pulmonary complication and shorten overall length of hospitalization [1, 10]. Large population based studies have confirmed the benefit of the VATS approach with the reduction of pulmonary complications by 3–4% [6, 11]. Recent large population based studies comparing VATS and robotic approaches have shown comparable rates of overall complication rates and length of stay [4, 12]. Although our study does not directly compare robotic to VATS approach, the overall reduction of pulmonary complication rate of 11%

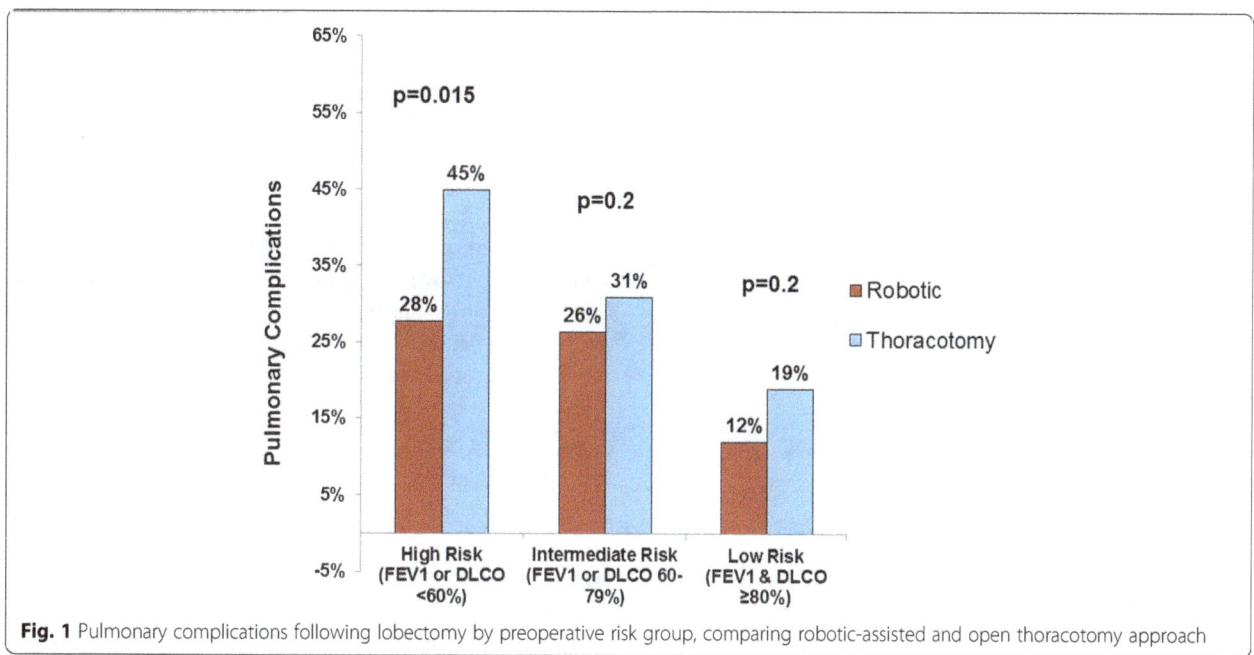

Fig. 1 Pulmonary complications following lobectomy by preoperative risk group, comparing robotic-assisted and open thoracotomy approach

compares favorably to the reported outcomes. This may be partly explained by the patient selection. In a recent study of the national STS database, Ceppa et al. showed that a VATS approach was associated with highest reduction in pulmonary complications for patients with impaired pulmonary function [6]. Our results confirm this finding, and show that the benefit of robotic approach is greatest for high-risk patients. High-risk patients are likely underrepresented in many current robotic lobectomy series, as surgeons may tend to select more straightforward cases when adopting new techniques [13]. One common concern has been the risk of postoperative air leak with a robotic approach, due to the lack of tactile feedback when manipulation diseased lungs, as well as the need for more dissection in the fissure, which could lead to increased risk of air leak. In this series we report a large number of high-risk patients undergoing robotic lobectomy, and demonstrate that the incidence of pulmonary complications can be significantly reduced using the robotic approach. Technical modifications that may have contributed to this result were cautious handling of the lung with the use of gauze rolls to avoid direct grasping. The risk of air leak may also be reduced in robotic lobectomy by improved visualization and precise dissection of the fissure with bipolar cautery, and the liberal use of staplers to divide the anterior and posterior fissure.

Lung cancer patients with poor pulmonary function present a challenge to thoracic surgeons. While lobectomy remains the best treatment for early stage lung cancer, alternative options are often considered for high-risk patients. In addition to sublobar resection, high-risk patients are also increasingly considered for

stereotactic radiation (SBRT) or ablation [14]. Crabtree et al. reported a comparison of two prospective clinical trials of high-risk patients with stage I lung cancer using sublobar resection (ACOSOG Z4032) and SBRT (RTOG 0236), and shown no difference in early mobidity in appropriately matched patients [15]. Selection criteria for the ACOSOG Z4032 and the currently enrolling JoLT Stablemates (former Z4099), which is directly comparing sublobar resection with SBRT, define high-risk patients by using preoperative pulmonary function tests as major criteria and age and cardiovascular comorbidities as minor criteria [16]. However, there remains significant debate on the appropriate risk stratification. Several studies have questioned these empiric ACOSOG criteria by showing acceptable outcomes following lobectomy in so called high-risk patients [17–19]. A recent study by Taylor et al. examined high-risk patients undergoing VATS lobectomy and found similar early morbidity to normal risk patients and a 30-day mortality < 1% in carefully selected patients who fit the mentioned trial criteria [19]. Our results in lobectomy patients confirm that lobectomy can be safely performed in selected high-risk patients with marginal pulmonary function, and that the surgical approach should be weighed when determining if patients are appropriate for lobectomy to ensure optimal oncologic therapy for high-risk patients.

We do acknowledge several limitations of our study. Given the retrospective nature of this study, we cannot exclude that results have been biased by selection and confounding of unmeasured factors including surgeon preference of technique and experience. However, for the purpose of comparing pulmonary outcomes we have

Table 4 Comparison of high-risk patients undergoing robotic- and open lobectomy

Characteristics	Robotic Lobectomy (n = 82)	Open Lobectomy (n = 107)	p-value
Age > 75 years	18 (22%)	12 (11%)	0.05
Male Gender	38 (46%)	55 (51%)	0.44
Zubrod Score			
0–1	78 (94%)	100 (93%)	0.88
2+	5 (6%)	7 (7%)	
Pack years, median (IQR)	50 (25–67)	40 (30–66)	0.035
Active smoker	38 (46%)	33 (31%)	0.035
COPD	67 (81%)	58 (54%)	< 0.001
FEV1 [% predicted], mean ± SD	67.0 ± 17.9	62.8 ± 18.0	0.10
DLCO [% predicted], mean ± SD	53.6 ± 15.7	57.8 ± 16.6	0.08
BMI > 30 kg/m²	20 (24%)	33 (31%)	0.47
Hypertension	60 (72%)	71 (66%)	0.38
Coronary artery disease	47 (57%)	52 (49%)	0.27
Peripheral vascular disease	11 (13%)	10 (9%)	0.47
Prior cardiothoracic surgery	13 (16%)	26 (24%)	0.15
Preop. Chemotherapy	5 (6%)	7 (7%)	0.88
Lung Cancer	69 (83%)	90 (84%)	0.86
Outcomes			
Pulmonary Complication	23 (28%)	48 (45%)	0.015
Air Leak (> 5 days)	4 (5%)	16 (15%)	0.024
Atelectasis (req. bronchoscopy)	6 (7%)	24 (22%)	0.005
Pleural effusion (req. drainage)	1 (1%)	5 (5%)	0.17
Pneumonia	3 (4%)	12 (11%)	0.05
Respiratory Failure	10 (12%)	13 (13%)	
ARDS	0	3 (3%)	0.12
Pneumothorax	3 (4%)	6 (6%)	0.52
Initial vent support > 48 h	0	2 (2%)	0.21
Tracheostomy	0	6 (6%)	0.028
Other pulmonary event	3 (4%)	1 (1%)	0.32
Length of hospitalization [days] Median (IQR)	4 (4–7)	8 (5–12)	< 0.001
Major Complications	16 (19%)	26 (24%)	0.41
Mortality	1 (1%)	2 (2%)	0.73

risk-stratified patients based on preoperative pulmonary function, and specifically compared the subgroup of high-risk patients. High-risk patients in the robotic group actually included older and sicker patients, as this series reflects a liberal application of robotics for higher risk patients beyond the initial learning curve. The large number of patients in this study allowed for rigorous multivariate modeling of pulmonary complication to control for confounding. In this study we were unable to compare the robotic approach to the VATS approach due the practice pattern at our institution, which should be inbestigated in a future study. Furthermore, the study is limited to comparison of perioperative outcomes and does not examine differences in pain, dyspnea, and health related quality of life. Postoperative pain may be a significant factor in reducing postoperative pulmonary morbidity and shorten recovery. Patient reported outcomes, cost, and long term outcomes are important topics for future studies.

Conclusions

Robotic lobectomy may decrease risk of pulmonary complications as compared with traditional thoracotomy. Patients with poor pulmonary function have the potential to derive the most benefit from a robotic approach. Therefore, robotically assisted thoracic approaches should be considered when selecting high-risk patients requiring lobectomy.

Abbreviations
ACCP: American College of Chest Physicians; AJCC: American Joint Committee on Cancer; ARDS: Acute respiratory distress syndrome; BMI: Body mass index; CI: Confidence Interval; CR: Serum Creatinine level; COPD: Chronic obstructive pulmonary disease; DLCO: Diffusing capacity of the lung for carbon monoxide; FEV1: Forced expiratory volume in one second; FRC: Functional reserve capacity; Hgb: Hemoglobin level; IQR: Inter quartile range; OR: Odds ratio; SD: Standard deviation; STS: Society of Thoracic Surgeons; VATS: Video-assisted thoracoscopic surgery

Acknowledgements
The authors would like to thank Gisela Simon for her assistance with the STS data query.

Authors' contributions
PK had full access to all of the data in the study and takes responsibility for the integrity of the data and the accuracy of the data analysis. DD, SMB, and RM contributed substantially to the study design, data analysis and interpretation, and the writing of the manuscript. All authors read and approved the final manuscript.

Authors' information
All authors are practicing thoracic surgeons and full time faculty at The Ohio State University.

Competing interests
The authors declare that they have no competing interests.

References

1. Scott WJ, Allen MS, Darling G, et al. Video-assisted thoracic surgery versus open lobectomy for lung cancer: a secondary analysis of data from the american college of surgeons oncology group z0030 randomized clinical trial. J Thorac Cardiovasc Surg. 2010;139(4):976–81. discussion 981–973
2. Li WW, Lee TW, Lam SS, et al. Quality of life following lung cancer resection: video-assisted thoracic surgery vs thoracotomy. Chest. 2002;122(2):584–9.
3. Ramadan OI, Wei B, Cerfolio RJ. Robotic surgery for lung resections-total port approach: advantages and disadvantages. J Vis Surg. 2017;3:22.
4. Rajaram R, Mohanty S, Bentrem DJ, et al. Nationwide assessment of robotic lobectomy for non-small cell lung cancer. Ann Thorac Surg. 2017;103(4):1092–100.
5. Wei B, Cerfolio RJ. Robotic lobectomy and segmentectomy: Technical details and results. Surg Clin North Am. 2017;97(4):771–82.
6. Ceppa DP, Kosinski AS, Berry MF, et al. Thoracoscopic lobectomy has increasing benefit in patients with poor pulmonary function: a society of thoracic surgeons database analysis. Ann Surg. 2012;256(3):487–93.
7. Burt BM, Kosinski AS, Shrager JB, Onaitis MW, Weigel T. Thoracoscopic lobectomy is associated with acceptable morbidity and mortality in patients with predicted postoperative forced expiratory volume in 1 second or diffusing capacity for carbon monoxide less than 40% of normal. J Thorac Cardiovasc Surg. 2014;148(1):19–28. dicussion 28–29 e11
8. Brunelli A, Kim AW, Berger KI, Addrizzo-Harris DJ. Physiologic evaluation of the patient with lung cancer being considered for resectional surgery: diagnosis and management of lung cancer, 3rd ed: American college of chest physicians evidence-based clinical practice guidelines. Chest. 2013; 143(5 Suppl):e166S–90S.
9. Kozower BD, O'Brien SM, Kosinski AS, et al. The society of thoracic surgeons composite score for rating program performance for lobectomy for lung cancer. Ann Thorac Surg. 2016;101(4):1379–86. discussion 1386–1377
10. Oparka J, Yan TD, Ryan E, Dunning J. Does video-assisted thoracic surgery provide a safe alternative to conventional techniques in patients with limited pulmonary function who are otherwise suitable for lung resection? Interact Cardiovasc Thorac Surg. 2013;17(1):159–62.
11. Paul S, Altorki NK, Sheng S, et al. Thoracoscopic lobectomy is associated with lower morbidity than open lobectomy: a propensity-matched analysis from the sts database. J Thorac Cardiovasc Surg. 2010;139(2):366–78.
12. Kent M, Wang T, Whyte R, Curran T, Flores R, Gangadharan S. Open, video-assisted thoracic surgery, and robotic lobectomy: review of a national database. Ann Thorac Surg. 2014;97(1):236–42. discussion 242-234
13. Mahieu J, Rinieri P, Bubenheim M, et al. Robot-assisted thoracoscopic surgery versus video-assisted thoracoscopic surgery for lung lobectomy: can a robotic approach improve short-term outcomes and operative safety? Thorac Cardiovasc Surg. 2016;64(4):354–62.
14. McMurry TL, Shah PM, Samson P, Robinson CG, Kozower BD. Treatment of stage i non-small cell lung cancer: What's trending? J Thorac Cardiovasc Surg. 2017;154(3):1080–7.
15. Crabtree T, Puri V, Timmerman R, et al. Treatment of stage i lung cancer in high-risk and inoperable patients: comparison of prospective clinical trials using stereotactic body radiotherapy (rtog 0236), sublobar resection (acosog z4032), and radiofrequency ablation (acosog z4033). J Thorac Cardiovasc Surg. 2013;145(3):692–9.
16. Fernando HC, Timmerman R. American college of surgeons oncology group z4099/radiation therapy oncology group 1021: a randomized study of sublobar resection compared with stereotactic body radiotherapy for high-risk stage i non-small cell lung cancer. J Thorac Cardiovasc Surg. 2012; 144(3):S35–8.
17. Sancheti MS, Melvan JN, Medbery RL, et al. Outcomes after surgery in high-risk patients with early stage lung cancer. Ann Thorac Surg. 2016;101(3):1043–50. Discussion 1051
18. Donahoe LL, de Valence M, Atenafu EG, et al. High risk for thoracotomy but not thoracoscopic lobectomy. Ann Thorac Surg. 2017;103(6):1730–5.
19. Taylor MD, LaPar DJ, Isbell JM, Kozower BD, Lau CL, Jones DR. Marginal pulmonary function should not preclude lobectomy in selected patients with non-small cell lung cancer. J Thorac Cardiovasc Surg. 2014;147(2):738–44. Discussion 744-736

30

Diagnostic accuracy of low-dose dual-source cardiac computed tomography as compared to surgery in univentricular heart patients

Narumol Chaosuwannakit[1]* and Pattarapong Makarawate[2]

Abstract

Background: To evaluate the ability of low radiation dose dual-source computed tomography (DSCT) to depict the features of morphological univentricular heart and to define accuracy by comparing findings with surgery.

Methods: Low radiation dose dual-source cardiac computed tomography (CCT) of 33 cases of functional univentricular heart preliminary diagnosis by echocardiography compared with the results of surgery were retrospectively analyzed (aged 1 day to 4 years, median 5 months). The appropriate dose reduction strategies and iterative reconstruction were applied.

Results: Thirty three univentricular heart patients were classified into three types according to Anderson's classification method, including 16 cases (48.5%) univentricular of right ventricular type with rudimentary chamber of left ventricle, 11 cases (33.3%) univentricular of left ventricular type with rudimentary chamber of right ventricle and 6 cases (18.2%) univentricular heart of indeterminate type without rudimentary chamber. The extracardiac malformation such as hypoplastic aortic arch, coronary artery fistula, total anomalous pulmonary venous returns or hypoplastic lung were presented frequently. The overall sensitivity and specification of cardiac CT was 100% compared to the results of surgery. The procedural dose-length product was 18 ± 5 mGy-cm, and unadjusted and adjusted radiation doses were 0.25 and 0.64 mSv, respectively.

Conclusion: Cardiac CT can diagnose accurately and be performed with a low radiation exposure in patients with the functional univentricular heart disease. The aorta, pulmonary artery and lung can be evaluated completely and simultaneously as well. Cardiac CT is an effective advanced non-invasive imaging modality to comprehensive evaluation the functional univentricular heart patients, particularly if cardiac MRI poses a high risk or is contraindicated.

Keywords: Univentricular heart, Single ventricle congenital heart disease, Cardiac CT, Dual-source CT

Background

Functional univentricular heart disease is a spectrum of severe congenital heart disease, with multiple anatomic variations but similar surgical treatment strategies. V Functional univentricular heart disease is anatomically defined as (1) connection of both atria to the same ventricle (2:1 connection) or as (2) connection of both to atria separate ventricles, one of which is hypoplastic (1:1 connection) [1, 2].

With the advent of advanced palliative and corrective surgical procedures, Functional univentricular heart disease patients are living longer into adulthood compared to two or three decades ago [3], and they are more frequently undergoing imaging to assist in clinical and surgical management. However, interpreting an imaging examination of a functional univentricular heart disease patient is a daunting task, not only because of unusual anatomy and varied post operative appearances but also because of the rarity of the functional univentricular heart disease that makes it difficult for the imaging specialist to maintain diagnostic proficiency.

* Correspondence: narumol_chao@yahoo.com
[1]Radiology Department, Faculty of Medicine, Khon Kaen University, Khon Kaen 40000, Thailand
Full list of author information is available at the end of the article

Echocardiography and cardiac magnetic resonance imaging (CMR) are the main imaging modalities used in adult patients with complex congenital heart disease. However, cardiac CT offers complementary imaging and can be performed safely in unwell patients with single ventricle physiology. Echocardiography is insufficient for evaluation of the thoracic vasculature or for reproducible estimation of ventricular function [4, 5]. Cardiac MRI (CMR) is commonly performed for these indications, but it requires relatively long imaging times, deep sedation, or anesthesia in young children. Many older patients have metallic implants with an artifact that degrades magnetic resonance imaging (MRI) quality [6]. In addition, it is relatively contraindicated in those with pacemakers and defibrillators as these devices have been known to cause an imaging artifact [7]. Recent findings of cerebral gadolinium deposits suggest that MRI use be carefully considered when angiography is needed [8–10]. Cardiac CT has been shown to be accurate for the evaluation of anatomy and function for most indications of congenital heart disease (CHD), [11] but there has not been a report on image quality, nor has a correlation been made with interventional findings, in a cohort of single-ventricle patients across all stages of palliation.

Methods

Patient population

This retrospective study included 33 functional univentricular heart disease patients who underwent both cardiac CT and surgery, between February 2013–December 2016. The indications for cardiac CT were pre-operative evaluation of complex congenital heart and functional univentricular heart disease patients which is considered appropriate indications for cardiac CT, based on the expert consensus document of the Society of Cardiovascular computed tomography [11]. Exclusion criteria for cardiac CT included the presence of renal failure, and a history of allergic reaction to iodine-containing contrast agents. The present study was approved by the Ethics Committee of the Faculty of Medicine, Khon Kaen University, Khon Kaen, Thailand, and informed consent was obtained from all patients The IRB protocol number of this study is 800001189.

Dual-source cardiac CT (CCT) scanning protocol

No sedation versus sedation with free breathing versus intubation, IV site and gauge, and adverse procedural events were determined from patient records. Nearly all patients could be performed cardiac CT with limited or no anaesthesia and with quiet respiration. Imaging was performed by using a second-generation dual-source CT scanner (Somatom Definition; Siemens Healthcare, Forchheim, Germany) with temporal resolution = 75 ms. The radiation dose is kept to minimum by reducing the kilovoltage and tube current appropriately. For children weighing less than 10 kg, 10–19 kg and 20–30 kg, we use 80 kV and 80

mAs, 80 kV and 100 mAs, and 100 kV and 120 mAs, respectively. Other cardiac CT parameters were as follows: number of X-ray tubes, two; collimation, 128 detector rows of 0.5 mm each, with double sampling by using rapid alteration of the focal spot in the longitudinal direction (z flying focal spot). Prior to scanning, the pitch was set automatically by the scanner software. Depending on heart rate, pitch was set between 0.2 and 0.43. Automated dose regulation methods such as CARE dose 4D (Siemens Healthcare) may be used to reduce the radiation. A bolus of iodinated contrast material (350 mg/mL, Omnipaque; GE Healthcare) at a dose of 1.5 ml/kg with dual-head power injector at a rate of 1.5–2.0 ml/s for a 22-gauge cannula, 3.0 ml/s for a 20- gauge cannula and 4.0–5.0 ml/s for a 18-gauge cannula followed by a 10–20 ml of saline flush at a same rate to that of the contrast injection. For timing purposes, an automated bolus-tracking software was used, starting the scan automatically 6 s after contrast agent density in the descending aorta reached a predefined threshold of 130 HU. The entire volume of the heart and pulmonary arteries was covered during one breath-hold in approximately 5 s with simultaneous recording of the ECG trace. Patients were scanned in the supine position. Cardiac CT is performed from the thoracic inlet level to L1–L2. When there is suspicion of anomalous pulmonary venous drainage, the scan can be extended down to the lower border of the liver.

Cardiac CT image analysis

Cardiac CT image analysis was performed by two cardiovascular and thoracic radiologists in consensus (with a respective 11 and 10 years of experience in examining cardiovascular and thoracic CT scans) and blinded to the clinical data and the results of surgery. First, axial all image data are evaluated using a 3D post processing workstation with Syngo software (Siemens Healthcare). Various image reformatting techniques including curved planar reconstruction, maximum intensity projection (MIP), minimum intensity projection, and volume-rendering technique (VRT) are used to get all the clinically relevant information. Curved planar reformatting and MIP are primarily used to evaluate curved structures such as the pulmonary arteries and major aortopulmonary collateral arteries (MAPCAs). Minimum intensity projection is used to evaluate the airway and lung parenchyma. For 3D reformatting of the complex anatomy, VRT is used. Thin-section multiplanar reformatting is used for quantitative analysis of the structure in question.

Cardiac surgery result analysis

Cardiac surgery result analysis was performed by an experienced cardiologist blinded to cardiac CT results by retrospectively reviewed operative notes.

Radiation dose parameters

The scanner platform, contrast, imaging sequence, CT dose–volume index, milligray (mGy), scan dose–length product (mGy-cm, 16 cm phantom), scan length, tube potential, and tube current were recorded for each scan. Individual scan and cumulative procedural dose–length products in mGy-cm were recorded.

Radiation dose estimation

Procedural dose–length product was used to estimate the radiation dose. An unadjusted radiation dose in milliSievert (mSv) was calculated by multiplying the dose– length product with the standard chest conversion factor given as scan dose–length product $\times 0.014$ [12]. For patients < 18 years of age, conversion factors were further calculated by age as follows: 0.039 for ≤ 0.50 years; 0.026 for 0.51–2.50 years; 0.018 for 2.51–7.50 years; and 0.014 for patients > 7.50 years [13, 14].

Statistical analysis

Continuous data were expressed as mean $\pm$ SD. Statistical analyses were performed using SPSS software version 16 (SPSS, Inc., Chicago, IL, USA). A significance level of $p < 0.05$ was considered a statistically significant result and all reported p-values were two-sided. Means were compared using unpaired t-test, and Mann-Whitney rank sum was used when data was not normally distributed.

Results

Thirty-three patients (20 boys, 13 girls; aged 1 day to 4 years, median 5 months) were included in this study over a period of 44 months. The mean time interval between cardiac CT and surgery was 1 ± 10 months (range, 3 days–14 months) and there were no clinical events between the 2 studies in any patient. Patient demographic data and cardiac CT scan information are lists as Table 1.

In patient analysis, out of 33 cardiac CT examinations, none of them was of non-diagnostic image quality. Thirty three univentricular heart patients were classified into three types according to Anderson's classification method, including 16 cases (48.5%) univentricular of right ventricular type with rudimentary chamber of left ventricle (Fig. 1), 11 cases (33.3%) univentricular of left ventricular type with rudimentary chamber of right ventricle (Fig. 2) and 6 cases (18.2%) univentricular heart of indeterminate type without rudimentary chamber.

Of the 33 patients, significant unexpected findings were two hypoplastic aortic arch (Fig. 3), three coronary artery fistula (Fig. 2), ten pulmonary atresia, one infracardiac type total anomalous pulmonary venous returns (Fig. 4) and one hypoplastic left lung were presented. Ten patients were scanned without sedation, 22 patients were scanned with minimal to moderate sedation, and one patient was intubated during the scan. The patient who was intubated

Table 1 Patient demographic data and cardiac CT information

Characteristic	Value
Age at scan (months), mean $\pm$ SD (range)	5 ± 8 (0–48)
Men, n (%)	20 (60.6%)
Height (cm), mean $\pm$ SD	90.8 ± 23
Weight (kg), mean $\pm$ SD	3 ± 10
Patient sedation	
• No sedation, n (%)	10 (30.3)
• Sedation with free breathing, n (%)	22 (66.6)
• Intubation, n (%)	1 (3.1)
Dose-length product (mGy-cm), mean $\pm$ SD (range)	18 ± 5 (15–21)
Unadjusted radiation dose (milliSievert), mean (range)	0.25 (0.21–0.29)
Adjusted radiation dose (milliSievert), mean (range)	0.64 (0.49–0.82)

for general anesthesia for multiple concurrent procedures including brain CT and cardiac CT.

The procedural dose-length product was 18 ± 5 (15–21) mGy-cm, and unadjusted and adjusted radiation doses were 0.25 (0.21–0.29) and 0.64 (0.49–0.82) mSv, respectively.

All patients underwent subsequent staged palliation. No patient had additional advanced diagnostic studies before initial surgical palliation. No discrepancy was found of opinion regarding the classification of univentricular heart disease at time of surgery compared to cardiac CT findings. The overall sensitivity and specification of CTA was 100% compared to the results of surgery.

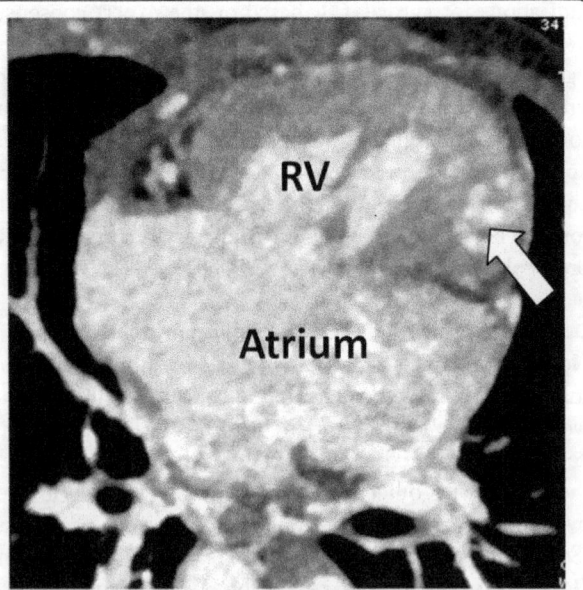

Fig. 1 Cardiac CT of a 2 days old infant showing single atrium (Atrium), univentricular right ventricle (RV) and rudimentary left ventricle (arrow)

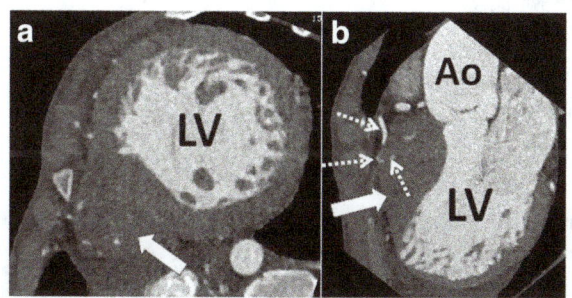

Fig. 2 Cardiac CT of a 1 month old boy showing univentricular left ventricle (LV) and rudimentary right ventricle (**a** and **b**; arrows). Coronary artery fistula from right coronary artery draining into the rudimentary right ventricle was found (**b**; dashed arrows)

Discussion

CT is a robust alternative diagnostic modality for diagnosis of functional univentricular heart disease. In a significant number of patients in our cohort who had previous echocardiography, cardiac CT was able to provide additional information on extracardiac findings such as hypoplastic aortic arch, infracardiac type total anomalous pulmonary venous returns and hypoplastic left lung. For highly select indications, the risk profile may sometimes be in favour of using cardiac CT compared with other diagnostic methods when risks from anaesthesia are considered. Univentricular heart patients are exposed to relatively high cumulative radiation levels during staged palliation [15, 16]. A single institution reports a median cumulative effective radiation dose of 25.7 mSv from birth to 33 months of age, of which 78% was from catheterization [15]. Another study of cumulative radiation dose for patients with all forms of congenital

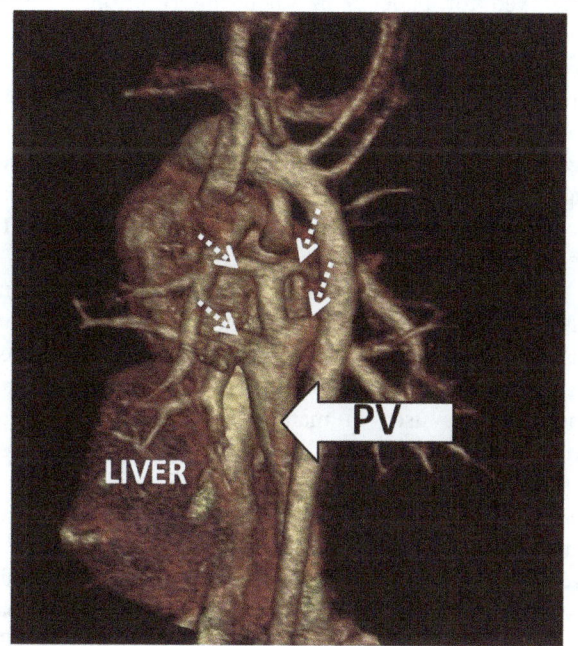

Fig. 4 Cardiac CT of a 1 year old univentricular left ventricle patient showing infracardiac type total anomalous pulmonary venous returns (dashed arrows) which draining into portal vein (arrow). (PV; portal vein)

heart disease showed that 5.3% of patients received over 20 mSv/year with a median follow-up time of 4.3 years [17].

A recent study directly comparing radiation doses from diagnostic catheterization ($n = 50$ cases) and computed tomography angiography ($n = 50$ cases) in children with congenital heart disease has shown 15-fold less radiation from CT angiography, although this was not specific to patients with single-ventricle heart disease [18]. Other studies using older CT scanner showing doses for CT angiography ($n = 21$) that are twofold higher than those in diagnostic cardiac catheterization ($n = 117$) [18]. These results show that the radiation dose from CT varies considerably depending on the type of scanner used and the aggressiveness of dose reduction. The image quality necessary for evaluation of coronary lesions in adult patients is rarely required for congenital applications, and patient-specific dose reduction must be implemented if a diagnostic strategy utilising CT is to be implemented. The standard diagnostic protocol at a majority of centers remains invasive catheterization before surgical palliation, despite data showing a favorable risk profile for non-invasive evaluation [3]. Non-invasive assessment before surgical palliation has shown similar operative outcomes compared with invasive catheterization involving lower risk as measured by radiation exposure, vascular access complications, length of anesthesia, and adverse events [19–21].

Our practice now uses CT preferentially for evaluation of anatomy before surgical palliation. Catheterization is

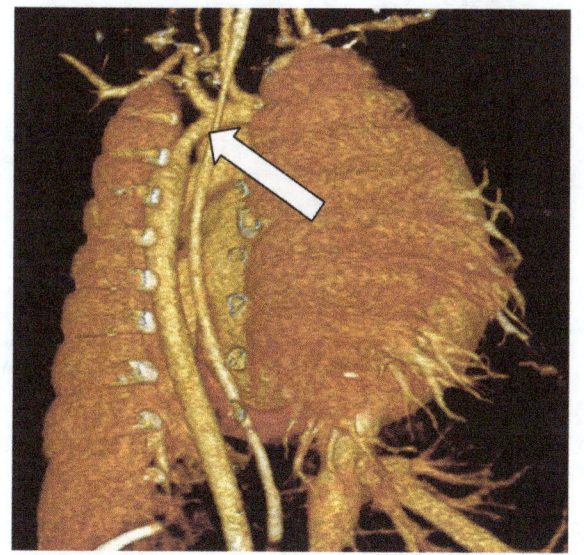

Fig. 3 Cardiac CT of a 1 month old univentricular right ventricle patient showing hypoplastic aortic arch (arrow)

preserved for patients in whom intervention is likely considered on the basis of echocardiography or clinical examination, and for patients with poor ventricular function and severe valve regurgitation in whom hemodynamics are considered relevant to clinical management. Some experts now propose a non-invasive algorythm for evaluation before surgical palliation in patients with single-ventricle heart disease considered to be at a low risk for requiring intervention [22–24].

Cardiovascular MRI is the most commonly used non-invasive advanced imaging modality in congenital heart disease but deep sedation or general anesthesia is required in young children, scan times are relatively long, and gadolinium is used in many patients for angiography. Anesthesia poses increased risk for patients with complex congenital heart disease undergoing MRI evaluation, and there is concern that repeated anesthesia exposure of young patients may have adverse neurological effects [25–34]. Gadolinium deposits have been found in brain tissue after repeated dosing in both children and adult patients, the significance of which is not yet known [35–38]. Risk assessment of non-invasive modalities should include assessment of risk from anesthesia and iodinated or gadolinium-based contrast exposure in addition to radiation exposure and vascular-access requirements.

Cardiac CT is an alternative imaging modality that can be used as part of the non-invasive imaging modality when cardiac MRI is considered to pose a high risk or when there is an imaging artifact [39, 40]. When anesthesia is needed, a single breath-hold is required for data acquisition and the length of anesthesia will be relatively short.

Despite promising initial results, our study has potential limitations. The findings from the present study are retrospective and limited to single-center experience, the generalizability of the present results is limited. The present result is also limited by the number of patients, therefore, the interpretation of sensitivity may be limited.

Conclusion

Cardiac CT can diagnose accurately and be performed with a low radiation exposure in patients with the functional univentricular heart disease. The aorta, pulmonary artery and lung can be evaluated completely and simultaneously as well. Cardiac CT is an effective advanced non-invasive imaging modality to comprehensive evaluation the functional univentricular heart patients, particularly if cardiac MRI poses a high risk or is contraindicated.

Abbreviations
CCT: Cardiac computed tomography; CHD: Congenital heart disease; CMR: Cardiac magnetic resonance imaging; CT: Computed tomography; MAPCAs: Major aortopulmonary collateral arteries; mGy: Milligray; MIP: Maximum intensity projection; MRI: Magnetic resonance imaging; mSv: Millisievert; VRT: Volume-rendering technique

Acknowledgements
The authors would like to thank the Faculty of Medicine for its support.

Funding
This study has not been funded by any research grant.

Authors' contributions
NC and PM participated in design of the study. NC collected data throughout the study with analysis and interpretation of data completed by PM assisted with the recruitment of all patients from clinics. All authors read and approved the final manuscript and gave consent for publication.

Competing interests
The authors declare that they have no competing interests.

Author details
[1]Radiology Department, Faculty of Medicine, Khon Kaen University, Khon Kaen 40000, Thailand. [2]Cardiology Unit, Internal Medicine Department, Faculty of Medicine, Khon Kaen University, Khon Kaen, Thailand.

References
1. Wilkinson JL, Anderson RH. Anatomy of functionally single ventricle. World J Pediatr Congenit Heart Surg. 2012;3(2):159–64. https://doi.org/10.1177/2150135111421508. indexed in Pubmed: 23804770
2. Jacobs ML, Mayer JE. Congenital heart surgery nomenclature and database project: single ventricle. Ann Thorac Surg. 2000;69(4 Suppl):S197–204. indexed in Pubmed: 10798438
3. Feinstein JA, Benson DW, Dubin AM, Cohen MS, Maxey DM, Mahle WT, et al. Hypoplastic left heart syndrome: current considerations and expectations. J Am Coll Cardiol. 2012;59(1 Suppl):S1–42. https://doi.org/10.1016/j.jacc.2011.09.022. indexed in Pubmed:22192720
4. Banka P, McElhinney DB, Bacha EA, et al. What is the clinical utility of routine cardiac catheterization before a Fontan operation? Pediatr Cardiol. 2010;31:977–85. https://doi.org/10.1007/s—246-010-973603. indexed in Pubmed:20503042
5. Stern KW, McElhinney DB, Gauvreau K, Geva T, Brown DW. Echocardiographic evaluation before bidirectional Glenn operation in functional single-ventricle heart disease: comparison to catheter angiography. Circ Cardiovasc Imaging. 2011;4:498–505. https://doi.org/10.1161/CIRCIMAGING.110.963280. indexed in Pubmed:2219272
6. Garg R, Powell AJ, Sena L, Marshall AC, Geva T. Effects of metallic implants on magnetic resonance imaging evaluation of Fontan palliation. Am J Cardiol. 2005;95:688–91. https://doi.org/10.1016/j.amjcard.2004.10.053. indexed in Pubmed:15721124
7. Cronin EM, Mahon N, Wilkoff BL. MRI in patients with cardiac implantable electronic devices. Expert Rev Med Devices. 2012;9:139–46. https://doi.org/10.1586/erd.11.73. indexed in Pubmed:22404775
8. Ramalho J, Semelka RC, Ramalho M, Nunes RH, AlObaidy M, Castillo M. Gadolinium-based contrast agent accumulation and toxicity: an update. AJNR Am J Neuroradiol. 2016;37:1192–8. https://doi.org/10.3174/ajnr.A4615. indexed in Pubmed:26659341
9. Kanda T, Oba H, Toyoda K, Kitajima K, Furui S. Brain gadolinium deposition after administration of gadolinium-based contrast agents. Jpn J Radiol. 2016; 34:3–9. https://doi.org/10.1007/s11604-015-0503-5. indexed in Pubmed: 26608061
10. Kanda T, Matsuda M, Oba H, Toyoda K, Furui S. Gadolinium deposition after contrast-enhanced MR imaging. Radiology. 2015;277:924–5. https://doi.org/10.1148/radiol.15150025. indexed in Pubmed:25742194
11. Han BK, Rigsby CK, Hlavacek A, et al. Computed tomography imaging in patients with congenital heart disease part I: rationale and utility. An expert consensus document of the Society of Cardiovascular Computed Tomography (SCCT): endorsed by the Society of Pediatric Radiology (SPR)

and the North American Society of Cardiac Imaging (NASCI). J Cardiovasc Comput Tomogr. 2015;9:475–92. https://doi.org/10.1016/j.jcct.2015.07.004. indexed in Pubmed:26272851

12. Halliburton SS, Abbara S, Chen MY, et al. SCCT guidelines on radiation dose and dose-optimization strategies in cardiovascular CT. J Cardiovasc Comput Tomogr. 2011;5:198–224. https://doi.org/10.1016/j.jcct.2011.06.001. indexed in Pubmed:21723512

13. AAPM Task Group 23 of the Diagnostic Imaging Council CT Committee. The measurement, reporting, and Management of Radiation Dose in CT, AAPM report 96. College Park: American Association of Physicists in Medicine; 2008. p. 1–25. ISBN: 978-1-888340-73-0

14. AAPM Task Group 204. Size-Specific Dose Estimates (SSDE) in pediatric and adult body CT examinations, AAPM report no.204; 2011. p. 1–23. ISBN: 978-1-936366-08-8

15. Downing TE, McDonnell A, Zhu X, et al. Cumulative medical radiation exposure throughout staged palliation of single ventricle congenital heart disease. Pediatr Cardiol. 2015;36:190–5. https://doi.org/10.1007/s00246-014-0984-5. indexed in Pubmed:25096904

16. Johnson JN, Hornik CP, Li JS, et al. Cumulative radiation exposure and cancer risk estimation in children with heart disease. Circulation. 2014;130: 161–7. https://doi.org/10.1161/CIRCULATIONAHA.113.005425. indexed in Pubmed:24914037

17. Glatz AC, Purrington KS, Klinger A, King L, Huda W, Hlavacek AM. Cumulative exposure to medical radiation for children requiring surgery for congenital heart disease. J Pediatr. 2014;164:789–94; e10. https://doi.org/10.1016/j.jpeds.2013.10.074. indexed in Pubmed:24321535

18. Watson TG, Mah E, Schoepf UJ, King L, Huda W, Hlavacek AM. Effective radiation dose in computed tomographic angiography of the chest and diagnostic cardiac catheterization in pediatric patients. Pediatr Cardiol. 2013;34:518–24. https://doi.org/10.1007/s00247-009-1436-x. indexed in Pubmed:19997730

19. Brown DW, Gauvreau K, Powell AJ, et al. Cardiac magnetic resonance versus routine cardiac catheterization before bidirectional glenn anastomosis in infants with functional single ventricle: a prospective randomized trial. Circulation. 2007;116:2718–25. https://doi.org/10.1161/CIRCULATIONAHA.107.723213. indexed in Pubmed:18025538

20. Brown DW, Gauvreau K, Powell AJ, et al. Cardiac magnetic resonance versus routine cardiac catheterization before bidirectional Glenn anastomosis: long-term follow-up of a prospective randomized trial. J Thorac Cardiovasc Surg. 2013;146:1172–8. https://doi.org/10.1016/j.jtcvs.2012.12.079. indexed in Pubmed:23380513

21. Han BK, Vezmar M, Lesser JR, et al. Selective use of cardiac computed tomography angiography: an alternative diagnostic modality before second-stage single ventricle palliation. J Thorac Cardiovasc Surg. 2014;148:1548–54. https://doi.org/10.1016/j.jtcvs.2014.04.047. indexed in Pubmed:24914037

22. Fogel MA. Is routine cardiac catheterization necessary in the management of patients with single ventricles across staged Fontan reconstruction? No! Pediatr Cardiol. 2005;26:154–8. https://doi.org/10.1007/s00246-004-0960-6. indexed in Pubmed:15868320

23. Fogel MA, Pawlowski TW, Whitehead KK, et al. Cardiac magnetic resonance and the need for routine cardiac catheterization in single ventricle patients prior to Fontan: a comparison of 3 groups: pre-Fontan CMR versus cath evaluation. J Am Coll Cardiol. 2012;60:1094–102. https://doi.org/10.1016/j.jacc.2012.06.021. indexed in Pubmed:4395971

24. Prakash A, Khan MA, Hardy R, Torres AJ, Chen JM, Gersony WM. A new diagnostic algorithm for assessment of patients with single ventricle before a Fontan operation. J Thorac Cardiovasc Surg. 2009;138:917–23. https://doi.org/10.1016/j.jtcvs.2009.03.022. indexed in Pubmed:19660367

25. Ramamoorthy C, Haberkern CM, Bhananker SM, et al. Anesthesia related cardiac arrest in children with heart disease: data from the Pediatric Perioperative Cardiac Arrest (POCA) registry. Anesth Analg. 2010;110: 1376–82. https://doi.org/10.1213/ANE.0b013e3181c9f927. indexed in Pubmed:20103543

26. Girshin M, Shapiro V, Rhee A, Ginsberg S, Inchiosa MA Jr. Increased risk of general anesthesia for high-risk patients undergoing magnetic resonance imaging. J Comput Assist Tomogr. 2009;33(2):312–5. https://doi.org/10.1097/RCT.0b013e31818474b8. indexed in Pubmed:19346867

27. Dorfman AL, Odegard KC, Powell AJ, Laussen PC, Geva T. Risk factors for adverse events during cardiovascular magnetic resonance in congenital heart disease. J Cardiovasc Magn Reson. 2007;9:793–8. https://doi.org/10.1080/10976640701545305. indexed in Pubmed:17891617

28. Rappaport B, Mellon RD, Simone A, Woodcock J. Defining safe use of anesthesia in children. N Engl J Med. 2011;364:1387–90. https://doi.org/10.1056/NEJMp1102155. indexed in Pubmed:21388302

29. Hays SR, Deshpande JK. Newly postulated neurodevelopmental risks of pediatric anesthesia. Curr Neurol Neurosci Rep. 2011;11:205–10. https://doi.org/10.1016/j.juro.2012.11.090. indexed in Pubmed:23178900

30. Wilder RT, Flick RP, Sprung J, et al. Early exposure to anesthesia and learning disabilities in a population-based birth cohort. Anesthesiology. 2009;110: 796–804. https://doi.org/10.1097/01.anes.0000344728.34332.5d. indexed in Pubmed:19293700

31. Flick RP, Katusic SK, Colligan RC, et al. Cognitive and behavioral outcomes after early exposure to anesthesia and surgery. Pediatrics. 2011;128:1053–61. https://doi.org/10.1542/peds.2011-0351. indexed in Pubmed:21969289

32. DiMaggio C, Sun LS, Kakavouli A, Byrne MW, Li G. A retrospective cohort study of the association of anesthesia and hernia repair surgery with behavioral and developmental disorders in young children. J Neurosurg Anesthesiol. 2009;21:286–91. https://doi.org/10.1097/ANA.0b013e3181a71f11. indexed in Pubmed:19955889

33. Fogel MA, Weinberg PM, Parave E, et al. Deep sedation for cardiac magnetic resonance imaging: a comparison with cardiac anesthesia. J Pediatr. 2008;152: 534–9. https://doi.org/10.1016/j.jpeds.2007.08.045. indexed in Pubmed:18346511

34. Odegard KC, DiNardo JA, Kussman BD, et al. The frequency of anesthesia-related cardiac arrests in patients with congenital heart disease undergoing cardiac surgery. Anesth Analg. 2007;105:335–43. https://doi.org/10.1213/01.ane.0000268498.68620.39. indexed in Pubmed:17646487

35. Miller JH, Hu HH, Pokorney A, Cornejo P, Towbin R. MRI brain signal intensity changes of a child during the course of 35 gadolinium contrast examinations. Pediatrics. 2015;136:1637–40. https://doi.org/10.1542/peds.2015-2222. indexed in Pubmed:26574593

36. Kanda T, Oba H, Toyoda K, Furui S. Recent advances in understanding gadolinium retention in the brain. AJNR Am J Neuroradiol. 2016;37:E1–2. https://doi.org/10.3174/ajnr.A4586. indexed in Pubmed:26494697

37. Roberts DR, Holden KR. Progressive increase of T1 signal intensity in the dentate nucleus and globus pallidus on unenhanced T1-weighted MR images in the pediatric brain exposed to multiple doses of gadolinium contrast. Brain and Development. 2016;38:331–6. https://doi.org/10.1016/j.braindev.2015.08.009. indexed in Pubmed:26345358

38. Kanda T, Fukusato T, Matsuda M, et al. Gadolinium-based contrast agent accumulates in the brain even in subjects without severe renal dysfunction: evaluation of autopsy brain specimens with inductively coupled plasma mass spectroscopy. Radiology. 2015;276:228–32. https://doi.org/10.1148/radiol.2015142690. indexed in Pubmed:25942417

39. Han BK, Lesser JR. CT imaging in congenital heart disease: an approach to imaging and interpreting complex lesions after surgical intervention for tetralogy of Fallot, transposition of the great arteries, and single ventricle heart disease. J Cardiovasc Comput Tomogr. 2013;7:338–53. https://doi.org/10.1016/j.jcct.2013.10.003. indexed in Pubmed:24331929

40. Khairy P, Van Hare GF, Balaji S, et al. PACES/HRS expert consensus statement on the recognition and management of arrhythmias in adult congenital heart disease. Heart Rhythm. 2014;30(10):1–63. https://doi.org/10.1016/j.cjca.2014.09.002. indexed in Pubmed:25262867

31

Prosthesis-patient mismatch after mitral valve replacement: a single-centered retrospective analysis in East China

Armah M Akuffu, Haige Zhao, Junnan Zheng* and Yiming Ni

Abstract

Background: Prosthesis–patient mismatch (PPM) may affect the clinical outcomes of patients undergoing mitral valve replacement (MVR) surgery. We aimed to investigate the incidence of PPM of the mitral position in our center and analyze the possible predictors of PPM as well as its effect on short-term outcomes.

Methods: We retrospectively examined all consecutive patients with isolated or concomitant MVR at our center from 2013 to 2015. PPM was defined as an indexed effective orifice area (iEOA) of ≤1.2 cm2/m2. After inclusion and exclusion, a total of 1067 patients were analyzed. The baseline information were collected and compared between the two groups. Multivariate logistic regression analysis was conducted to determine the preoperative predictors of PPM as well as the effect of PPM on early mortality.

Results: A total of 1067 patients were included in the study. PPM was detected in 15.9% of the patients while 12 patients (1.12%) met the criteria for severe PPM. Patients with PPM compared to the non-PPM patients had higher age, larger body surface area and were more likely to be male and obese. Logistic regression analysis showed that higher age, larger BSA, bioprosthesis and smaller left ventricle end-diastolic diameter were predictors of PPM. There were no significant differences between the PPM and non-PPM groups regarding post-operative complications. Logistic regression analysis showed that PPM was not a risk factor of short-term mortality ($P = 0.654$). Also, there were no significant differences regarding short–/mid-term heart function between the PPM and non PPM groups ($P = 0.902$).

Conclusions: Our results demonstrated that higher age, bioprosthesis, larger BSA and smaller left ventricle size were associated with mitral PPM. However, PPM was not associated with poorer early outcomes after MVR surgery. In eastern of China, the prevalence of mitral valve stenosis is high; therefore, whether the standard PPM criteria are suitable for patients of this district needs to be further verified.

Keywords: Prosthesis-patient mismatch, Mitral valve replacement, Effective orifice area, Short-term mortality

Background

The phenomenon of prosthesis-patient mismatch (PPM) was initially described by Rahimtoola and Murphy about 40 years ago [1, 2]. Currently, PPM is considered a condition in which the effective orifice area (EOA) of the implanted valve prosthesis does not match the patient's body size.

PPM of the aortic position has been proved to be associated with poorer outcomes including long- and short-term cardiac death [3–5]. However, PPM following mitral valve replacement (MVR) has still been less investigated.

In recent years, PPM after MVR has attracted more and more attention from researchers. Researches has shown that the EOA of mitral valve prosthesis is often too small in relation to body size, thus, normally functioning mitral prosthesis often has relatively high transvalvular gradients similar to those found in mild to moderate mitral valve stenosis patients [6–10].

In East Asia, where rheumatic mitral valve stenosis is very common, the mitral valve annulus in patients is

* Correspondence: zhengjunnan@zju.edu.cn
Department of Cardiothoracic Surgery, the First Affiliated Hospital of
Zhejiang University, No.79 Qingchun Road, Hangzhou 310003, China

relatively small; therefore more patients meet the standard of mitral PPM [11]. We aim to investigate the incidence of PPM of the mitral position in our center and analyze the possible predictors of PPM as well as its effect on short-term outcomes. We will also discuss the eligibility of the current PPM standard for this population.

Methods

Patient population and data collection

We retrospectively reviewed all consecutive patients who underwent elective isolated or concomitant MVR at our center, the Department of Cardiothoracic Surgery, the First Affiliated Hospital, Zhejiang University, School of Medicine, from January 2013 to December 2015. Written informed consent waivers obtained from the Hospital Review Board were completed by all patients.

We analyzed all consecutive patients aged more than 18 years undergoing isolated MVR or MVR concomitant with other non-valve-replacement procedures. Patients with incomplete clinical data or patients who received MVR due to failed mitral valvuloplasty were excluded (Fig. 1).

In total, 1067 patients were included in this study. Baseline, intraoperative and outcome data were prospectively collected and validated, which were queried retrospectively. 30-month postoperative follow-up was conducted for discharged patients at the outpatient clinic. Patients who did not show up at the visit were contacted by telephone.

PPM definition and EOA Index (EOAI) calculation

Body surface area (BSA) of the patients was calculated using the Dubois formula. The EOA of the mitral valve prosthesis was derived from in vitro measurements provided by the manufacturers and from scientific publications, as outlined in Table 1.

EOAi (also called indexed effective orifice area, iEOA) was obtained with EOA divided by BSA. Mitral PPM was defined as EOAi ≤ 1.2 cm^2/m^2. EOAi ≤ 0.9 cm^2/m^2 was considered severe mitral PPM.

Other definitions were listed as follows. Chronic renal insufficiency: serum creatinine ≥ 2 mg/dl. Peripheral arterial disease: claudication, carotid stenosis > 50% or previous/planned intervention on the abdominal aorta, limb arteries or carotids. Coronary artery disease: $\geq 50\%$ reduction in one or more coronary vessels in single or multiple plane angiographic images. Emergency surgery: operation required within 24 h of onset of symptoms. Postoperative renal failure: increase in baseline creatinine greater than 2 mg/dl.

Surgical technique and prosthesis application

The operation records of all patients were reviewed. A total of 868 mechanical valve prostheses and 199 bioprostheses were implanted. The following prostheses were used in as followings:

Mechanical prosthesis: CarboMedics Orbis Universal (CarboMedics, Inc., Austin, TX, USA) ($n = 679$); St Jude Master (St Jude Medical, Inc., St Paul, MN, USA) ($n = 154$); ATS open pivot (ATS Medical, Inc., Minneapolis,

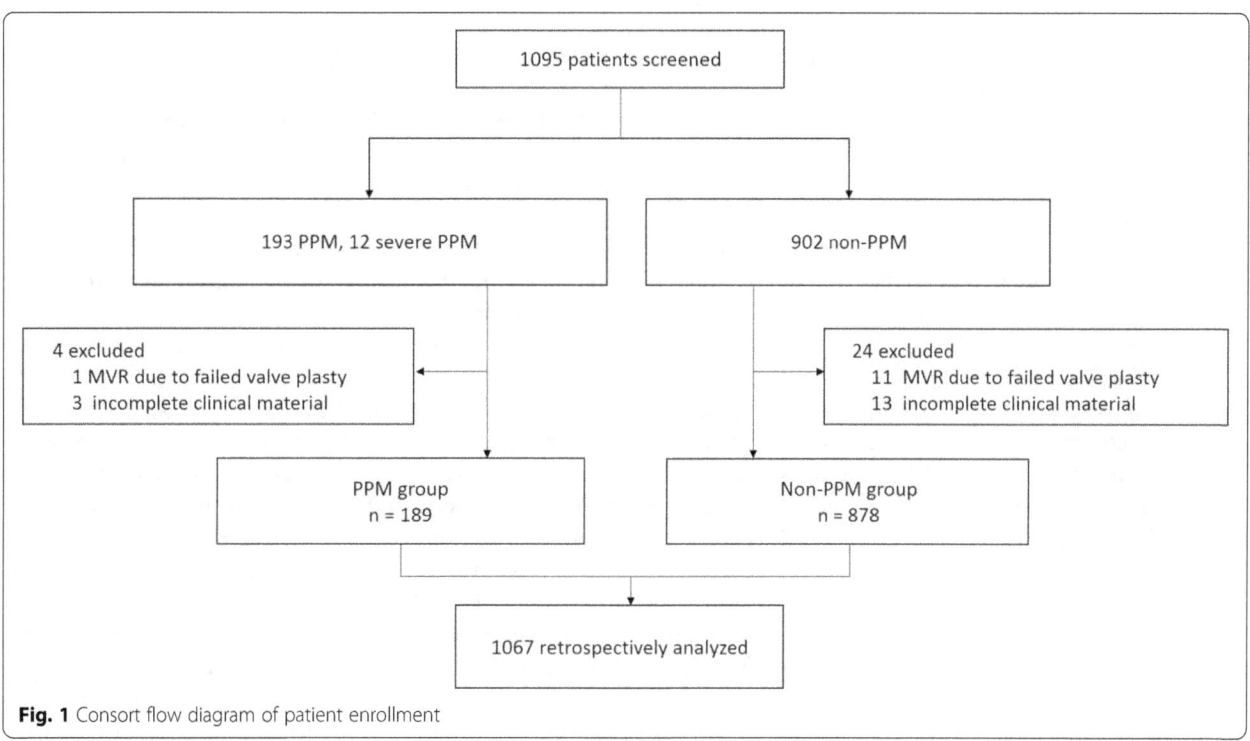

Fig. 1 Consort flow diagram of patient enrollment

Table 1 In vivo effective orifice area values (cm^2) corresponding to each valve

Valve prosthesis	patients	23 mm	25 mm	27 mm	29 mm	31 mm	33 mm	Ref
Mechanical	868							
CarboMedics Orbis Universal	680	1.8	2.2	2.2	2.4	2.4	2.3	[12]
St.Jude Master series	154	1.0	1.5	1.8	1.8	2.0	2.0	[13, 21]
ATS open pivot	33	–	1.8	2.8	2.8	2.9	2.9	[22]
Bioprosthesis	199							
Medtronics Hancock II	110	–	1.5	1.8	1.9	2.6	2.6	[12]
Medtronics Mosaic	5	–	1.5	1.7	1.9	1.9	–	[13]
St. Jude Bicor Stented	45	–	1.4	1.5	2.3	2.2	2.3	[23]
Carpentier-Edwards perimount	39	–	1.7	1.9	2.3	2.8	2.7	[12]

Ref: reference

MN, USA) ($n = 33$); Bioprosthesis: Hancock II Porcine Bioprosthesis (Medtronic, Inc., Minneapolis, MN, USA) ($n = 110$); Mosaic Porcine Bioprosthetic Valves (Medtronic, Inc., Minneapolis, MN, USA) ($n = 5$); Bicor Stented Bioprosthesis (St Jude Medical, Inc., St Paul, MN, USA) ($n = 45$); Carpentier-Edwards perimount (Baxter Healthcare Corp., Edwards Division, Santa Ana, CA, USA) ($n = 39$).

An isolated or concomitant MVR was performed in all patients. Concomitant procedures included tricuspid valvuloplasty, coronary artery bypass grafting, atrial septum defect repair and/or other procedures. Standard anesthesia and cardiopulmonary bypass methods were implemented. Most of the patients were approached through a full median sternotomy followed by an antegrade 4:1 cold blood cardioplegia for myocardial protection. Antegrade plus retrograde cardioplegia was applied for patients with coronary stenosis. Intermittent perfusion of cold blood cardioplegia was maintained at a frequency of once every 20 min.

After consulting with the patients preoperatively, the final decision of the type of prosthesis was made by the surgeons during operation, taking into consideration the preoperative information and intraoperative findings. When performing the MVR, sub-valvular structures were preserved as much as possible.

Statistical analysis

The Kolmogorov-Smirnov test was used to verify the distribution of all the quantitative variables. Gaussian distributed continuous variables were presented as mean ± standard deviation (SD), while non-Gaussian distributed variables were presented as medians (interquartile range). Categorical variables were expressed as an absolute number (percentage). Pearson's χ2 test was used for descriptive, univariate statistics, such as the comparison of portions, while the Student's unpaired t-test was used for normally distributed data comparisons. Otherwise, the Mann-Whitney U test was otherwise used for comparison of non-Gaussian distributed variables. Two-tailed

P-values were derived from the calculated test statistics, and $P \leq 0.05$ was considered statistically significant. Binary multivariate logistic regression analysis was performed to study the factors affecting PPM as well as mortality. IBM SPSS Statistics 20.0 software (IBM, Armonk, NY, USA) was used to analyze the data.

Results

Preoperative data and baseline information

A total of 1067 patients were included in this study. Mitral PPM was detected in 17.71% (189/1067) of the patients and only 12 (1.12%) patients met the criteria for severe PPM.

Compared with the non-PPM group, patients with PPM were older, taller and heavier and had a higher prevalence of male gender, hypertension, smoking history, coronary heart disease, and had a lower prevalence of mitral stenosis (Table 2).

Patient characterize, PPM and valve prosthesis size

We analyzed the association among age, weight, height, BSA and valve size (Fig. 2). Krusal-Wallis analysis showed that weight, height and BSA are significantly associated with valve size ($P < 0.01$). In summary, larger mitral bioprosthetic valves were implanted in the taller and more obese patients.

Also, the PPM rate of each size of the prostheses was analyzed (Fig. 3). The results showed that the PPM rate of mechanical valve prostheses was considerably lower compared with bioprostheses (10.6% vs 48.5%, respectively, $P < 0.001$). As for the mechanical prostheses, there were no significant differences regarding the PPM occurrence of each valve size, whereas, the PPM rate of the 25 mm bioprosthesis was higher than that of the 27 mm and 29 mm bioprostheses ($P < 0.01$).

On the other hand, the PPM rate also differed among different brands of prostheses. As for mechanical prostheses, according to our data, PPM rate was highest (55.8%, 86/154) in patients underwent MVR with

Table 2 Preoperative patient baseline information

preoperative information	total (n = 1067)	PPM group (n = 189)	non-PPM group (n = 878)	P value
Age, y	56(48–62)	63(55–67)	54(46–61)	< 0.001
Male	379(35.5%)	89(47.1%)	290(33.0%)	< 0.001
Height, cm	160.72 ± 7.82	163.26 ± 7.87	160.17 ± 7.71	< 0.001
Weight, kg	57.72 ± 10.33	62.42 ± 10.23	56.70 ± 10.07	< 0.001
BMI, kg/m^2	22.29 ± 3.67	23.34 ± 2.86	22.07 ± 3.79	< 0.001
BSA, m^2	1.57 ± 0.16	1.64 ± 0.17	1.55 ± 0.16	< 0.001
Smoking history	123(11.5%)	32(16.9%)	91(10.4%)	0.016
Diabetes	102(9.6%)	22(11.6%)	80(9.2%)	NS
Hypertention	192(18.0%)	47(24.9%)	145(16.5%)	0.009
Cerebrovascular accident	34(3.2%)	6(3.2%)	28(3.2%)	NS
Coronary heart disease	22(2.1%)	9(4.8%)	13(1.5%)	0.009
NYHA functional class (≥ III)	400(37.5%)	77(40.7%)	323(36.8%)	NS
Atrial fibrillation	533(50.0%)	92(48.7%)	441(50.2%)	NS
Previous cardiac surgery	54(5.1%)	8(4.2%)	46(5.2%)	NS
Previous MI	1(0.1%)	0(0.0%)	1(0.1%)	NS
Mitral stenosis	786(76.7%)	128(67.7%)	658(74.9%)	0.036
MR (moderate to severe)	470(44.0%)	88(46.5%)	382(43.5%)	NS
LVEF	62.11 ± 8.48	62.23 ± 8.95	62.09 ± 8.38	NS
LVdD, mm	50(45–56)	51(46–58)	50(45–56)	NS
LAD, mm	51.36 ± 12.04	51.36 ± 11.93	51.36 ± 12.07	NS
Emergency surgery	2(0.2%)	0(0.0%)	0(0.0%)	NS
Aspirin within 5 days	29(2.7%)	9(4.8%)	20(2.3%)	NS
Clopidogrel within 5 days	19(1.8%)	6(3.2%)	13(1.5%)	NS

BMI body mass index, *BSA* body surface area, *NYHA* New York Heart Association, *MI* myocardial infarction, *MR* mitral valve regurgitation, *LVEF* left ventricular ejection fraction, *LVdD* left ventricular diastolic diameter, *LAD* left atrial diameter, *NS* not significant

St. Jude Master Mechanical prostheses. And PPM rate was considerably low regarding CarboMedics mechanical prosthesis (0.9%, 6/679) and ATS open pivot mechanical prostheses (0.0%, 0/33). As for bioprosthesis, our results showed that PPM rate was high in patients using Medtronic Mosaic porcine bioprosthesis (80.0%, 4/5) or St. Jude Bicor bioprosthesis (82.2%, 37/45), whereas patients underwent MVR with Carpentier-Edwards Perimount bioprosthesis (17.7%, 5/38) and Medtronic Hancock II (45.4%, 50/110) showed lower rate of PPM.

Operative data

As shown in Table 3, there were no significant differences between PPM and non-PPM patients regarding cardiopulmonary bypass (CPB) time. However, we found that there is an average five-minute cross-clamp time reduction in the PPM group.

Not surprisingly, remarkably more patients with a PPM were implanted with a bioprosthetic mitral valve. And as for patients who received a bioprosthesis, the prevalence of mitral stenosis was higher for mismatch

patients (58.3% vs 41.7%, P = 0.019), whereas patients of mechanical prostheses did not differ in the prevalence of mitral stenosis, whether PPM or not (77.4% vs 79.4%, P > 0.05).

As for combined procedures, there were more combined coronary artery bypass grafting (CABG) and surgical ablation for atrial fibrillation in the PPM group.

Factors affecting PPM

According to a multivariate binary logistic regression analysis including all preoperative and intraoperative variables, higher age (P = 0.011), larger BSA (P < 0.001), smaller left ventricular diastolic diameter (LVDd) (P < 0.001) and bioprosthesis (P < 0.001) were factors affecting mitral PPM (Table 4).

Postoperative outcomes and factors affecting postoperative mortality

There were no obvious differences between the two groups regarding early post-operative complications including blood transfusion, ventilation time, reintubation, intensive care unit (ICU) time, postop stroke, postop

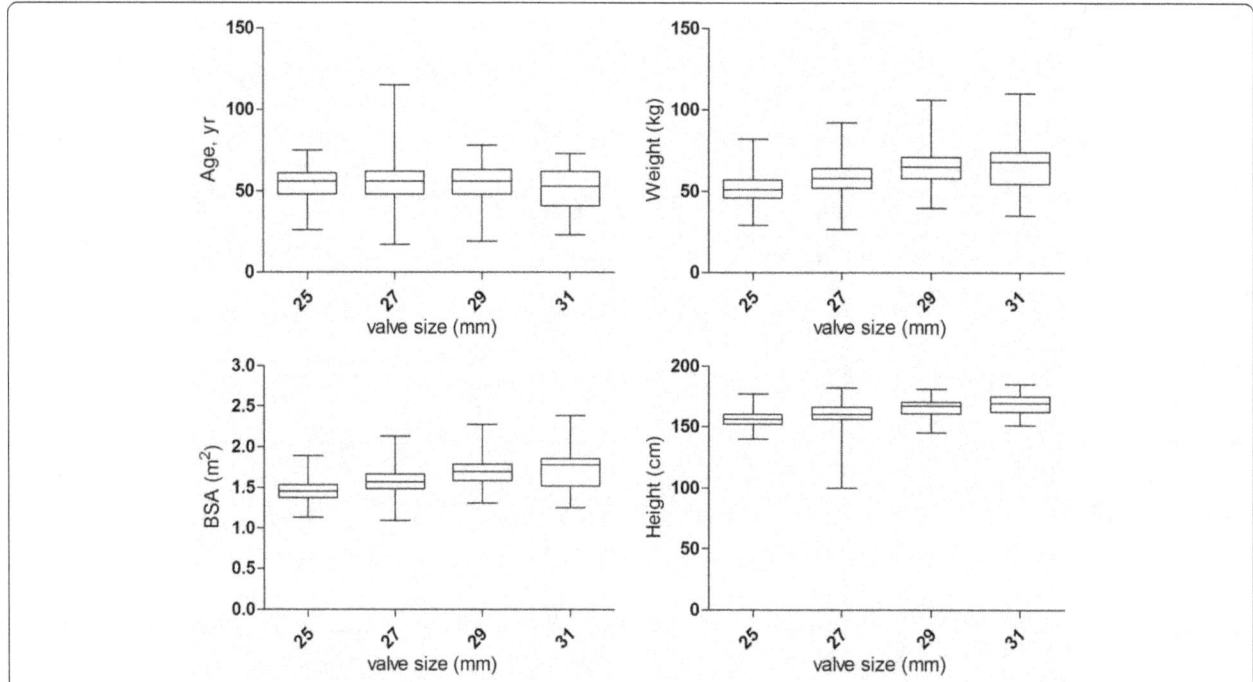

Fig. 2 Boxplot showing distribution of age (NS), weight ($P < 0.01$), height ($P < 0.01$), and body surface area ($P < 0.01$), respectively, according to aortic valve size implanted

atrial fibrillation and short-term mortality. Also, there were no other reoperation for valve-rated complications including PPM or other cardiac disease during hospital-stay except that two patients underwent emergency percutaneous coronary intervention for acute myocardium ischemia. Interestingly, we found that there was a small increase in hospitalization expense as well as a slightly prolonged hospital stay for the PPM patients (Table 5).

Altogether there were nine patients died within 30 days after surgery. Among them, five patients died due to malignant arrhythmia or cardiac arrest, two patient died of sever systematic infection, one patient died of uncontrollable bleeding and one patient died because of stroke. Among these short-term deaths, 2 patients underwent

MVR with Hancock II bioprostheses, whereas 7 patients were replaced with CarboMedics mechanical prostheses.

Logistic regression analysis showed that smoking history and preoperative low left ventricular ejection fraction (LVEF) were independent factors predicting post-operative short-term all-cause mortality. However, PPM was not a risk factor for short-term mortality (Table 6).

Mid-term follow-up

During mid-term follow-up, two patients underwent re-operative for stuck of the mechanical prostheses (both CarboMedics Mechanical prostheses). Both of the patients had an irregular medication history of Warfarin.

Mid-term deaths occurred in eight patients who all underwent MVR with a mechanical prosthesis, adding to the previously mentioned nine short-term deaths. Cumulative mid-term overall survival is 0.986 for both PPM and non-PPM patients (Fig. 4), and there were no significant difference regarding mid-term mortality for the two groups (SE 0.037, Log-rank $p = 0.847$). All the later occurring eight deaths were coagulation-related death. The overall mortality at 30 months was approximately 1.6% (Table 7). During follow-up, about 9.2% of the patients presented compromised cardiac functions with New York Heart Association (NYHA) functional classes III to IV. However, there were no significant differences between the PPM and non-PPM patients.

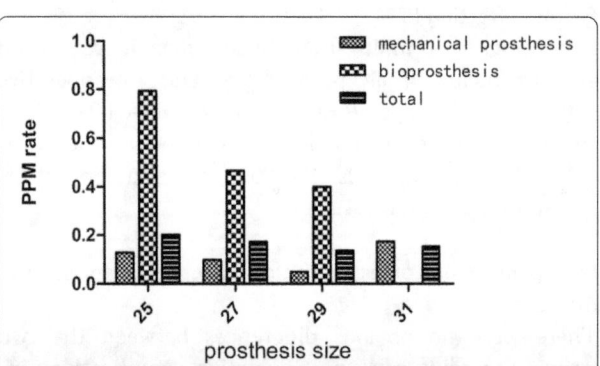

Fig. 3 The PPM rate of each valve size for bioprostheses and mechanical prostheses respectively

Table 3 Intraoperative data

	total	PPM group n = 189	non-PPM group n = 878	P value
First time surgery	1013(94.9%)	181(95.8%)	832(94.7%)	NS
CPB time (min)	83(70–92)	83(70–89)	83(70–93)	NS
Cross-clamp time (min)	50(41–62)	45(40–55)	50(41–63)	< 0.001
Bioprosthesis	199(18.7%)	96(50.8%)	103(11.7%)	< 0.001
Combined procedure				
Tricuspid valve plasty	277(26.0%)	38(20.1%)	239(27.2%)	NS
CABG	28(2.6%)	11(5.8%)	17(1.9%)	0.005
AFRA or Maze surgery	106(9.9%)	30(15.9%)	76(8.7%)	0.005
Others	139(13.0%)	30(15.9%)	109(12.4%)	NS

CPB cardiopulmonary bypass, CABG coronary artery bypass grafting surgery, AFRA atrial fibrillation radio frequency surgery, NS not significant

Discussion

PPM occurrence and its risk factors

Although highly variable, PPM rates for mitral position in most of the literature ranged from 20 to 70% [11–16]. However, the incidence of PPM after MVR in our single-centered cohort was 17.7% and only 1.2% of the cases met the criteria for severe PPM.

We performed logistic regression analysis and found that larger BSA, higher age, implantation of bioprosthesis and smaller LVDd were risk factors for PPM. Besides BSA, EOA was the only variable defining the EOAi which determined the occurrence of PPM. Bioprosthesis possessed smaller EOA compared with mechanical prosthesis of the same valve size, leading to an increased rate of PPM. Also, bioprostheses were more prone to late degenerative calcification, which may further decrease its EOA. Thus, the more common use of bioprosthesis for degenerative mitral regurgitation might explain the lower prevalence of mitral stenosis of the PPM group in the preoperative data. As for LVDd, it was an indirect reflection of the mitral annulus diameter, which was another decisive factor in choosing prosthesis size, affecting the EOA of the prosthesis implanted. Higher age was then associated with more bioprosthesis implantation, thus leading to the increase in PPM occurrence. Hence, the difference of patient baseline characteristics between the PPM and non-PPM patients in hypertension and coronary heart disease could be explained by the higher age and obesity of the PPM patients.

Table 4 Logistic regression analysis for prosthesis-patient mismatch

Factors	mean or %	OR	95% CI	P value
Age	54	1.029	1.006–1.051	0.011
BSA (m²)	1.57	152.111	45.261–511.208	< 0.001
LVDd (mm)	51.26	0.964	0.944–0.984	< 0.001
bioprosthesis	18.7%	7.539	4.632–12.273	< 0.001

OR odds ratio, CI confidence interval, BSA body surface area, LVDd left ventricular diastolic diameter

In the Asian population, especially the eastern Chinese population, mitral stenosis and small size mitral prosthesis implantation might generally be considered to occur more frequently than in Western populations due to rheumatic causes associated with a small annulus. However, due to rheumatic etiology, the episode age of these patients was considerably younger than patients with valvular degeneration as predominant causes in Western countries. Thus, a larger ratio of patients of this population were implanted with mechanical mitral prostheses which possessed larger EOA than bioprosthesis. Also, patients of this population had a smaller body surface area than those in Western populations, leading to a further reduction in PPM occurrence. The aforementioned factors altogether help explain the low PPM rate in our study population.

PPM and patient outcomes

Since its first description in 1978 by Rahimtoola [1], PPM after MVR has been suggested to potentially correlate with poor clinical outcomes including late tricuspid regurgitation and persistent pulmonary hypertension [11, 14, 17], similar to the outcomes of residual mitral stenosis. However, there were also reports suggesting that PPM did not affect survival after MVR [18, 19].

In our analysis, no impact of PPM on patient mortality was detected either in the postoperative short-term period or in the mid-term follow-up. Our findings are consistent with several large sample multi-centered analyses [15, 19]. Our results showed that smoking history and low preoperative LVEF were associated with higher short-term mortality, but not PPM.

Interestingly, our study showed that cross-clamp times were shorter in patients with PPM, with an average shortened time of 5 min. This might be explained because less time was spent suturing the mitral prosthesis due to the smaller mitral annulus diameter of the PPM patients. The longer hospitalization time of the PPM patients shown in the results might be due to the their

Table 5 Postoperative outcomes

	total	PPM group	non-PPM group	P
Perioperative transfusion	269(25.2%)	47(24.9%)	222(25.3%)	NS
Ventilation time (hr)	21(20–23)	21(20–23)	21(20–23)	NS
Reintubation	3(0.3%)	0(0.0%)	3(0.3%)	NS
Duration of first time ICU	72(72–96)	72(72–96)	72(72–96)	NS
Reentering ICU	2(0.2%)	2(1.1%)	0(0.0%)	NS
Chest tube output (ml)	545.88 ± 365.82	555.15 ± 295.51	543.87 ± 379.47	NS
Reoperation for bleeding	18(1.7%)	1(0.5%)	17(1.9%)	NS
Sternal wound infection	3(0.3%)	0(0.0%)	3(0.3%)	NS
Cerebral infarction	5(0.5%)	0(0.0%)	5(0.6%)	NS
Postoperative stroke	1(0.1%)	0(0.0%)	1(0.1%)	NS
Newly onset AF	3(0.3%)	0(0.0%)	3(0.3%)	NS
Mortality within 30 days	9(0.8%)	2(1.1%)	7(0.8%)	NS
Hospitalization expense (USD)	13,726 (11632–16,030)	14,446 (12538–17,010)	13,628 (11509–15,775)	0.032
Length of stay (d)	14(12–18)	15(13–19)	14(12–18)	0.011

ICU intensive care unit, *AF* atrial fibrillation, *NS* not significant

higher average age and because their recovery time might be longer than in younger patients. Also, the elevated hospitalization expense could be explained by higher price of the bioprosthesis which was more common in the PPM group.

Clinical implication for east Asian population

Currently, the most precise parameter in characterizing PPM is the EOAi [20], which is defined as the EOA of the prosthesis divided by the patient's BSA. EOAi is in fact the only parameter found to consistently correlate with the postoperative gradient; therefore it is the most widely used. In Western countries, the predominant cause of mitral valve disease is degenerative mitral valve regurgitation. For this population, patients with mitral valve diseases usually have a larger left ventricle volume (left ventricular diastolic diameter) than the eastern Asian population; therefore, implantation of a large size prosthesis to avoid PPM will not have an obvious effect on left ventricular function. Hence, the parameter of EOAi has high feasibility in characterizing PPM for Western populations.

However, in a rheumatic population such as the eastern Asian population, the incidence of mitral valve stenosis is

much higher than mitral valve regurgitation [11]. A larger proportion of this population has small left ventricle size, with part of the patients' LVDd even smaller than the mitral annulus diameter. For these patients, implantation of a large sized prosthesis might compromise the effective cardiac muscular contraction of the left ventricle, causing

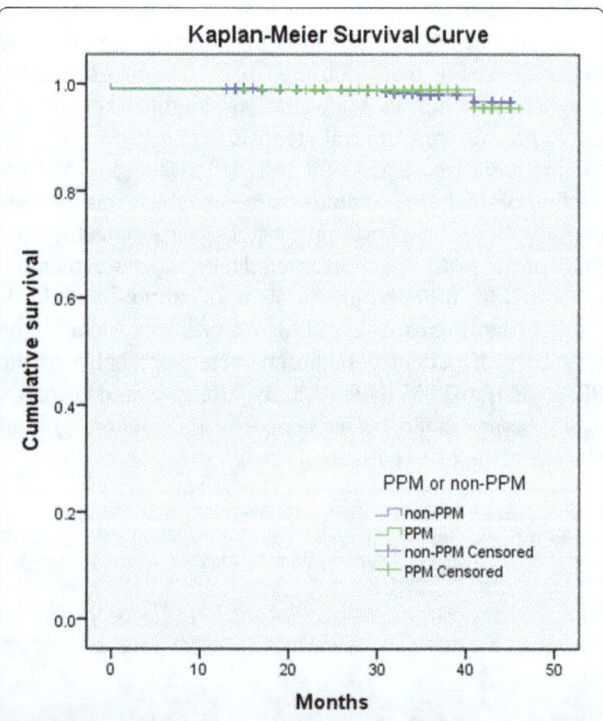

Fig. 4 Kaplan-Meier cumulative mid-term survival, Prosthesis-patient mismatch (PPM) vs non prosthesis-patient mismatch

Table 6 Logistic regression model for postoperative 30-day global mortaliy

Factors	mean or %	Odds ratio	95% CI	P value
smoking history	11.5%	3.199	0.729–14.041	0.004
preoperative LVEF	62.11	0.955	0.887–1.029	0.001
PPM	17.7%	1.138	0.226–5.743	0.654

CI confidence interval, *LVEF* left ventricular ejection fraction

Table 7 Mid-term follow-up information

	Total	PPM group	non-PPM group	P value
Follow-up time (months)	31(23–35)	32(24–35)	31(23–33)	$P = 0.362$
NYHA functional class (III-IV)	9.2%	9.0%	9.6%	$P = 0.902$
Mortality	17(1.6%)	3(1.6%)	14(1.6%)	$P = 0.994$

NYHA New York Heart Association

left ventricular systolic dysfunction or, even worse, increase the risk of left ventricular rupture.

In our opinion, whether the current PPM standard is suitable for a rheumatic population such as the eastern Chinese is worth further exploration. Our results showed that there were no differences regarding the PPM occurrence of each valve size in the mechanical prosthesis. In our future study, we hope that we can explore a more precise parameter in predicting PPM then the current one, hence providing a more accurate prediction of patient outcomes for patients who underwent MVR in our population.

Limitations of the study

There are limitations of the study which must be recognized. First, this is a retrospective analysis, and, as an inherent disadvantage, the recorded differences in patient outcomes could have originated from smaller recorded or unrecorded differences between PPM and non-PPM patients. Second, in our study, EOA was predicted by reference tables, which might not reflect the actual in vivo values of the EOAi. Moreover, this is a single-centered short/mid-term study, and sample size and follow-up time were limited. Therefore, a randomized prospective multi-centered clinical trial with a long follow-up time is needed to study the effect of mitral PPM on longer-term patient outcomes.

Conclusions

Our results demonstrated that higher age, bioprosthesis, larger BSA and smaller left ventricle were associated with mitral PPM. However, PPM was not associated with poorer early outcomes after MVR surgery. In eastern China, the prevalence of mitral valve stenosis is high; therefore, whether the standard PPM criteria are suitable for patients of this district needs to be further verified.

Abbreviations

AF: Atrial fibrillation; AFRA: Atrial fibrillation radio frequency surgery; BMI: Body mass index; BSA: Body surface are; CABG: Coronary artery bypass grafting; CABG: Coronary artery bypass grafting; CI: Confidence interval; CPB: Cardiopulmonary bypass; EOA: Effective orifice area; EOAi (iEOA): Effective orifice area index; ICU: Intensive care unit; LAD: Left atrial diameter; LVDd: Left ventricular diastolic diameter; LVEF: Left ventricular ejection fracture; LVESV: Left ventricular end-systolic volume; MR: Mitral valve regurgitation; MVR: mitral valve replacement; NS: Not significant; NYHA: New York Heart Association; OR: Odd ratio; PHM: Prosthesis-patient mismatch; PPM: Prosthesis-patient mismatch; SD: Standard deviation

Acknowledgements

The authors would like to thank the anesthetists, intensivists, heart surgeons, nursing staff, perfusionists and the laboratory department at the First Affiliated Hospital, Zhejiang University for the collection and management of the data presented in this report.

Authors' contributions

AA and JZ analyzed and interpreted the patient data, and wrote the paper. HZ and YN prepared the tables and figure, and were major contributors in writing the manuscript. JZ drafted the final manuscript. All authors read and approved the final manuscript.

Competing interests

The authors declare that they have no competing interests.

References

1. Rahimtoola SH. The problem of valve prosthesis-patient mismatch. Circulation. 1978;58(1):20–4.
2. Rahimtoola SH, Murphy E. Valve prosthesis--patient mismatch. A long-term sequela. Br Heart J. 1981;45(3):331–5.
3. Hong S, Yi GJ, Youn YN, Lee S, Yoo KJ, Chang BC. Effect of the prosthesis-patient mismatch on long-term clinical outcomes after isolated aortic valve replacement for aortic stenosis: a prospective observational study. J Thorac Cardiov Sur. 2013;146(5):1098–104.
4. Fuster RG, Montero Argudo JA, Albarova OG, et al. Patient-prosthesis mismatch in aortic valve replacement: really tolerable? Eur J Cardiothorac Surg. 2005;27(3):441–9 discussion 9.
5. Guo L, Zheng J, Chen L, et al. Impact of prosthesis-patient mismatch on short-term outcomes after aortic valve replacement: a retrospective analysis in East China. J Cardiothorac Surg. 2017;12(1):42.
6. Dumesnil JG, Honos GN, Lemieux M, Beauchemin J. Validation and applications of mitral prosthetic valvular areas calculated by Doppler echocardiography. Am J Cardiol. 1990;65(22):1443–8.
7. Dumesnil JG, Yoganathan AP. Valve prosthesis hemodynamics and the problem of high transprosthetic pressure gradients. Eur J Cardiothorac Surg. 1992;6(Suppl 1):S34–7 discussion S8.
8. Leavitt JI, Coats MH, Falk RH. Effects of exercise on transmitral gradient and pulmonary artery pressure in patients with mitral stenosis or a prosthetic mitral valve: a Doppler echocardiographic study. J Am Coll Cardiol. 1991; 17(7):1520–6.
9. Rosenhek R, Binder T, Maurer G, Baumgartner H. Normal values for Doppler echocardiographic assessment of heart valve prostheses. J Am Soc Echocardiogr. 2003;16(11):1116–27.
10. Dumesnil JG, Pibarot P. Prosthesis-patient mismatch: an update. Curr Cardiol Rep. 2011;13(3):250–7.
11. Lee SH, Chang BC, Youn YN, Joo HC, Yoo KJ, Lee S. Impact of prosthesis-patient mismatch after mitral valve replacement in rheumatic population: does mitral position prosthesis-patient mismatch really exist? J Cardiothorac Surg. 2017;12(1):88.
12. Lam BK, Chan V, Hendry P, et al. The impact of patient-prosthesis mismatch on late outcomes after mitral valve replacement. J Thorac Cardiovasc Surg. 2007;133(6):1464–73.
13. Magne J, Mathieu P, Dumesnil JG, et al. Impact of prosthesis-patient mismatch on survival after mitral valve replacement. Circulation. 2007; 115(11):1417–25.
14. Li M, Dumesnil JG, Mathieu P, Pibarot P. Impact of valve prosthesis-patient mismatch on pulmonary arterial pressure after mitral valve replacement. J Am Coll Cardiol. 2005;45(7):1034–40.
15. Jamieson WR, Germann E, Ye J, et al. Effect of prosthesis-patient mismatch on long-term survival with mitral valve replacement: assessment to 15 years. Ann Thorac Surg. 2009;87(4):1135–41 discussion 42.
16. Aziz A, Lawton JS, Maniar HS, Pasque MK, Damiano RJ Jr, Moon MR. Factors affecting survival after mitral valve replacement in patients with prosthesis-patient mismatch. Ann Thorac Surg. 2010;90(4):1202–10 discussion 10-1.

17. Angeloni E, Melina G, Pibarot P, et al. Impact of prosthesis-patient mismatch on the regression of secondary mitral regurgitation after isolated aortic valve replacement with a bioprosthetic valve in patients with severe aortic stenosis. Circ Cardiovasc Imaging. 2012;5(1):36–42.

18. Sakamoto H, Watanabe Y. Does patient-prosthesis mismatch affect long-term results after mitral valve replacement? Ann Thorac Cardiovasc Surg. 2010;16(3):163–7.

19. Shi WY, Yap CH, Hayward PA, et al. Impact of prosthesis--patient mismatch after mitral valve replacement: a multicentre analysis of early outcomes and mid-term survival. Heart. 2011;97(13):1074–81.

20. Pibarot P, Dumesnil JG. Prosthesis-patient mismatch: definition, clinical impact, and prevention. Heart. 2006;92(8):1022–9.

21. Bitar JN, Lechin ME, Salazar G, Zoghbi WA. Doppler echocardiographic assessment with the continuity equation of St. Jude Medical mechanical prostheses in the mitral valve position. Am J Cardiol. 1995;76(4):287–93.

22. Cohn LH, Edmunds LH. Cardiac surgery in the adult. 3rd ed. New York: McGraw-Hill Medical; 2008.

23. Borracci RA, Rubio M, Sestito ML, Ingino CA, Barrero C, Rapallo CA. Incidence of prosthesis-patient mismatch in patients receiving mitral Biocor(R) porcine prosthetic valves. Cardiol J. 2016;23(2):178–83.

32

Sternal instability measured with radiostereometric analysis. A study of method feasibility, accuracy and precision

Rikke Falsig Vestergaard[1,3*], Kjeld Søballe[2,3], John Michael Hasenkam[3] and Maiken Stilling[2,3]

Abstract

Background: A small, but unstable, saw-gap may hinder bone-bridging and induce development of painful sternal dehiscence. We propose the use of Radiostereometric Analysis (RSA) for evaluation of sternal instability and present a method validation.

Methods: Four bone analogs (phantoms) were sternotomized and tantalum beads were inserted in each half. The models were reunited with wire cerclage and placed in a radiolucent separation device. Stereoradiographs ($n = 48$) of the phantoms in 3 positions were recorded at 4 imposed separation points. The accuracy and precision was compared statistically and presented as translations along the 3 orthogonal axes. 7 sternotomized patients were evaluated for clinical RSA precision by double-examination stereoradiographs ($n = 28$).

Results: In the phantom study, we found no systematic error ($p > 0.3$) between the three phantom positions, and precision for evaluation of sternal separation was 0.02 mm. Phantom accuracy was mean 0.13 mm (SD 0.25).
In the clinical study, we found a detection limit of 0.42 mm for sternal separation and of 2 mm for anterior-posterior dislocation of the sternal halves for the individual patient.

Conclusion: RSA is a precise and low-dose image modality feasible for clinical evaluation of sternal stability in research.

Keywords: Sternum, Wound healing, Bone healing

Background

The median sternotomy has been the preferred way to gain access to mediastinal organs since the dawn of thoracic surgery. The procedure is quick and efficient, and has only two major complications: sternal infection (1–3% of patients) and non-union (2–8% of patients). Sternal non-union is usually a result of primary dehiscence, poor wound healing, or premature overexertion [1].

Some patients have a higher risk of developing sternal instability than others, i.e. patients suffering from morbid obesity, COPD, diabetes mellitus, smoking, and osteoporosis. Few patients are diagnosed with non-union, but up to 56% [2] experience chronic postoperative pain, which might be an indicator of underdiagnosed sternal non-unions.

The clinical diagnosis of sternal instability is determined by manual palpation by a physician and the radiological diagnosis may be confirmed by Computed Tomography (CT). Both methods are correlated with a high degree of intra- and inter-observatory variance. We have previously shown the relative intra-observer variance of radiological evaluation of sternal CT to be a mean – 9.32% (SD ± 16.18), and the relative inter-observer variance to be mean – 14.29% (SD ± 14.88) [3].

We propose the use of a radiostereometric analysis (RSA), which is a low-dose image diagnostic modality, to diagnose sternal instability in clinical studies following cardiac surgery). RSA was developed in 1974 [4] and is today considered the gold standard for evaluation of prosthesis migration in hip and knee arthroplasty [5]. RSA has also been used to assess fracture stability and

---
* Correspondence: rikke.vestergaard@clin.au.dk
[1]Dept. of Cardio-Thoracic Surgery, Aarhus University Hospital, Skejby, Palle Juul-Jensens Boulevard 99, 8200 Aarhus N, Denmark
[3]Dept. of Clinical Medicine, Aarhus University, Incuba/Skejby, Bygning 2, Palle Juul-Jensens Boulevard 82, 8200 Aarhus N, Denmark
Full list of author information is available at the end of the article

healing [6]. The safety of RSA is proven through years of use and 99.5% of the beads are stable 6 weeks after implantation [7].

One millimeter radiopaque tantalum beads are used to mark the two fractures pieces. In a pair of x-ray images (stereoradiographs), the three-dimensional bead-positions are reconstructed, resulting in an accurate calculation of the pose of the two fracture pieces. This technique quantifies micromotion with a reported accuracy that ranges between 0.05 and 0.5 mm for translations [8]. Accuracy in this range is certainly sufficient for evaluation of sternal instability [9, 10].

The aim of this study was to investigate the feasibility of RSA in evaluation of the motion between the two sternal halves after median sternotomy and to implement the technique in a clinical population.

Methods

Phantom study

Four bone analog phantoms (20pcf density, Sawbones Europe AB, Malmö, Sweden) were subjected to a midline sternotomy. In each sternal half we placed 8 tantalum beads (diameter = 1 mm) by use of a bead-gun (Wennbergs Finmek AB, Gunnilse, Sweden). The sternal halves were reunited using six standard single cerclages. The cerclages were placed to mimic the metal-obscurance seen from wire cerclages in patients. A custom-made separation device for the sternum was built of radiolucent materials, to enable radiographic exposure of the components in all directions (Fig. 2). Images were made with the sternum in 3 different positions to mimic the expected maximal change in motion and angulation of the sternum during a breathing cycle: 1) neutral (sternum perpendicular to the platform), 2) caudal end of sternum elevated to a 15° angle (inspiration), 3) cranial end of sternum elevated to a 15° angle (expiration). The 3 positions were repeated at 4 different separation points (0 mm, 1 mm, 2 mm, 3 mm separation). Twelve radiographs per saw bone were recorded, resulting in 48 stereoradiographs in total.

According to the induced separation of the sternal halves, the difference in means of the measured phantom translations between the 4 separation points should approximate 1 mm in each of the three position groups (neutral, cranial tilt, caudal tilt). We evaluated the accuracy as the measured mean and standard deviation in each of the 3 position groups (neutral, cranial and caudal tilt) in order to show if 1 mm measurements were susceptible to variation in position of the sternum. We further evaluated the translation precision (mm) for each orthogonal axis as the combined mean difference (Mean$_{diff}$) and SD of the mean differences (SD$_{diff}$) of the 3 phantom tilt positions and 4 sternal separations. The Mean$_{diff}$ express systematic errors and the SD$_{diff}$ express the precision of the method. A low SD$_{diff}$ show high precision.

Clinical study

This study was approved by The Central Denmark Regions Committee on Biomedical Research Ethics as it adheres to the Helsinki Declaration II, and all participants gave their informed consent to participate in this study with the intent to publish.

In the clinical study, approximately 10 tantalum beads (ø = 1 mm) were inserted with a bead gun (Wennbergs Finmek AB, Gunnilse, Sweden) in each sternal half during thoracic surgery. 6 weeks after surgery we recorded double-examination stereoradiographs in full inspiration and in full expiration of 7 sternotomized patients ($n = 28$ stereoradiographs). The clinical precision is presented for each orthogonal axis as the coefficient of repeatability (CR) = standard deviation of the mean differences × 1.96. The CR can be perceived as a detection limit for assessment of patient individual migration between th[5]e two sternal halves.

RSA set-up

To accurately calculate the positions of the tantalum beads in the saw bones we used a uniplanar focused-grid carbon calibration box (Box 24, Medis Specials, Leiden, the Netherlands) with calibration markers in two layers and film cassettes placed side by side under the calibration

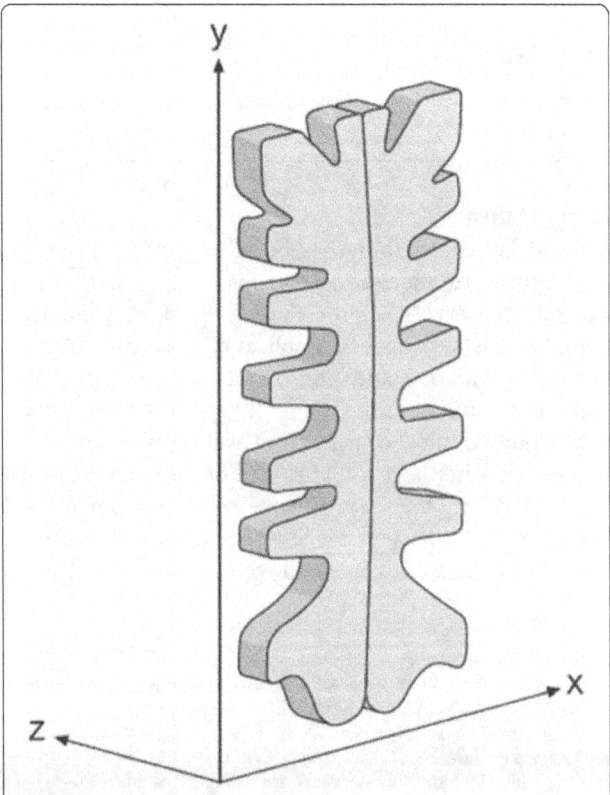

Fig. 1 Schematic drawing of axes relating to the anatomy of the sternum

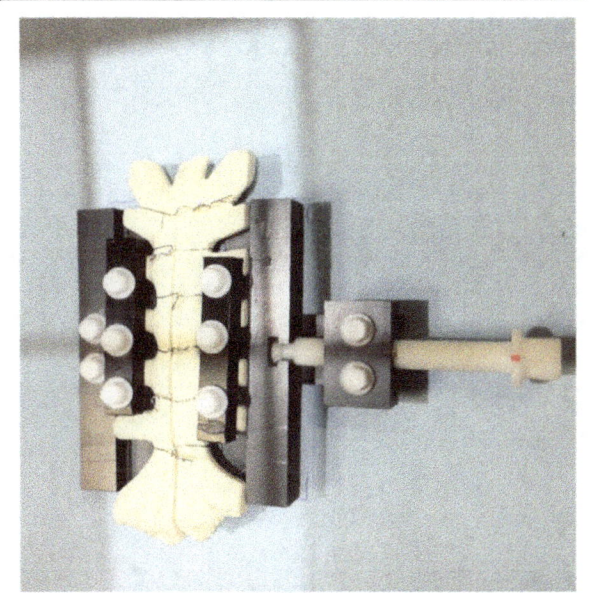

Fig. 2 Photograph of the sternal sawbone after median sternotomy and with wire-cerclage placed in the custom-made fixture device

box. The calibration box was positioned underneath the x-ray table. The calibration box coordinate system defined the translations (mm) in the frontal plane (the x-axis and y-axis) and in the out-of-plane (the z-axis) (Fig. 1).

A standard RSA setup of two synchronized ceiling-fixed x-ray tubes (Arco-Ceil/Medira; Santax Medico, Aarhus, Denmark), angled toward each other at a 40° angle were used. All stereoradiographs were fully digitalized (FCR Profect CS; Fujifilm, Tvedbæk, Denmark) and were stored without compression. The stereoradiographs that we used for analysis were scaled to 2080 × 2529 pixels (grayscale BMP file-format).

Analysis of stereoradiographs

RSA analysis was carried out with model-based RSA 3.31 software (RSAcore, Leiden, The Netherlands) by one observer (RFV) and the software computed the relative sternal motion. The left sternal half was defined as a rigid body (fixed reference) and the right sternal half was defined as the migrating object (Fig. 2). Migration was measured between the 2 sternal halves with the phantoms in 3 different positions (neutral, and 15° cranial or caudal tilt) along the 3 orthogonal axes (x, y, and z-axis) at each of the 4 separation points (0, 1, 2 and 3 mm separation).

Statistics

The measured signed translations in the phantom study followed a Gaussian distribution, and therefore statistical comparisons of the means was done with Students paired ttest, and comparison of variations were performed with an f-test. The primary endpoint of the phantom and clinical study was precision of measured migration along the X-axis (frontal plane motion of the sternal halves).

Results

Phantom study

We found no systematic error with similar means ($p > 0.3$) between the three phantom positions (Table 1). The combined precision measure of 0.02 mm for assessment of sternal separation (x-axis) in the 3 positions and 4 distractions was very good (Table 1).

The accuracy for measurement of sternal separation (mean difference for the 3 positions on the x-axis) was − 0.13 mm, since the mean of 0.87 mm approximated the intended 1 mm separation of the jig. There was some underestimation (mean 0.47 mm) for the first separation interval (0–1 mm) and a slight overestimation (0.08 mm) for the two other separation intervals (1–2 mm, 2–3 mm) (Table 2).

Clinical study

The mean difference of patient double examination in assessment of sternal separation was 0.07 mm, and the precision (detection limit in individual patients) in terms of the CR was 0.42 mm (Table 3).

Discussion

In clinical research, we should always aim at using the diagnostic tests, which inflict the least danger to the patient, without compromising accuracy and precision, and at a reasonable price. In this study we aimed to investigate the feasibility and validity RSA as a low-dose image modality alternative to CT for evaluation of sternal healing in clinical research.

In the phantom study, we showed the accuracy of the RSA measurements to be acceptable (measurement error of 0.13 mm) with small and statistically non-significant mean differences and variances. Likewise, the precision was at submillimeter level and similar to phantom studies of orthopaedic prostheses [9, 10]. Further, there was no

Table 1 Phantom precision

Phantom study (n = 4 phantoms)	X-axis (sternal separation)	Y-axis (proximal-distal translation)	Z-axis (anterior-posterior translation)
Sternum Mean_diff (mm)	0.00	0.00	−0.07
SD_diff (mm)	0.02	0.04	0.31

The combined mean difference (Mean_diff) and standard deviation of differences (SD_diff) for the 3 phantom tilt positions and 4 sternal separations of the 4 phantoms. The Mean_diff express systematic errors and the SD_diff express the precision of the method

Table 2 Phantom Accuracy

Phantom Position / Axes	X axis (sternal separation) Mean (SD)	Y axis (proximal-distal translation) Mean (SD)	Z axis (anterior-posterior translation) Mean (SD)
Neutral			
Separation 0–1 mm	0.52 (0.35)	−0.11 (0.16)	−0.53 (0.52)
Separation 1–2 mm	1.05 (0.1)	−0.36 (0.14)	0.04 (0.12)
Separation 2–3 mm	1.06 (0.13)	−0.41 (0.15)	−0.29 (0.22)
Mean neutral	0.88 (0.25)	0.29 (0.13)	−0.26 (0.23)
15° Cranial tilt			
Separation 0–1 mm	0.54 (0.34)	−0.03 (0.16)	−0.65 (0.32)
Separation 1–2 mm	1.09 (0.08)	−0.35 (0.07)	−0.06 (0.18)
Separation 2–3 mm	1.05 (0.1)	−0.35 (0.23)	−0.44 (0.77)
Mean 15° cranial tilt	0.89 (0.25)	−0.24 (0.15)	−0.38 (0.24)
15° Caudal tilt			
Separation 0–1 mm	0.52 (0.31)	0.19 (0.15)	−0.46 (0.43)
Separation 1–2 mm	1.04 (0.07)	0.37 (0.12)	−0.01 (0.16)
Separation 2–3 mm	1.03 (0.11)	0.44 (0.07)	−0.17 (0.37)
Mean 15° caudal tilt	0.86 (0.24)	0.33 (0.11)	−0.21 (0.19)

The measured difference in means with standard deviations of an approximated 1 mm x-axis phantom migration on the custom made jig. N = 4

systematic error between the 3 tested sternal positions of the phantom, which simulated the maximal expected clinical change in sternal angulation corresponding to inspiration and expiration.

In the clinical study, double examination stereoradiographs were recorded 6 weeks after surgery where stable tantalum beads in the sternal osteotomy are expected [7]. With repeat stereoradiographs at full inspiration and expiration, we found a clinical precision of less than 0.5 mm for measurement of sternal separation and of 2 mm for measurement of anterior/posterior translation of one sternal half. Dispite cerclage osteosynthesis, up to 2 mm sternal separation has been shown post-operatively at physiological strains [7, 8]. The precision of RSA is certainly sufficient to evaluate sternal instability and non-union at this criteria, as well as to compare the fixation potential of the many different new osteosynthesis techniques currently available to thoracic surgeons. The lower precision in the out-of-plane (Z axis) is a well-known limitation in RSA studies, but it is probably enhanced in our model as a result of tantalum beads being placed almost on a straight line in both the frontal and the sagittal plane [11]. However, this is inevitable because of the flat and narrow anatomy of the sternum.

The radiation dose of 0.8 mSv for RSA is considerably less than the approximate 7 mSv dose for CT. A further advantages of RSA is the lesser economic burden (image recording and analysis) of estimated 46 USD (double examination RSA) compared to approximately 296USD for CT [12]. A limitation of marker-based RSA is the invasive requirement of bead-insertion during surgery; however, the method has proven safe during decades [7]. Furthermore, the radiographic quality of RSA man be lower in patients with high BMI; however, we saw radiographic quality better than the expected standard for thoracic radiographs, and the high atom number of tantalum

Table 3 Clinical double examinations

Clinical position / Axes	X axis (sternal separation) Mean (SD)	Y axis (proximal-distal translation) Mean (SD)	Z axis (anterior-posterior translation) Mean (SD)
Inspiration (n = 7)	0.09 (0.24)	−0.16 (0.30)	0.53 (0.96)
Expiration (n = 7)	−0.13 (0.19)	−0.40 (0.36)	1.13 (1.22)
Combined (n = 14)	0.07 (0.21)	−0.55 (0.32)	0.67 (1.06)
CR (precision) (n = 14)	0.42 mm	0.63 mm	2.08 mm

Double examination results of 14 patient sterni recorded 6 weeks postoperative during inspiration and expiration (28 stereoradiographs). The mean express the change in sternal separation between inspiration and expiration, the SD express the clinical variation, and the CR (coefficient of repeatability = 1.96 x SD_{diff}) express the clinical precision of individual RSA for measurements of sternal instability

ensure marker-visibility even with a large soft-tissue bulk. Lastly, the wire-cerclage may occlude the tantalum beads; however, when 10 tantalum beads were inserted per sternum half we did not experience this as a problem for a sufficient marker geometry.

Conclusion

RSA is a low-dose image modality, which requires insertion of small tantalum beads during surgery and specialized radiographic equipment. The present study confirms the feasibility and precision of RSA for clinical assessment of sternal instability. To the extent of our knowledge, no one has previously used RSA for evaluation of sternal displacement and instability. Currently, RSA is probably the only high-precision, low-dose and safe-proven image modality that can quantify sternal micromotion following median sternotomy as an alternative to conventional CT.

Abbreviations

CT: Computed Tomography; RSA: Radiostereometric Analysis

Acknowledgements

We would like to thank Rikke Mørup in the Department of Clinical Research in Orthopedic Surgery for her assistance with RSA.

Author contribution

RFV and MS contributed to study design, carried out the data collection and analysis as well as writing and revising this manuscript. KS and JMH conceived of the study, and participated in its design and coordination and approved the final manuscript.

Competing interests

No financial support was given to this project and there are no conflicts of interest for any of the authors.

Author details

[1]Dept. of Cardio-Thoracic Surgery, Aarhus University Hospital, Skejby, Palle Juul-Jensens Boulevard 99, 8200 Aarhus N, Denmark. [2]Dept. of Orthopedic Surgery, Aarhus University Hospital, Tage Hansens Gade 2, 8000 Aarhus C, Denmark. [3]Dept. of Clinical Medicine, Aarhus University, Incuba/Skejby, Bygning 2, Palle Juul-Jensens Boulevard 82, 8200 Aarhus N, Denmark.

References

1. Song DH, Lohman RF, Renucci JD, Jeevanandam V, Raman J. Primary sternal plating in high-risk patients prevents mediastinitis. Eur J Cardiothorac Surg. 2004;26:367–72.
2. Eisenberg E, Pultorak Y, Pud D, Bar-El Y. Prevalence and characteristics of post coronary artery bypass graft surgery pain (PCP). Pain. 2001;92:11–7.
3. Vestergaard RF, Nielsen PH, Terp KA, Soballe K, Andersen G, Hasenkam JM. Effect of hemostatic material on sternal healing after cardiac surgery. Ann Thorac Surg. 2014;97:153–60.
4. Selvik G, Roentgen stereophotogrammetry. A method for the study of the kinematics of the skeletal system. Acta Orthop Scand Suppl. 1989;232:1–51.
5. Valstar ER, Gill R, Ryd L, Flivik G, Borlin N, Karrholm J. Guidelines for standardization of radiostereometry (RSA) of implants. Acta Orthop. 2005;76: 563–72.
6. Madanat R, Moritz N, Larsson S, Aro HT. RSA applications in monitoring of fracture healing in clinical trials. Scand J Surg. 2006;95:119–27.
7. Shah RP, MacLean L, Paprosky WG, Sporer S. Routine use of Radiostereometric analysis in elective hip and knee arthroplasty patients: surgical impact, safety, and bead stability. J Am Acad Orthop Surg. 2018;
8. Karrholm J, Roentgen stereophotogrammetry. Review of orthopedic applications. Acta Orthop Scand. 1989;60:491–503.
9. McGregor WE, Trumble DR, Magovern JA. Mechanical analysis of midline sternotomy wound closure. J Thorac Cardiovasc Surg. 1999;117:1144–50.
10. Losanoff JE, Jones JW, Richman BW. Primary closure of median sternotomy: techniques and principles. Cardiovasc Surg. 2002;10:102–10.
11. Ryd L. Micromotion in knee arthroplasty-a roentgen stereophotogrammetric analysis of tibia1 component fixation. Sweden: University Department of Orthopedics in Lund; 1986.
12. Stilling M, Larsen K, Andersen NT, Soballe K, Kold S, Rahbek O. The final follow-up plain radiograph is sufficient for clinical evaluation of polyethylene wear in total hip arthroplasty. A study of validity and reliability. Acta Orthop. 2010;81:570–8.

Permissions

List of Contributors

Amr A. Arafat, Elatafy E. Elatafy and Ahmed Elmahrouk
Cardiothoracic Surgery Department, Tanta University, Al-Geish Street, Tanta 31527, Gharbya, Egypt

Sahar Elshedoudy
Cardiology Department, Tanta University, Tanta, Egypt

Mahmoud Zalat
Cardiothoracic Surgery Department, Misr Children Hospital, Cairo, Egypt

Neamet Abdallah
Cardiology Department, Misr Children Hospital, Cairo, Egypt

M. Navaratnarajah, R. Rea, R. Evans, F. Gibson, C. Antoniades, A. Keiralla, M. Demosthenous, G. Kassimis and G. Krasopoulos
Oxford Heart Centre, John Radcliffe Hospital, Headley Way, Oxfordshire OX3 9DU, UK

L. Castro, S. Pecha, M. Linder, H. Reichenspurner and S. Hakmi
Department of Cardiovascular Surgery, University Heart Center Hamburg, Hamburg, Germany

J. Vogler, N. Gosau, C. Meyer and S. Willems
Department of Cardiology, Electrophysiology, University Heart Center Hamburg, Hamburg, Germany

Smita Sihag, Bao Le and Cameron D. Wright
Division of Thoracic Surgery, Massachusetts General Hospital, 55 Fruit Street, Founders 7, Boston, Massachusetts 02114, USA

Alison S. Witkin, Josanna M. Rodriguez-Lopez and Richard N. Channick
Division of Pulmonary and Critical Care Medicine, Massachusetts General Hospital, 55 Fruit Street, Boston, Massachusetts 02114, USA

Mauricio A. Villavicencio and Gus J. Vlahakes
Division of Cardiac Surgery, Massachusetts General Hospital, 55 Fruit Street, Cox 6, Boston, Massachusetts 02114, USA

Smita Sihag
Thoracic Surgery Service, Memorial Sloan Kettering Cancer Center, 12 75 York Avenue, C-881, New York, NY 10065, USA

Xiaopeng Wen, Shan Gao, Jinteng Feng, Shuo Li, Rui Gao and Guangjian Zhang
Department of Thoracic Surgery, First Affiliated Hospital of Xi'an Jiaotong University, #277 West Yanta Road, Xi'an, Shaanxi Province 710061, People's Republic of China

Jingtao Huang, Zhongwei Zhang and Tao Zhang
Department of Thoracic Surgery, Tianjin Nankai Hospital, No. 6 Changjiang Road, Nankai District, Tianjin 300100, China

Ann C. Gaffey, Carol W. Chen, Jennifer J. Chung, Jason Han, Christian A. Bermudez and Pavan Atluri
Division of Cardiovascular Surgery, Department of Surgery, Perelman School of Medicine, University of Pennsylvania, Silverstein 6, 3400 Spruce St, Philadelphia, PA 19104, USA

Joyce Wald
Division of Cardiology, Department of Medicine, Perelman School of Medicine, University of Pennsylvania, Philadelphia, USA

Dan Wei, Jie Han, Haibo Zhang, Yan Li, Chunlei Xu and Xu Meng
Department of cardiac surgery, Capital medical university affiliated Beijing anzhen hospital, Chaoyang District Anzhen Road No. 2, Beijing 100029, China

Fausto Biancari and Debora Brascia
Department of Surgery, University of Turku, Turku, Finland

Fausto Biancari
Department of Surgery, University of Oulu, Oulu, Finland

Fausto Biancari, Vesa Anttila and Juhani K. E. Airaksinen
Heart Center, Turku University Hospital and University of Turku, Hämeentie 11, 20521 Turku, PL 52, Finland

Angelo M. Dell'Aquila
Department of Cardiac Surgery, University Hospital, Münster, Germany

Saša D. Borović and Predrag S. Milojević
Dedinje Cardiovascular Institute, Belgrade, Serbia, 1 Heroja Milana Tepića Street, Belgrade 11000, Serbia

Milica M. Labudović Borović, Ivan V. Zaletel and Jelena T. Rakočević
2Institute of Histology and Embryology Aleksandar Đ. Kostić", Faculty of Medicine, University of Belgrade, 26 Višegradska Street, Belgrade 11000, Serbia

Vera N. Todorović
Faculty of Stomatology, University Business Academy in Pančevo, Novi Sad, Serbia

Jelena M. Marinković-Erić
Institute of Medical Statistics, Faculty of Medicine, University of Belgrade, Belgrade, Serbia

Britt Hofmann, Claudia Kaufmann, Markus Stiller, Thomas Neitzel, Rolf-Edgar Silber and Hendrik Treede
Department of Cardiac Surgery, University Hospital Halle, Ernst-Grube-Strasse 40, 06120 Halle, Germany

Andreas Wienke
Institute of Medical Epidemiology, Biostatistics and Informatics, Martin-Luther-University Halle-Wittenberg, 06097 Halle, Germany

Anna Gomes and Bhanu Sinha
Department of Medical Microbiology, University of Groningen, University Medical Center Groningen, Groningen, Netherlands

Jayant S. Jainandunsing
Department of Anesthesiology, University of Groningen, University Medical Center Groningen, Groningen, Netherlands

Sander van Assen
Department of Internal Medicine, Infectious Diseases, Treant Care Group, Hoogeveen, Netherlands

Peter Paul van Geel
Department of Cardiology, University of Groningen, University Medical Center Groningen, Groningen, Netherlands

Sandro Gelsomino, Daniel M. Johnson and Ehsan Natour
Department of Thoracic Surgery, Maastricht University Medical Center, Maastricht, Netherlands

Ehsan Natour
Department of Cardio-Thoracic Surgery, University of Groningen, University Medical Center Groningen, Groningen, Netherlands

Alexandr V. Bogachev-Prokophiev, Alexandr V. Afanasyev, Sergei I. Zheleznev, Vladimir M. Nazarov, Ravil M. Sharifulin and Alexandr M. Karaskov
Heart Valves Surgery Department, Meshalkin National Medical Research Center Ministry of Health Russian Federation, 15 Rechkunovskaya street, Novosibirsk, Russian Federation630055

Piergiorgio Muriana, Angelo Carretta, Paola Ciriaco, Alessandro Bandiera and Giampiero Negri
Department of Thoracic Surgery, San Raffaele Scientific Institute, Milan, Italy

Erkan Kaba, Mehmet Oguzhan Ozyurtkan and Tugba Cosgun
Department of Thoracic Surgery, Istanbul Bilim University Medical Faculty, 34381 Sisli, Istanbul, Turkey

Kemal Ayalp, Mazen Rasmi Alomari and Alper Toker
Department of Thoracic Surgery, Group Florence Nightingale Hospitals, Istanbul, Turkey

Nicola Oswald and Babu Naidu
1Institute of Inflammation and Ageing, University of Birmingham Laboratories, University of Birmingham, Queen Elizabeth Hospital Birmingham, Edgbaston, Birmingham B15 2TT, UK

John Hardman, Amy Kerr, Ehab Bishay, Richard Steyn, Pala Rajesh and Maninder Kalkat
Department of Thoracic Surgery, Heart of England NHS Foundation Trust, Bordesley Green East, Birmingham Heartlands Hospital, Birmingham B9 5SS, UK

Ming-Chun Ma, Tai-Jan Chiu, Wan-Yu Tien, Ya-Chun Lan, Yen-Yang Chen and Shau-Hsuan
Department of Hematology-Oncology, Kaohsiung Chang Gung Memorial Hospital and Chang Gung University College of Medicine, 123 Ta-Pei Road, Niaosong Dist, Kaohsiung, Taiwan, Republic of China

Hung-I Lu and Chien-Ming Lo
Department of Thoracic and Cardiovascular Surgery, Kaohsiung Chang Gung Memorial Hospital and Chang Gung University College of Medicine, Kaohsiung, Taiwan, Republic of China

Wan-Ting Huang
Department of Pathology, Kaohsiung Chang Gung Memorial Hospital and Chang Gung University College of Medicine, Kaohsiung, Taiwan, Republic of China

Chang-Han Chen
Institute for Translational Research in Biomedicine, Kaohsiung Chang Gung Memorial Hospital, Kaohsiung, Taiwan, Republic of China
Department of Applied Chemistry, and Graduate Institute of Biomedicine and Biomedical Technology, National Chi Nan University, Nantou, Taiwan, Republic of China
Center for Infectious Disease and Cancer Research, Kaohsiung Medical University, Kaohsiung, Taiwan, Republic of China

Yassar A. Qureshi, M. Muntzer Mughal and Borzoueh Mohammadi
Department of Oesophago-Gastric Surgery, University College London Hospital, 250 Euston Road, London NW1 2BU, UK

Sheraz R. Markar
Department of Surgery and Cancer, Imperial College London, London, UK

Jeremy George
Department of Thoracic Medicine, University College London Hospital, London, UK

Martin Hayward and David Lawrence
Department of Thoracic Surgery, University College London Hospital, London, UK

Thomas S. Metkus and Monica Mukherjee
Division of Cardiology, Johns Hopkins University School of Medicine, 600 N. Wolfe Street, Blalock 524 D2, Baltimore, MD 21287, USA

Alejandro Suarez-Pierre, Todd C. Crawford, Jennifer S. Lawton and Glenn J. Whitman
Division of Cardiac Surgery, Johns Hopkins University School of Medicine, Baltimore, MD, USA

Lee Goeddel and Jeffrey Dodd-o
Department of Anesthesia and Critical Care Medicine, Johns Hopkins University School of Medicine, Baltimore, MD, USA

Theodore P. Abraham
Division of Cardiology, Department of Medicine, University of California, San Francisco, 505 Parnassus Ave., Suite M344 San Francisco, San Francisco, CA, USA

Robert A. Sorabella, Anna Olds, Halit Yerebakan, Dua Hassan, Michael A. Borger, Michael Argenziano, Craig R. Smith and Isaac George
Division of Cardiothoracic Surgery, New York Presbyterian Hospital -Columbia University College of Physicians and Surgeons, 177 Fort Washington Ave, MHB 7GN-435, New York, NY 10032, USA

Hao Ma, Zhenghua Xiao, Jun Shi, Lulu Liu, Chaoyi Qin and Yingqiang Guo
Department of Cardiovascular Surgery, West China Hospital, Sichuan University, Chengdu 610041, China

Marco Zanobini, Claudia Loardi, Paolo Poggio, Gloria Tamborini, Fabrizio Veglia, Alessandro Di Minno, Veronika Myasoedova, Liborio Francesco Mammana, Raoul Biondi, Mauro Pepi, Francesco Alamanni and Matteo Saccocci
Department of Cardiac Surgery, Centro Cardiologico Monzino IRCCS, University of Milan, Via Parea, 4, 20138 Milan, Italy

Matteo Saccocci
Heart Center, University Hospital of Zürich, University of Zürich, Zürich, CH, Switzerland

Hiroshi Kubota, Hidehito Endo, Hikaru Ishii, Hiroshi Tsuchiya, Yusuke Inaba, Yu Takahashi and Katsunari Terakawa
Department of Cardiovascular Surgery, Kyorin University, 6-20-2, Shinkawa, Mitaka, Tokyo 181-8611, Japan

Andreas Moritz
Department of Anesthesiology, University Hospital of Erlangen, Krankenhausstrasse 12, 91054 Erlangen, Germany

Andrea Irouschek
Department of Anesthesiology, University Hospital of Erlangen, Krankenhausstrasse 12, 91054 Erlangen, Germany

Torsten Birkholz
Department of Anesthesiology, University Hospital of Erlangen, Krankenhausstrasse 12, 91054 Erlangen, Germany

Johannes Prottengeier
Department of Anesthesiology, University Hospital of Erlangen, Krankenhausstrasse 12, 91054 Erlangen, Germany

Horia Sirbu
Department of Thoracic Surgery, University Hospital of Erlangen, Krankenhausstrasse 12, 91054 Erlangen, Germany

Joachim Schmidt
Department of Anesthesiology, University Hospital of Erlangen, Krankenhausstrasse 12, 91054 Erlangen, Germany

David P. Taggart
Nuffield Department of Surgery, University of Oxford, John Radcliffe Hospital, Oxford, UK

Carolyn M. Webb
National Heart and Lung Institute, Imperial College London, London, UK

Carolyn M. Webb and Carlo Di Mario
Department of Cardiology, Royal Brompton Hospital, Sydney Street, London SW3 6NP, UK

Anthony Desouza and Rashmi Yadav
Department of Cardiothoracic Surgery, Royal Brompton Hospital, Sydney Street, London, UK

Keith M. Channon
Department of Cardiovascular Medicine, University of Oxford, John Radcliffe Hospital, Oxford, UK

Fabio De Robertis
Department of Cardiothoracic Surgery, Harefield Hospital, Middlesex, London, UK

Elizabeth M. Colwell
Cardiothoracic Surgery, Stanford University, 300 Pasteur Dr. Falk Cardiovascular Research Bldg, Stanford, CA 94305-5407, USA

Carlos O. Encarnacion
University of Maryland, Division of Cardiac Surgery, 110 S. Paca St. 7th floor, Baltimore, MD 21201, USA

Lisa E. Rein
Medical College of Wisconsin, 8701 Watertown Plank Road, Milwaukee, WI 53226, USA

Aniko Szabo
Division of Biostatistics, Institute for Health and Equity, Medical College of Wisconsin, 8701 W. Watertown Plank Road, Milwaukee, WI 53226, USA

George Haasler and David Johnstone
Division of Cardiothoracic Surgery, HUB for Collaborative Medicine, Medical College of Wisconsin, 8701 Watertown Plank Road, Milwaukee, WI 53226, USA

Mario Gasparri
Division of Cardiovascular and Thoracic Surgery, SSM Heath – St. Mary's Madison, Madison, WI 53715, USA

William Tisol
Aurora Medical Group CVTS, 2901 W Kinnickinnic River Pkwy Suite 501, Milwaukee, WI 53125, USA

Supomo Supomo
Department of Thoracic and Cardiovascular Surgery, Dr. Sardjito General Hospital, Faculty of Medicine, Public Health and Nursing, Universitas Gadjah Mada, Kesehatan St. Number 1, Sleman, Yogyakarta 55281, Indonesia

Handy Darmawan and Adika Zhulhi Arjana
Faculty of Medicine, Universitas Islam Indonesia, Yogyakarta, Indonesia

Lisa Verwijmeren, Peter Gerben Noordzij and Eric Paulus Adrianus van Dongen
Anesthesiology, Intensive Care and Pain Medicine, St. Antonius Hospital, Koekoekslaan 1, Nieuwegein 3430 EM, The Netherlands

Bas van Zaane and Linda Margaretha Peelen
Anesthesiology, Intensive Care and Emergency Medicine, University Medical Center Utrecht, Utrecht University, Heidelberglaan 100, Utrecht 3584 CX, The Netherlands

Linda Margaretha Peelen
Epidemiology, Julius Center for Health Sciences and Primary Care, University Medical Center Utrecht, Utrecht University, Heidelberglaan 100, Utrecht 3584 CX, The Netherlands

Peter J. Kneuertz, Desmond M. D'Souza, Susan D. Moffatt-Bruce and Robert E. Merritt
Department of Surgery, Thoracic Surgery Division, The Ohio State University Wexner Medical Center, Doan Hall N846, 410 W 10th Avenue, Columbus, OH 43210, USA

Narumol Chaosuwannakit
Radiology Department, Faculty of Medicine, Khon Kaen University, Khon Kaen 40000, Thailand

Pattarapong Makarawate
Cardiology Unit, Internal Medicine Department, Faculty of Medicine, Khon Kaen University, Khon Kaen, Thailand

Armah M Akuffu, Haige Zhao, Junnan Zheng and Yiming Ni
Department of Cardiothoracic Surgery, the First Affiliated Hospital of Zhejiang University, No.79 Qingchun Road, Hangzhou 310003, China

Rikke Falsig Vestergaard
Dept. of Cardio-Thoracic Surgery, Aarhus University Hospital, Skejby, Palle Juul-Jensens Boulevard 99, 8200 Aarhus N, Denmark

Kjeld Søballe and Maiken Stilling
Dept. of Orthopedic Surgery, Aarhus University Hospital, Tage Hansens Gade 2, 8000 Aarhus C, Denmark

Rikke Falsig Vestergaard, Kjeld Søballe, John Michael Hasenkam and Maiken Stilling
Dept. of Clinical Medicine, Aarhus University, Incuba/Skejby, Bygning 2, Palle Juul-Jensens Boulevard 82, 8200 Aarhus N, Denmark

Index

www.ingramcontent.com/pod-product-compliance
Lightning Source LLC
Chambersburg PA
CBHW080412190526
45161CB00003B/209